The
Keeler
Migraine
Method

The Keeler Migraine Method

A Groundbreaking, Individualized

Program from the Renowned

Headache Treatment Clinic

Robert Cowan, M.D.

AVERY   a member of Penguin Group (USA) Inc.   New York

Published by the Penguin Group
Penguin Group (USA) Inc., 375 Hudson Street, New York, New York 10014, USA • Penguin Group
(Canada), 90 Eglinton Avenue East, Suite 700, Toronto, Ontario M4P 2Y3, Canada (a division of Pearson
Canada Inc.) • Penguin Books Ltd, 80 Strand, London WC2R 0RL, England • Penguin
Ireland, 25 St Stephen's Green, Dublin 2, Ireland (a division of Penguin Books Ltd) • Penguin Group
(Australia), 250 Camberwell Road, Camberwell, Victoria 3124, Australia (a division of Pearson
Australia Group Pty Ltd) • Penguin Books India Pvt Ltd, 11 Community Centre, Panchsheel Park,
New Delhi–110 017, India • Penguin Group (NZ), 67 Apollo Drive, Rosedale,
North Shore 0632, New Zealand (a division of Pearson New Zealand Ltd) • Penguin Books
(South Africa) (Pty) Ltd, 24 Sturdee Avenue, Rosebank, Johannesburg 2196, South Africa

Penguin Books Ltd, Registered Offices: 80 Strand, London WC2R 0RL, England

Most Avery books are available at special quantity discounts for bulk purchase for sales promotions,
premiums, fund-raising, and educational needs. Special books or book excerpts also can be
created to fit specific needs. For details, write Penguin Group (USA) Inc. Special Markets,
375 Hudson Street, New York, NY 10014.

Library of Congress Cataloging-in-Publication Data

Cowan, Robert, M.D.
The Keeler migraine method : a groundbreaking, individualized treatment program
from the renowned headache clinic / Robert Cowan.
p.   cm.
Includes index.
ISBN 978-1-58333-322-8
1. Migraine.   I. Title.
RC392.C69   2008   2008033852
616.8'4912—dc22

Printed in the United States of America
3   5   7   9   10   8   6   4   2

BOOK DESIGN BY NICOLE LAROCHE

Undertaking a work as comprehensive as *The Keeler Migraine Method* has required incredible discipline, patience, and faith—on the part of the author's family. My wife, Mercedes, has been my intellectual, emotional, and practical partner for thirty years. This book, my career, and our family would never have happened without her. If this book helps you, thank her.

Clinical medicine does not develop in a vacuum. Without patients, there is no clinical progress. The incredible advances in headache medicine over the last fifteen years have been fueled as much by patients as by scientific investigation. Nowhere is this truer than at the Keeler Center. This book reflects the accumulated experience of the thousands of patients who have shaped my understanding of headache. This book is dedicated to all of you, with my deepest gratitude.

ROBERT P. COWAN, M.D., FAAN

Acknowledgments

Where to begin? With my parents, who blessed me with the genes of a migraine sufferer; my wife, who encouraged me to go to medical school; my professors, colleagues, and patients, who have educated me? The list could go to volumes! A few very specific acknowledgments are appropriate here: Katie Vecchio, fellow migraineur, extraordinary literary editor, and friend. This book would have been unreadable without her. Lucia Watson, my editor at Avery, whose focus, experience, and patience turned my sow's ear into a silk purse of a book. Felicia Eth, my agent, who saw the need for a book that offered a practical approach to headache management and found us a like-minded publisher. And finally, my colleague and friend Michael Harrington, M.D., whose passion for science and patient care has fueled the engine that created this work.

Contents

What Should a Good Migraine Book Do?

had migraines long before I became a doctor, long before I became a headache specialist. I spent many hours as you probably are right now—standing in front of a shelf full of migraine books, staring at the covers, paging through some, trying to decide which, if any, would help my headaches. Sometimes I ended up walking away in frustration. Other times, I bought two or three because I saw something in them that rang true for me. Sadly, a few months later, I found myself back in a bookstore, repeating the same futile ritual.

Why was it, with so many titles out there, that nothing seemed to give me the answers I was looking for? *Why do I get headaches? How can I avoid them? What can I do when they hit?* Many of the available books touch on some of these issues, but none of them seems to offer a comprehensive plan for taking care of a person with headaches. One book talks about diet. Another describes different kinds of headaches. Yet another gives a chiropractor's view. And so forth. I just wanted one book that covered all of it—the latest research, the best of Western and alternative medical treatments, and the lifestyle changes that I can implement to help minimize the frequency and severity of my headaches.

The fact is that the book I wanted, that my patients wanted, simply wasn't on the shelf. That is why I wrote *The Keeler Migraine Method*. In this book, I bring together the latest science and medicine, along with the best of natural and alternative therapies, and lay them out before you. I also help you learn to analyze your own headaches as well as your lifestyle, to help you and your physician design the best possible treatment plan for *your* headaches. While medicine does not provide any one-size-fits-all cure for migraines, the Keeler Method does teach you how to build a simple and effective management strategy to make your headaches less frequent and less severe.

The
Keeler
Migraine
Method

Introduction

The Keeler Method for Migraine Management

She sat across the desk from me, her arms and legs crossed, wearing an expression I could describe only as hostile. For more than thirty of her forty-four years, she had dealt with a long line of doctors for her headaches, and I was just the latest. So far, all I had done was introduce myself, and already I was in trouble. It didn't help that she looked a lot like my fourth-grade teacher. For a second, I thought about having her change into a gown in case she was packing a weapon. "Do you have a headache today?" I asked her, instead. "I can turn down the lights if you like."

She glared a moment longer, sizing me up. "I have a headache every day. But yes, that would be very nice." Her expression softened a bit. "I hate the fluorescents."

"Me too," I commented as I flicked the switch, "especially when I have a migraine."

She uncrossed her arms.

"You get headaches?"

Her resistance melted away as I explained to her, apparently for the first time, *why* fluorescent lights bother migraine sufferers, even when we don't have a headache. I told her that certain shades of sunglasses work better than others for light sensitivity, and mentioned that some recent research in Japan suggests that specific preventives are better for people with severe light sensitivity. She and I were developing what we doctors call a therapeutic relationship, meaning we were finding a common ground where we could work together on her headaches.

At least for the moment, she suspended the defenses that she'd developed during a lifetime of trying to convince doctors, coworkers, and even family members that her headaches are real, serious, and important. Over the next several months, we reworked some aspects of her lifestyle, changed her medication strategy, and gently educated her employer and her family. While she had suffered daily headaches and missed an average of four workdays per month, we reduced that to one weekly headache that she treated early and effectively with a different rescue medication.

Her case is pretty typical of the results we see at the Keeler Center, but every treatment plan we create is unique, custom fitted to each individual patient. That, in a nutshell, is why the Keeler plan is so successful.

When I tell patients that I, too, get headaches, it is not a ploy to gain their trust or sympathy (though this is often a beneficial consequence). I mention it as a simple reality. The fact is, I get migraines. Some days I may have to cancel their appointments because I have a headache. Migraines are just part of my world, and I have had some really bad ones. I know how they feel, how they can ruin too many days and can dominate your life. Like most migraine sufferers, I have tried on occasion to work through a migraine and ended up making a mess of things. During migraines, I have made bad decisions, missed major family events, gotten into fights with my wife, been short with my kids, and even thrown up in my host's bathroom once or twice. Twenty-five years ago, I even considered dropping out of medical school because of my headaches. I practice what I preach and, now, I doubt that I miss more than one or two days a year because of a headache. Today, for the most part, I know what causes my headaches, how to avoid them, and how to treat them when avoidance doesn't work. With the help of my patients, my research, and the many scientists and clinicians with whom I work, I have gotten a lot better at managing my own migraines, and most of these incidents are just painful memories. Now my headaches are a footnote rather than the focus of my life. And while the plan you develop with the Keeler Method will likely be different from mine, it should do the same for you as it has for me.

A Migraine Cure?

I would love to have titled this book *The Migraine Cure*, but the reality is, we're not there yet. Both patients and practitioners tend to look for and latch on to the notion of a cure, that one thing that will make it all go away. That is why there is such a proliferation of books, articles, and websites claiming to offer "the cure":

"Heal Your Headaches with Magnesium!"
"Magnets Cure Migraines!"
"Eat Away Your Headaches!"
"Pilates for Headache Health!"

The list is endless. Any one of these approaches may be perfect for a given patient, but in twenty-five years of caring for headache patients (fifty years, counting caring for myself), I have studied—and tried—dozens upon dozens of miracle cures. But I still get headaches and, unfortunately, so will you. The reality is, there is still no cure. A cure would not stay a secret for long. If we had a one-size-fits-all solution to headaches, it wouldn't be buried in a back-page ad in the *National Enquirer*, you wouldn't need to search the Internet for it, and you wouldn't hear it from your aunt in Omaha. Thirty million of us suffer from migraines, so a cure would be on the front page of *The New York Times*, Matt Lauer would be talking about it on the *Today* show, and the Internet would be lit up with references to major medical journals.

Brains are complicated, and so are the conditions that affect them. If every headache sufferer had the same triggers, responded the same way to every medication, and had readily predictable headaches, migraine management would be easy. It isn't. Still, I have yet to meet the headache sufferer who, with the help of the Keeler plan, does not experience a significant improvement in quality of life, usually through a reduction in the number, severity, and duration of headaches. That's why I wrote this book—because all headache patients are unique, and so are their headaches. This book will help you identify your unique migraine characteristics and teach you how to use this information to better manage your headaches.

Procrustes, the son of Poseidon, invited weary travelers to rest at his inn, and then broke their bones so that they would fit into a bed too small for them. Many doctors have a very "Procrustean" approach to headache treatment. They generate lists of foods that give some people headaches, asserting that avoiding those foods will prevent all headaches. They simply prescribe one drug after another, hoping one will work, and they try the same therapies in the same order, on patient after patient. Sometimes these measures work, sometimes not, because, aside from the pain, my headaches are probably not exactly like yours. What works for me might not work for you, and vice versa.

Until very recently (about the last fifteen years), headache was the "poor relation" in neurology. Until the last ten years or so, we had no fellowship programs (special postresidency training) in headache and, even today, there are only a few programs. Indeed, through *seven years* of training in medical school and residency, headaches were covered in a few *hours*, with the emphasis on secondary headaches (those headaches that are a symptom of something else, like brain tumors or ruptured blood vessels). Even today, federal funding for headache research is less than $15 million per year. Headache sufferers and their treating physicians know the frustration in treating a condition about which they know little and for which there is minimal support, either from the medical community or from society at large. When the treating physician is also a headache sufferer, this frustration is multiplied.

If migraine were like an infection, we could draw some blood, put it in a petri dish, see which infectious agent caused the problem, and pick the right drug to knock it out. But migraine is not an infection. Migraine is a disorder of sensory processing. People with migraine often feel pain after stimuli that typically do not bother nonmigraineurs. Migraine sufferers have symptoms in common, starting with the pain (although some forms of migraine do not have pain as a component). What triggers the pain, however, varies from individual to individual. This is the focus of clinical research. We endeavor to identify the unique features in migraineurs that will lend insight to the common underlying causes of head pain. For example, recent research suggests that people who experience their headaches as "exploding" may have a different response to certain treatments from the response of those whose headaches are described as imploding. While this has yet to be verified, it is an exciting clinical observation that can teach us a great deal about the nature of head pain and its treatment.

Since all headache sufferers have their own unique triggers, they each need their own unique management plan to address those triggers as well as the pain and other symptoms that result. This means that one of the biggest problems for migraine sufferers today is with our health care system. While the medical community is extraordinarily good at dealing with acute and life-threatening conditions (like major trauma, cancer, and pneumonia), it is not set up to treat chronic, episodic, progressive diseases—like asthma, depression, diabetes, obesity, heart disease, and migraine.

When a physician's schedule only allots seven minutes to take a headache sufferer's history, examine the patient, and design a treatment plan, it is impossible to provide ample customization to prevent and treat that patient's migraines. But without that level of customization, the plan is doomed from the outset. Instead, patients and their doctors perform endless experiments with drug after drug, or get referrals to psychiatrists, neurologists, or pain specialists. The fortunate ones may find their way to headache specialists, yet often even these superspecialists are overworked and overwhelmed. In the end, patients often feel that they have not been heard, their questions have not been answered, and they have no plan. Still, they have a new prescription and a follow-up visit in three months, when, one hopes, they will get some relief.

We shouldn't blame the doctors, the emergency room staff, or anyone else who is honestly trying to help. Most of them weren't trained for this and, almost always, these practitioners are doing the best they can. Even so, the greatest challenge in implementing your treatment plan can often be to enlist effective support from your doctor, your insurance company, your benefits counselor, and everyone else involved in your health care.

The Keeler Center for the Study of Migraine

When I was the chief of the Headache and Facial Pain Section at the University of Southern California (USC), I learned a great deal about how to improve care for headache sufferers. I also began to understand what would be required to care for headache sufferers effectively. I came to envision the perfect headache clinic, a facility that offered both traditional and alternative treatment modalities. It would have a close affiliation with a cutting-edge research institution committed to applying state-of-the-art scientific investigation to the problems of headache pathophysiology and treatment. This clinic would be free of economic constraints, so any headache sufferer who needed help could get access, regardless of their ability to pay for it. And I wanted it all housed in a friendly environment with skilled nurse practitioners, physical therapists, psychologists, biofeedback technicians, yoga instructors, nutritionists, and patient educators—all working with patients to improve their lives, given the reality that, at least for the present, headaches *are* a part of life. My years trying to care for and understand headaches in a traditional medical environment convinced me that such a model was the only option. At the time, it was all a fantasy, unless I won the lottery. Since I didn't play the lottery, this seemed unlikely.

With the dawn of a new millennium, the fates conspired to make my fantasy a reality. First, I met Michael Harrington, M.D., Ch.B., FRCP, formerly of the National Institutes of Health (NIH) and the California Institute of Technology (Caltech), and presently director of the molecular neurology program at the prestigious Huntington Medical Research Institutes (HMRI) in Pasadena, California. Dr. Harrington came to present grand rounds at USC, and offered the most innovative approach to the study of a variety of neurological disorders that I had ever encountered. Unfortunately, migraine was not on his radar. But after his lecture, we talked. And talked and talked. Before long, we wrote a proposal for NIH funding. We received the funding and began to research migraines.

The next bit of good fortune came from the family of the late Fred Keeler, a very successful businessman and philanthropist in Ojai, California. When Mr. Keeler passed away, his family wanted to honor his memory by continuing his good works in the community. The family generously funded the Keeler Migraine Center in Ojai. Essentially, they gave me carte blanche—and the resources—to create a state-of-the-art clinical facility as well as the advice and expertise of a remarkable assembly of people to guide the fiscal, administrative, and creative efforts that would guarantee the clinic's success.

Located just inland from Santa Barbara, California, the Keeler Migraine Center treats patients suffering from some of the most difficult and severe headaches in the world. One of the most renowned clinics in the country, the center is a refuge for headache sufferers. It is quiet, the colors are soothing, the pace is calm. As medical director, I work with a team of specialists, the best minds with the most powerful treatment options and newest resources, to practice at the cutting edge of migraine management. Closely affiliated with Dr. Harrington and HMRI's molecular neurology program, we focus our efforts on helping patients overcome their migraines. At the Keeler Center, we study new and innovative approaches, and integrate the latest science with treatments dating back thousands of years and crossing many cultures, so we can offer every scientifically proven tool—including traditional and alternative modalities—to treat chronic headaches.

Comprising physicians, scientists, and many others, the Keeler team integrates the latest research discoveries and cutting-edge science into our treatment plans. Not only do we have our own laboratories investigating the biology and chemistry of migraines, but we also actively incorporate discoveries from other researchers into our treatment strategies.

Making the Study of Headache a Priority

Today, we know a great deal about why we get headaches, how to prevent them, and how to take care of them when they break through our defenses. We know that migraine is a genetic disease with a clear (if incompletely understood) biological basis. We know that migraine is a chronic condition, which does not mean that patients always have a headache, but that they are always *susceptible* to getting one, just as an asthmatic is always susceptible to an asthma attack. We also have a much better understanding of what triggers, worsens, and alleviates headaches. We even have medicines that are not simply generic painkillers, but that work specifically for migraines.

There is still a lot we don't know. We don't know if migraines start in the cortex (the "thinking" part of the brain) or if they start in the brain stem, where "unconscious" processing takes place. We don't know if people who have an aura or warning before their migraines have a different condition from those of us whose headaches come on without warning. We don't know why chocolate triggers headaches in one patient but not in the next. Nor do we know if having migraines places you at increased risk for other medical conditions, particularly neurological ones. Migraine is a very complicated puzzle. But it is one that is coming together quickly.

Since the 1940s, the scientific underpinnings of migraine had not changed much, until the introduction of the triptans. With the introduction of sumatriptan in 1993 and the ensuing infusion of money from drug companies, an explosion in research funding and clinical fellowships in studying headache followed, and as a result, our understanding of and ability to care for migraine changed dramatically.

Today, we have an awareness of the basic pathophysiology of migraines that simply did not exist as recently as 2007. Drugs now in development could revolutionize our current rescue and prevention strategies. We are learning about the microenvironment of the brain and its interactions with the outside world and the rest of the body. Even our understanding of migraine pain has become much more sophisticated. We now know that headache pain proceeds in several distinct phases, each of which can (and should) be addressed differently. Pain begins peripherally in the nerves that mediate sensation in the head, and then proceeds into the central nervous system where, if left unchecked, it eventually becomes a vicious cycle of inflammation. We have a better understanding of how to recognize where in this pain cycle a patient is at any given moment, and how best to treat the pain.

Despite the recent explosion of information, the science of migraine is still in its infancy. The Keeler Center works closely with the HMRI molecular neurology lab to understand the basic science of migraine by examining the spinal fluid of headache sufferers. Through a combination of private and federal funding (from the National Institutes of Health), our laboratory, under the direction of my colleague Dr. Harrington, uses chromatography and other sophisticated technologies to study the spinal fluid of hundreds of volunteers. Eventually, this research will yield information about diet, medication, and genetics that will dramatically improve the lives of those suffering from debilitating migraines.

Our approach to research is a little like that of a private detective who goes through a subject's garbage looking for clues. In our case, the subject is migraines, and the garbage is the spinal fluid, which carries the products of brain metabolism (its garbage, so to speak) off to the veins and eventually to the kidneys for excretion in the urine. Since spinal fluid can be obtained only through an invasive spinal tap, we hope eventually to access this information from more obtainable fluids such as blood, urine, saliva, and even tears. We are interested in understanding the basic biology of headache; developing an easy test to determine if a given headache is a migraine (for which certain medications will be effective); learning the effect of dietary alterations, such as changing the ratio of omega-3 fatty acids to omega-6 fatty acids; and developing novel drugs that work at specific sites in the brain to prevent or stop a migraine. We already have promising data in each of these areas.

Our laboratory research has already helped our patients at the Keeler Center in many ways. Many of our treatment protocols, dietary recommendations, and lifestyle modifications are based on research from our laboratories and the research of the laboratories of our colleagues across the country and around the world.

For example, recent work has shown that migraine has two stages and that triptans are effective primarily in the first stage but considerably less so in the second. A phenomenon called cutaneous allodynia helps us identify when the first stage is ending and the second stage beginning. Basically, cutaneous allodynia refers to that time in a headache when the skin and skin appendages, such as hair and teeth, become very sensitive, even painful to the touch. For most migraineurs, this occurs between thirty minutes and two hours into a headache and can last for hours, often beyond the end of the pain phase of the headache. In terms of treatment, this is very helpful information because it

- explains why triptans are often not effective if taken late in a headache;
- gives valuable guidance as to when to take a triptan;
- indicates when it is too late and probably useless to take a triptan, which is expensive medication.

Another example of recent scientific progress influencing migraine treatment comes from our own laboratory, where we identified a particular prostaglandin found in high concentration in the spinal fluid of migraineurs compared to nonmigraineurs. This prostaglandin is associated with sleep. This lends insight into the healing magic of sleep for migraineurs, and also gives us a tool for managing migraines through the medical manipulation of the prostaglandin pathway. We are also studying dietary manipulations.

By closely following the scientific literature and meeting with the scientists and clinicians in the group on a regular basis, we continually upgrade and modify our treatment strategies as our understanding of headaches continues to evolve.

The Keeler Method for Migraine Management

Most of us have ideas about how to take care of our headaches. Most patients try to avoid situations they think might cause a headache, and sometimes go to the emergency room when things get really bad. For the most part, these are partial solutions or desperate measures. They do not constitute a plan. But thirty million Americans suffer from headaches. They can't all come to Ojai—nor do they need to.

This book outlines my general principles as well as specific steps you can take to develop your own unique treatment plan, your own strategy to guide you away from a life dominated by headaches. This is the Keeler Migraine Method, the culmination of more than twenty years of caring for people with headaches, myself and thousands of others.

The Keeler Migraine Method is different. **The Keeler Method offers each patient a customized, personalized, workable plan for managing their headaches.** This approach works much better than trial-and-error medications, chiropractic adjustments, purges, purgatives, electroshock, or any other treatment out there. We combine many tiny adjustments and interventions that, when taken together, dramatically reduce the number of headaches you get as well as the severity of the pain and other symptoms when headaches do occur. *The Keeler Method provides a philosophy of migraine management to help patients understand their headaches and use that understanding to create an antimigraine environment.*

Most headache sufferers can control their headaches with some education, a few simple self-assessment tests, and the help of a good and willing physician. This book will help you understand the source of your headaches, show you how to isolate *your* specific triggers, and give you pointers on how to communicate effectively with your doctor. Here, you will learn the most current strategies for treating migraines, from the newest scientific discoveries to tried-and-true clinical medicine and alternative therapies, too. This book describes every aspect of the treatment plans we use to successfully treat our patients at the Keeler Center.

Every migraineur (a person whose headache meets the criteria for being migraine) presents unique sets of triggers and pain patterns. That's why the Keeler program does not include lists of forbidden foods, rigid diets, or blanket edicts about things you must avoid. The reality is that triggers differ from person to person, and *anything* can be a trigger. Triggers can be:

- dietary
- hormonal
- psychological
- environmental
- chronobiologic (sleep-related)
- psychosocial

- medicinal (medication-related)
- medical (due to other health conditions)

In Chapter 3, I explain much more about the vast array of triggers that can cause migraines. However, some generalizations *do* seem to apply to many migraine sufferers. From these observations, we have developed a philosophy that guides our treatment strategies:

> When we understand the individual migraine sufferer's unique triggers, we can influence disruptions to the lifestyle patterns associated with each trigger and gain control of the headaches.

Migraineurs do not do well with chaos. Put another way, migraines thrive on change. All individuals have a unique set of responses to disruptions to their environment, and migraines can be one of these responses. So each migraineur has specific lifestyle elements to which that person is especially sensitive, and changes in *these* areas of life are more likely to trigger that individual's migraines. The key, then, to effective migraine management is for individual migraineurs to understand their personal sensitivities and to create strategies to minimize disruption of those patterns. Whether we are talking about sleep schedules or meal timing or an exercise routine, we encourage patterned behavior whenever possible and, when a change is unavoidable (such as plane travel, a big party, or tax season), we try to anticipate that disruption and take extra headache precautions. This philosophy is at the heart of the Keeler Migraine Method and this book.

It's not a magic formula. But when you understand the importance of careful observation, keeping a routine, and clever planning (facilitated by the self-assessment tools in this book), you can understand your headaches and create your own formula for controlling them. For example, Jeri is a twenty-year-old college junior who has had headaches since her early teens. For the most part, they were Tylenol headaches, meaning she could knock them out with a couple of Tylenol. Over the last couple of years, her headaches became more of a problem and were now affecting her academic and social life. We had her keep a headache diary for one month. When she came back to the clinic, she said that her headaches were no longer a problem. Just from her own observation, she realized that her headaches were linked to her erratic sleep pattern, caffeine consumption, and inconsistent exercise. With a little organization and awareness, she was back on track.

While we have yet to cure our first migraine, my patients will tell you that their headaches have never been better, that they are less frequent, less severe, and of shorter duration. More important, their *lives* have never been better. They miss fewer workdays. They attend more family events. They can exercise, go out to dinner, and maybe even have a drink or two. They have regained control of their lives. While they still get migraines, headaches are no longer the focus of their lives. They are a footnote. So while some patients (such as those who suffer from chronic daily headaches) should see a headache specialist, and every headache sufferer should be under the care of a physician, every migraine sufferer can significantly improve their life by following the Keeler Migraine Method.

Constructing Your Keeler Migraine Method Treatment Plan

Every migraine patient is unique, and so is every treatment plan, but all of our treatment strategies have three parts: lifestyle modification, prevention, and rescue. Many new patients tell me that "nothing works," or "only one thing works." But nearly always, these migraineurs have not experienced such a comprehensive treatment program.

The Antimigraine Lifestyle

Generally, migraineurs need a healthy rhythm in their lives. But creating a healthy rhythm is the last thing we want to think about after a headache. People do not want to think about their headaches when they are without headaches. We are far more interested in getting on with our lives and making up for the time we have lost to headaches. We frantically take advantage of these good days, rushing about, making up for lost time, and avoiding anything that might break the delicate, pain-free balance. And when we do have a headache, we just want to lie down, never mind developing a migraine prevention strategy. Between these two states, that pretty much covers all the time there is, and doesn't leave any opportunity for planning. As a result, we live in a constant cycle of headache, catch-up, tiptoe, trigger.

It is clear that migraineurs do better when their lives are more patterned, but often the nature of the headache sufferer's life resists patterning. This is the challenge. How do we break the cycle and create a fresh behavior pattern?

The Keeler Method starts with our most basic patterns: sleeping, eating, and physical activity. For most migraineurs, keeping regular hours, eating regular meals, and exercising regularly can work wonders with their headaches. So we want to work toward living an antimigraine lifestyle. This alone can often solve a multitude of problems—migraine-related and otherwise.

While the antimigraine lifestyle thrives on patterns, it does *not* need to be boring. Too many migraineurs avoid special events, parties, travel, and other pleasures for fear of getting a headache. But with creative anticipation and strategic planning, you can effectively manage most situations and stop letting headaches decide how and where you spend your time.

Lifestyle modification is the process of analyzing your behaviors, activities, relationships—everything—in order to identify those components that may contribute to your headaches. Once we identify them, we can figure out how to modify lifestyle such that the quality remains but the headaches diminish. This is a decision-making process. It involves:

- eliminating those activities that serve no positive purpose;
- avoiding those that can be avoided without significant loss;
- modifying those that are important enough to hold on to.

While these decisions and the changes they require can be the most difficult part of putting a migraine treatment plan into action, over the long run, *lifestyle modification has the biggest impact on headache frequency, severity, and duration.* And the payback is a vastly improved quality of life.

Lifestyle modification means understanding your headaches and how they affect you, and then using that information to make decisions about having wine with dinner, or going to the gym, or just scheduling your day. This knowledge won't limit you, it will empower you.

An Ounce of Prevention

Not every headache sufferer needs a daily preventive medication, but for some migraineurs, prevention is mandatory. For most headache sufferers, though, my rule of thumb is that *the patient should be on a preventive if headaches substantially interfere with life.* This would be a simple rule, yet surprisingly, migraineurs often do not realize how much headaches interfere with their lives. Without a diary or an observant companion, we migraineurs tend to woefully underestimate both the frequency and severity of our headaches and, between headaches, most of us feel quite normal. Though there may be compelling evidence that we are *not* perfectly normal, we perceive that we only need medical attention when we have a headache, so we need to learn from the people around us the extent to which headaches interfere with our lives. For example, you may feel that, because you get only one or two headaches per month, your life is relatively unaffected, but your spouse may point out that, for fear of getting a headache, you avoided eight social events and three of your kid's soccer games, and you did not go to the gym last month. Thus, your family, friends, and even coworkers can help you gain further insight into how your headaches truly affect you and those you care about.

There are a few other important points to keep in mind about prevention. When we talk about prevention, usually we are referring to preventive medications, but nonmedication preventives are also important. Prevention includes many options, from daily prescription medications to nutraceuticals and herbs to lifestyle modifications such as diet, yoga, massage, exercise, biofeedback, and a variety of modalities. These choices are based on personal preference, lifestyle, side effects, other medical concerns, and, most important, what works.

To the Rescue

When most of us think of headache treatment, we tend to think of solutions to get us out of pain. In migraine management, we call this "rescue." Whether the rescue consists of finding a cool, dark place where we can curl up, the strongest painkiller in the cabinet, or the closest emergency room, we just want rescue from the pain when it is bad. While the Keeler Method teaches us how to prevent, avoid, and modify, we are migraine sufferers, and we are going to get headaches. So rescue is a big part of the plan, and it will remain so until a cure is found.

In the Keeler Method, our rescue goals follow two principles:

- Safety—Never use a rescue that can have bad consequences down the road.
- Preparedness—Be armed with backup alternatives in case the first rescue doesn't provide enough relief.

As a result, Keeler management plans involve designing medication strategies that will rescue you from the pain, and "layering" these strategies so that you know what to do when plan A doesn't work.

Flexible and adaptable to your unique headache patterns, the Keeler Migraine Method incorporates the latest scientific research with a systematic treatment approach. It integrates traditional with alternative strategies and proven methods with cutting-edge treatment into one plan. Now you can learn more about these techniques and apply them to *your* headaches. In the next chapters, I lead you step by step through the Keeler Method and help you develop your own personalized plan to regain control of your headaches—and your life.

PART ONE

Understanding Headache: Get Educated, Get Better

Chapter 1

Why Humans Get Headaches

Whether they are a creationists or Darwinian evolutionists, most people believe that there is some sense, some order to the universe, and that there must be an explanation for why things are the way they are. So, most of us would like to believe that migraines are not just some cruel joke or fluke of design (although you might make that argument for the famously underdesigned knee and the disproportionately large avocado pit). It is more reasonable to assume that migraines, like many human afflictions, are merely one extreme of a necessary and usually workable design, whether evolved or intelligently designed. The fact is, our pain protects us and serves a valuable function for the survival of our species.

How Pain Protects Us

Through sensation, we perceive and interact with the world. Sight, smell, hearing, taste, and touch all provide our brains with valuable information, and we, in turn, interpret and respond to that input. For example, in response to something noxious, we perceive an uncomfortable sensation and, in response to a painful stimulus, we usually withdraw. When our ancestors created fire, no doubt several of them immediately stuck their hands into the fire to see what it felt like. (I suspect I am directly descended from some of these people.) Those who failed to learn from the pain might have continued to make unhealthy mistakes and died off, but those who learned to avoid painful stimuli would have survived. For a stimulus like heat, sharp objects, or toxic fumes, the response is fast and uniform throughout the species. Presumably, humans without such a response did not survive into modern times. For the rest of us, today, the pain mechanism alerts us to dangers in the environment, and we learn to avoid them. As a species, pain has actually served us well. But what is the pain signal that alerts us, as a species, to avoid more subtle environmental threats? You do not have to be a headache sufferer to know that if you go from sea level to a high-altitude ski resort, then immediately hit the slopes without acclimatizing, you will get a headache. Most people will get a headache when subjected to extreme altitude, heat, or noxious fumes, and our response will be to relocate, if possible, to a more convivial climate.

Imagine a group of our ancestors migrating along the edge of a desert. When they find that they do not feel well (the most sensitive of their tribe experiencing headaches, for example), the tribe is less likely to settle in that environment. The same would be true for a group traveling at high altitude or downwind of active volcanoes spewing sulfuric gases. *More keenly attuned to environmental insults than the rest of the tribe, migraineurs acted as sentinels for a society struggling to find a safe environment in an unsettled world.* So perhaps the migraineurs among us helped our ancestors realize that they shouldn't live at twelve thousand feet altitude or in the middle of the desert. (The ones who didn't make the connection are no longer with us.) In the same way, our modern migraineurs shy away from a hostile stimulus in response to pain. While our ancestors moved to more temperate climates, we migraineurs have learned to retreat to a safe environment that is devoid of stimulus, where it is cool, dark, and quiet.

But we are modern, busy people, just trying to deal with life despite our migraines. Why should we bother to understand their "theoretical" cause? In fact, understanding the evolutionary utility of migraines—their purpose in humans and advantage to our species—is a crucial step in gaining control over your headaches, because this understanding gives you a frame of reference from which you can evaluate your world and identify your triggers. Once you understand that migraines are your response to something disruptive in the internal or external environment, you can begin to address your own specific migraines effectively.

As with all aspects of human development, our pain response is subject to infinite individual variation. Some of us are genetically more comfortable in cold weather, others in warmer weather. Some of us describe ourselves as having high or low thresholds for pain. But generally, *migraineurs likely represent a subgroup of humans who are more sensitive to environmental extremes than the general population.* Indeed, if an extreme environment is one that is hostile to a comfortable existence, then *our* definition of "extreme" is more narrowly defined than it is for the general population.

The fact is, anyone can get a migraine. Anyone. Even someone who "never" gets headaches will get a typical migraine when exposed to an environment that is hostile enough. For the lucky ones, it takes a powerful stimulus to produce a headache. These are the folks who get a rare migraine after camping for three days without sleep on the side of a sulfur-spewing volcano at twenty thousand feet. Others of us are much more sensitive. Never mind breathing sulfur for three days or hiking through a blistering-hot desert, we will get a migraine just walking past the perfume counter in a department store, spending an afternoon in the sun, or flying in an airplane at high altitude.

Through our senses, the brain gets billions and billions of bits of data from the outside world and, at the same time, it gets billions and billions of bits of data from our body's internal environment. The brain's job is to make sense of all this information, deciding which information requires action, what to file for later, and what to discard. One of the brain's main functions is to recognize threats and respond appropriately. Migraine brains are generally more sensitive to these inputs, and can "overreact" to a relatively innocuous stimulus, like a fluorescent light or loud music.

In fact, I know a wonderful neurologist who argues that migraineurs are further along the evolutionary path than nonmigraineurs. Because of our heightened sensitivity to hostile elements in the environment, we are better equipped to act as the sentinels of civilization. Whether this is true or not, it provides a clue as to why humans get headaches. Yes, it is quite a burden for a guy with a migraine. But once we understand why *people* get headaches, we have a frame of reference to consider why we *as individuals* get headaches.

This raises an interesting correlate question: If the migraineur's set point for physically reacting to a hostile environment is too low, are there individuals in the population whose set point is too *high*? In fact, there are. A "risk taker" gene has actually been identified in individuals who seem impervious to dangerous environments. So migraineurs may be at the other end of the spectrum and, given natural selection, perhaps this is a safer—though more painful—place to be.

If we assume that headaches, like other forms of pain, are a natural mechanism that the body uses to *inform* us that we are in a hostile environment, then we can also assume that those of us who more frequently get headaches are more sensitive to hostile environments. Once we understand how *really* hostile environments (like arid deserts and high-altitude mountains) can give any human headaches, we can begin the process of weeding out those triggers in the environment that we find worsen our *individual* headaches. Then, and only then, can we develop strategies to avoid, modify, or prevent those triggers and the headaches they cause.

The interaction between our brains and our environment is at the very heart of migraine management. The underlying problem in migraine is a problem in the parts of the brain that tell us when we are in a hostile environment. Is the perfume counter at Nordstrom's truly toxic? To the species as a whole, probably not (though who really knows?), but it can certainly be hostile enough to some migraineurs. Migraine is likely the result of an impaired sensory system, but just as logically, migraine might represent a more highly evolved sensory system. Either way, *for migraineurs to manage well, they need to deal with those aspects of the environment that their brains perceive as hostile.*

But the "environment" includes not only the *external* environment but our *internal* environment as well. While the world around us teems with potential headache triggers, a whole host of migraine triggers can also bombard us from within. From hormonal fluctuations and circadian rhythms to the foods we eat and medications we take, triggers are everywhere, inside and out. They are the key to migraine and its prevention. Because each migraineur is unique, so, too, is the constellation of triggers that can result in each migraineur's headache.

How Are Migraineurs "Different"?

A traditional way to understand diseases is to understand the normal function that has gone awry. For example, our bodies use insulin to help utilize sugar when the sugar level in the blood is too high, but when the body doesn't produce enough insulin to store away the sugar, the person gets diabetes. Similarly, our airways change size according to changes in air temperature or particulate composition, but when this system over-reacts to nonthreatening changes (like exercise or cold), asthma results. Most chronic diseases work this way, resulting from either a loss of function (as in diabetes) or a gain of function (as in asthma).

So what about migraine? What normal system goes bad in people with migraine? Many headache specialists believe the problem is in the way our brains process stimuli. The pain system alerts the brain to the fact that there is something hostile in the environment. In the "normal," nonmigrainous person, it takes a strong assault, like high altitude, noxious fumes, or extreme heat, to produce migraine-like pain. Just as the insulin system fails for some people, there are those, at the extremes of regulation, who have problems with headaches.

We do not know why migraineurs' brains have an overly sensitive response to changes in the environment. But we do know that when a noxious stimulus reaches the trigeminal nerve (the cranial nerve that mediates sensation in the head), it triggers the release of vasoactive peptides, chemicals that create changes in the diameter of blood vessels in the meninges, the membrane that lines the brain. It also causes other changes in the brain stem, the deepest part of the brain. Then, in the "thinking" part of the brain, the cortex, the sensitivity of nerve-firing changes, and this change radiates across the cortex—at least in those patients who have aura (a visual or other sensory "warning" before the actual head pain begins), and probably others as well—in a slow wave known as cortical spreading depression (not to be confused with clinical depression, which is an entirely different story).

Well-designed controlled studies have demonstrated that migraineurs, *even when they don't have a headache,* are more sensitive to sensory input than people who do not experience migraines. Another way to put it is that headache sufferers have a more "reactive" brain. Recent studies have also shown that the migraineur's brain becomes increasingly more sensitized to input, both during a headache and over years of intermittent headaches. This phenomenon is called "windup." Seen in other pain syndromes, this is the main argument for early and consistent treatment of headaches to prevent or minimize this process.

Of course, for those of us who are migraineurs, it is tempting to promote the theory that we are evolutionarily more advanced than our insensitive, nonmigrainous cohabitants, but this is not likely the case. Usually, migraineurs' responses to certain environmental stimuli are what anthropologists call "maladaptive," meaning that they are not particularly useful. While we are not exactly X-Men, neither are we neurotic. Migraine is *not* an imaginary, "psychiatric," or "emotional" condition, but rather a chronic disease much like asthma or diabetes, and it is largely determined by our genetics. Migraine is also manageable, particularly when we understand the system that has the problem.

Still, without the mechanism that results in our headaches, we as a species would not have survived and flourished. Humans need the pain response to interact safely with the world. Those humans whose pain response is significantly reduced or absent tend not to do as well in the world; at the other end of the spectrum are we "sensitive" souls for whom relatively mild noxious stressors can lead to headaches. And who knows? It may turn out that avoiding those toxic perfumes, dark chocolates, and unprotected days at the beach will ultimately ensure our survival as a species. It may turn out that migraineurs, not the meek, shall inherit the Earth!

Why We Get Headaches

Rarely, a headache is a symptom of something else (like a brain tumor, burst blood vessel, or infection). Much more commonly, though, the headache is not caused by another disease or condition but is the primary problem. Either way, all headaches have one thing in common:

they all cause a particular nerve pathway in the head to fire. The trigeminal nerve sends pain messages from the face, head, sinuses, and lining of the brain into the brain for processing. If a tumor presses on the blood vessels of the lining of the brain, this pressure will activate the trigeminal nerve, which will then send a pain message to the brain and create a headache. If the nerve itself happens to have an overly sensitive response threshold, the result is the same: the brain gets a pain message, and the headache will feel like a migraine, a perceived pain resulting from stimulation of nerves in the trigeminal pathway.

Whether the pain is triggered by a food, sinus congestion, or tension, it is still the trigeminal nerve that communicates that pain to the brain. Complicating an already complex picture, the rare "sinus headache" and the very common migraine can share a number of features, which can complicate both the diagnosis and the treatment of these headaches. This is also true of tension-type headaches. Studies suggest that as much as 40 percent of such migraineurs are misdiagnosed—the triggers being mistaken for the type of headache they cause.

The overwhelming majority of headache sufferers have headaches because of a genetic predisposition to migraines. Ours is a genetic disease. Though the inheritance pattern is not as straightforward as it is for blue eyes or red hair, headaches run in families. Of course, this is not true for every headache sufferer, but it is for most. In fact, recent research has traced a very rare form, familial hemiplegic migraine, to a specific gene. But as yet, no gene has been identified for the more common forms of migraines. Still, it is very unusual to find someone with migraine headaches without a family history of migraines. Indeed, family history is very important in making the diagnosis of migraines, and when patients come into the clinic with no headaches in their family history, it is a red flag that their headaches may be something other than migraines, and we are more likely to look for alternative explanations for the pain. It is not the only diagnostic factor, to be sure, but is certainly an important one.

Fortunately, not every child of migraineurs gets headaches. In my family, both of my parents had migraines and my sister and I get them, but my older brother does not. And while my son does not get migraines, sadly, my daughter does.

Other than our genetic susceptibility, we do not know why thirty million Americans get migraines and 190 million do not. By looking at the epidemiology of migraines, we can learn a lot. We know that migraines are most prevalent in women between the ages of twenty-one and fifty, and approximately three times more common in women than in men. Slightly more common among middle- and lower-middle-class economic groups, migraines are present in all socioeconomic strata and all industrialized countries, without a geographical bias. While the data are hard to collect, migraines are probably just as common in developing countries. This tells us that there are many factors involved in determining who gets migraines, but it is clear that migraines do not respect gender, geography, or socioeconomic status, except by degree.

We do know a little bit more about what actually goes on in your brain when you get a migraine. Very real biochemical changes take place in the brains of migraineurs during a headache. We have been able to show that there is a spreading wave of decreased firing across the brain during a migraine. We have even been able to record video of changes in blood vessel diameter and increased metabolism in certain areas of the brain stem and cortex. We also know that the brain chemistry of migraineurs, even between headaches, differs from that of nonmigraineurs. In our own lab, when we compare the spinal fluid of migraine sufferers with that of nonmigraineurs, we find significant differences in the makeup of the fluid. Several neurotransmitter systems—serotonin, dopamine, and gamma-aminobutyric acid (GABA)—are involved in the migraine process, and prostaglandins, vasoactive peptides (like calcitonin gene-related peptide [CGRP], substance P, and neurokinin A), and fatty acids (the omega-3 to omega-6 ratio) all play significant roles. We are discovering that neuropeptides like orexin, grehlin, and adiponectin all influence migraines. While we do not know the underlying biochemical abnormality, several theories relating to the way we regulate sodium in the brain, the way electrical charges move through brain tissue, and the way in which the hypothalamus, fat cells, and neurotransmitters are distributed have all been invoked as possible "first events."

While we still do not know whether migraine begins in the cortex (the more highly evolved, "thinking" part of the brain) or in the brain stem (the more phylogenetically primitive, "automatic" part), we have learned much about how a headache spreads once it has begun. Both the neocortex and brain stem are involved, and an electrically measurable wave of change moves across the brain during a migraine. This process is called cortical spreading depression. We have imaged the brain during migraine and seen an abnormal level of activity in specific areas, including a part of the brain stem called the nucleus caudalis basalis as well as the hypothalamus and parts of the frontal lobes. We know a great deal about the chemistry of these areas of the brain, and this has given us valuable insight into how we might modify the migraine process.

We are also learning how the brain functions during a migraine, and the way in which migraines begin—often with a triggering event from outside the brain—and then progress to a pain cycle that is quite independent of external (or extra-cerebral, internal) stimuli. In other words, there appear to be two phases to a migraine headache, the first tied to the brain's response to the trigger(s) and the second involving a central (in the brain) feedback loop that perpetuates the pain, even after the trigger has been removed.

Recent research has shown that repairing a small hole between the left and right sides of the heart, a patent foramen ovale (PFO), may cause some migraines to improve. In about 25 percent of people, this hole has been left open after birth. Anecdotal reports have claimed that migraineurs who had this "hole in the heart" repaired saw dramatic improvement in their migraines. A controlled trial, called MIST 1, was conducted to see if closing the hole would "cure" migraines, but the study was negative—no cure. Unfortunately, this study was designed to measure complete *elimination* of headaches, rather than a reduction. However, a second study is under way, looking not for a "cure," but for *improvement*. If the hole was just one of many migraine triggers, we might expect that closing it could reduce headache frequency and/or severity in these patients.

Mounting evidence indicates that headache sufferers' brains are different from other people's brains, even between headaches and even when there is no hint of a headache. As we have found in our lab, the composition of spinal fluid in migraine sufferers is different from that of people who don't easily get headaches, and this means that their brains are, too. For example, prostaglandin D2, which is involved in sleep, is markedly increased in migraineurs' spinal fluid between headaches, and it spikes even higher during a headache. Omega-3 fatty acids are lower during migraines, and sodium levels are abnormal as well. Most migraineurs will also attest to the fact that even between headaches they feel more sensitive to certain stimuli such as fluorescent lights and loud sounds.

So the acute pain may just be the loudest expression of a chronic condition. To change your thinking on this, consider whether you would ask "When does a diabetes start?" or "Do you have an asthma?" Certainly, diabetics and asthmatics *always* have these conditions but can have crises or "attacks" when things get out of control. The same is probably true for migraine sufferers. This important notion changes the way we think about living with the condition. For example, even when things are under great control, diabetics will not go for Twinkies unless they have their insulin close by. Similarly, a migraineur, even between headaches, should be mindful of the triggers that can erupt into a migraine crisis.

Other recent studies suggest that molecules released by fat cells may contribute to the transformation of episodic migraines into chronic daily headaches. Considerable evidence also points to the overuse of rescue medicines as one possible culprit in this transformation to chronic daily headaches, and still other research points to a chronic inflammatory process in the blood vessels. Finally, it appears that migraines, left untreated, will become more frequent and severe. We do not know whether these many observations represent a variety of medical conditions whose outward appearance is a migraine, or whether these are all contributing factors in a single medical condition—migraines. A recent theory is that migraine is part of a larger syndrome of dysregulation of the body's biorhythms (sleep, hunger, exercise), and there is mounting evidence to support this. However, the underlying primary disorder has yet to be identified.

Whether migraine turns out to be a single medical condition or one manifestation of another, more diverse condition, we know that the results entail head pain, light sensitivity, nausea, and other symptoms that can come and go, more or less frequently and with varying severity. Until we know what the underlying abnormality is and how to correct it, our charge as headache physicians and headache sufferers is to reduce the frequency, duration, and severity of headaches as much as possible.

Chapter 2

What Is a Headache?

A t least once a day a patient tells me, "Some of my headaches are so bad they must be migraines." Or the flip side: "Oh, I get headaches, but they're not bad. Not like *migraines* or anything." Other patients start out by telling me that they have three kinds of headaches, or that they get "regular" headaches and "migraines too," or that they have allergies and also get "sinus headaches."

While it is true that an unlucky few have common migraine as well as hypnic headache, or both hemicrania continua and cluster headaches, such cases are extremely rare. What most of us construe as "different headaches" are actually different *presentations* of one headache type, and that is usually migraine.

It is the rare day when I see two headache patients with similar presentations. But the popular misconception is that "migraine" is doctorspeak for a severe, big-league headache and that a mild headache is not a migraine. Wrong, wrong, wrong, wrong, wrong. Migraine is a particular kind of headache. While I have never seen a "good" migraine, there are definitely "bad" migraines, severe migraines, mild migraines, and slight migraines. The overwhelming majority of headache patients have one kind of headache and, usually, that is migraine. Migraine is by far the most common kind of headache. I believe triggers cause the confusion. What many people think of as different kinds of headaches are actually different *triggers* for the same kind of headache: migraine.

If everyone's headaches had the same triggers, responded the same way to treatments, and had a common cause, there would be little need for the Keeler Method. Instead, headaches—and their diagnosis and treatment—can be quite complex. This chapter catalogs many of the features of migraine—normal and not—and discusses headache diagnosis. Of course, whether you have migraines or another kind of headache, particularly a rare or dangerous kind, your physician should diagnose your headache. But the information in this chapter can be a useful guide in those discussions.

Every Headache Is a Migraine Until Proven Otherwise

A very famous physician, Sir William Osler, proposed a basic principle that has stood for nearly a century now. It is called "parsimony of diagnoses." Basically, he said that before you give someone two diagnoses, make sure you can't explain everything with one. A corollary to this is: "Common things are common." The great majority of headaches that come to medical attention are migraines. Certainly, TMJ syndrome, muscle tension, sleep apnea, and temporal arteritis are all capable of causing headaches, but in a headache practice *every headache is migraine until proven otherwise*.

Sometimes it is easy to prove otherwise. If a man walks into my office, says his head hurts, and happens to have an axe embedded in his forehead, my first thought will not be migraine (although statistically, he may well be a migraineur). But when someone comes in and says, "I have had headaches all my life and now they are getting out of control," I think migraine, not sinus or tension or tumor. Certainly, other disorders and diseases can cause headaches, yet in a headache practice, I assume headaches are migraines unless I have reason to think they're not. When I examine a patient and take a history, I can confirm the diagnosis and focus on a treatment plan.

Not only is migraine the most common kind of headache, but the word actually refers to a particular kind of headache. The International Headache Society defines migraine as:

A one-sided headache that is throbbing, moderate or severe, and associated with nausea and/or vomiting or sensitivity to light and/or sound, lasting from four to seventy-two hours.

That sounds simple enough. Still, it can be tricky to determine what kind of headache you have, or even what kind of migraine you have. People who have some but not all of the above features are termed "probable migraine" for purposes of diagnosis. But it is important to sort this out because management can vary greatly for the different types, including migraine with aura, hemiplegic migraine, basilar migraine, and my personal favorite, late-life migrainous accompaniments. See pages 46–50 for more on these.

For most people, from headache to headache, the pain and things that come with it will stay remarkably similar, varying little except in intensity. But from person to person, migraines vary a great deal. In addition to different triggers, different people have vastly different headache patterns. Usually, when we talk about different kinds of headaches, we are talking about different causes, different qualities of pain, or differences in other features. These distinctions help because they can enable us to distinguish one headache from another, which is useful in developing a treatment strategy.

The term "headache" gets tossed around quite a bit. My parents even used to refer to me as "quite a headache." Famous as an excuse to get out of anything from unwelcome sexual encounters to family reunions, headaches have been touted as the harbinger of serious medical conditions such as stroke and brain tumor, and trivialized as a neurotic bit of "kvetching." But I have yet to meet the headache sufferer who would willingly trade a visit from her most dreaded in-law for a headache. Still, even today, I am frequently asked whether headaches are physical or psychological. Migraine sufferers might not be surprised that this question usually comes from migraineurs' spouses, parents, and children. But those of us with headaches, and those of us who study those of us with headaches, know *without a doubt* that headaches have a clear biological basis. Interestingly, the scientific distinction between the physical and the psychological has blurred as we discover the *physical* underpinnings, including the genetic basis, abnormal proteins, and functional imaging abnormalities. Emotion and psychology, however, *do* have roles in migraines. Tension and emotional strain are perhaps the most common triggers for headaches (as well as for ulcers, irritable bowel syndrome, diabetes, asthma, and congestive heart disease). To question the "organicity" of migraines in the present day makes as much sense as questioning the organicity of heart failure.

Still, migraines can be very hard to understand. They have no obvious outward sign; there's no measurable blood test or proof from an imaging study like an X-ray or a CAT scan. They seem to come out of the blue and disappear just as mysteriously. However, most people who live with migraineurs do learn to recognize a certain facial expression, body posture, or behavior that shouts headache, as clearly as if there were a sign on their foreheads. And the fact that triptan drugs are effective in treating many patients' migraines but are useless for other pains such as broken arms, postsurgical pain, or low-back pain, strongly suggests that migraine is a unique, biological disease.

To help migraineurs and our loved ones understand this, it helps if they learn more about what the heck headaches are. Obviously, a headache is a pain in the head. It is also a pain in the you-know-what, if you are someone who gets headaches or lives with, works with, or cares for someone with headaches. But to doctors, headache simply means a pain in the head. We use the term *cephalalgia* to describe the condition, without interpreting it and without implying the cause, severity, duration, or medical significance of the head pain. It is a useful if somewhat pedantic term because the one thing every headache sufferer has in common, regardless of the headache type, is pain. Without it, there is nothing to talk about.

A headache is simply a perceived pain resulting from stimulation of nerves in the trigeminal pathway. It is no more mysterious than arm pain from touching a hot frying pan or foot pain from stubbing your toe. But headaches are different. Often, the causes are less obvious, the pain lasts longer, and they sometimes have some strange accompaniments. So a lot of myths and mystery persist about the significance of different headaches, even the most common types, and to sort them out, a doctor who is tasked with diagnosing a headache needs to consider a few options.

Headache Diagnosis

We classify migraine headaches into types, subsets with certain characteristic features. Some common and others quite rare, various kinds of migraines present differently and have distinguishable features that can aid both your diagnosis and your management. Understanding the various migraine forms—as well as other headaches—will help you and your doctor sort through the specifics of your headache pattern. This information should help you recognize an unusual headache that calls for help, a situation that merits a doctor visit, or a headache that demands a trip to the emergency room. Since some of these are potentially dangerous conditions, you should use this information to start a discussion with a physician who can best diagnose your headaches.

Headache can be a secondary condition or a primary disorder. Quite rare, secondary headaches are a *symptom* of something else, such as an underlying disease or condition, or another process in the body, like a brain tumor, burst blood vessel, or infection. Very common, however, are primary headaches, when the headache itself is the problem, and it is not caused by another disease or condition. These include migraine, cluster, tension-type, and a few others.

Frequently, when we refer to different *kinds* of headaches, we are talking about different *causes* for the headaches, as well as different qualities of the pain and possibly other distinguishing features. For most people, from headache to headache, the pain and the things that accompany it are remarkably similar. Some people have common migraine headaches and others have cluster headaches, but usually each person's migraine or cluster will vary little (except in intensity) from headache to headache.

Diagnostic Tests

These days, not every patient presenting with long-standing, relatively stable headaches needs to undergo diagnostic tests, like a spinal tap or imaging scans. Sure, you might want to discuss these tests, and your provider may well consider them, but your doctor doesn't necessarily need to order them.

In some situations, a doctor will need to do a spinal tap, or lumbar puncture. In this procedure, we extract a sample of cerebrospinal fluid (CSF), which can tell us a great deal about what is going on inside the brain, much as going through someone's trash can tell a lot about the person who threw it out. CSF surrounds the brain, fills a series of connected chambers deep inside the brain, and flows around the spinal cord, so it informs us about the chemistry of the brain and its environment.

For example, if there is an infection in the brain, it will also be present in the spinal fluid. When we examine CSF under a microscope, we can see bacteria, if present, and we can usually identify the bacteria and test antibiotics on them to see if they will effectively kill the bacteria. So if a headache looks like a symptom of a central nervous system infection, such as meningitis or encephalitis, we need to do a spinal tap.

Spinal fluid analysis can also help a doctor confirm or rule out whether a blood vessel has ruptured. This is called a subarachnoid hemorrhage, which results from head trauma or a ruptured aneurysm (a long-standing weak area in an artery). CSF is normally blood free, but if a vessel has ruptured, a measurable amount of blood mixes into the spinal fluid and aids this diagnosis.

The third and final reason for examining spinal fluid is the possibility that increased pressure is causing a headache. Spinal fluid is constantly being produced and reabsorbed. When the balance of the fluid is disturbed, say by a blockage or problem with production or reabsorption, a headache can result. The most common cause of this is called benign intracranial hypertension, or pseudotumor cerebri (named more than a hundred years ago when, without brain imaging, doctors diagnosed tumors and operated but found no tumors). In this condition, removing the spinal fluid often brings instant, though temporary, relief.

It is increasingly rare to encounter a headache sufferer who has not had at least one MRI or CAT scan, also called a CT scan. In many cases, this is largely due to medico-legal concerns rather than medical decision making. In general, it is probably not a bad thing to have an imaging study at some point during the first evaluation of a headache and, certainly, if the character of the headache changes or if there is recent head trauma, imaging is appropriate. However, frequently, patients will have CT scans *every* time they come to the emergency room with a headache. From a medical point of view, this is clearly excessive.

Emergency room doctors are concerned about potentially life-threatening headaches, including ruptured blood vessels in the brain or, commonly, headaches caused by head trauma. CT scans are better than standard MRI at picking up blood in the brain. So when emergency room physicians are unsure of the cause of a new headache, they often order CT scans.

MRI is more sensitive than CT scans for evaluating masses such as brain tumors, abnormal collections of blood vessels, and certain cysts. The headache specialist is the best judge of whether a particular headache history necessitates an MRI as part of the workup, which might also include blood tests, spinal fluid analysis, and other tests. However, in the emergency room, the need for MRI for headaches is extremely rare. Usually, this decision can be left to the primary care doctor or neurologist at a follow-up appointment *after* the ER visit.

Recent studies in patients with chronic daily headaches have suggested that changes in the brain's blood vessels resemble the spasms we see in vasculitis or inflammation of the brain vessels. If larger studies confirm these findings, it may become the standard of practice to order MRI or CT angiography in selected patients. Those patients with abnormal findings would be treated with a calcium channel blocker, such as nimodipine, which is relatively specific for cerebral blood vessels.

The Stages of Migraine

To define a headache by the degree of pain is not really productive. Some migraineurs say that once the pain is really rolling, it is almost too late to do anything but ride it out, so a more important issue is *when* to treat a headache. This is also trickier. But if you approach headache as an underlying disease like asthma or diabetes rather than as an isolated incident such as stroke or heart attack, you are more likely to begin to manage your life in a way that will reduce the probability of going into migraine crisis. Indeed, if we could learn to view stroke and heart attack the same way, we could probably manage these conditions better as well.

Along the time continuum, a typical migraine follows four phases:

- prodrome
- aura
- headache (including a complex of symptoms)
- postdrome

Prodrome

With good evidence, we are beginning to understand that migraines begin hours *or even days* before the pain sets in. This first phase is called the prodrome, and different people experience it differently. I tend to yawn a lot for a day or two before the headache begins. Other early symptoms include cravings (often for carbohydrates), increased sensitivity to light or sound, and fluid retention. Often, we attribute these early symptoms to changes in the hypothalamus, which regulates sleep, body temperature, appetite, and water balance, and is active in controlling mood and how we respond to pain.

Aura

About one in five migraine sufferers experiences an aura after the prodrome, and it is still controversial as to whether migraines with aura and migraines without aura are different presentations of the same condition.

Usually a transient episode that lasts from five to twenty minutes in most people, an aura represents a "dysfunction" in one part of the brain. Though the most common auras are visual, they are not *eye* problems but *brain* problems. Such changes tell one of the great stories in migraine exploration. Early on, the visual changes were thought to be the result of blood vessel constriction in the eyes. Later, researchers felt that they were due to blood vessel constriction in the part of the brain that interprets images. Today, however, evidence suggests that these changes result from an abnormality in the brain itself, rather than in the blood vessels. Even the people who get visual auras experience considerable variability. Flashes of light or blind spots are the most common presentations, but visual auras can also be intensely colorful, geometric forms; perceptions that surroundings are larger or smaller than they really are; or even bizarre visual distortions, as Lewis Carroll experienced. The migraine-suffering author described such scenes in *Alice in Wonderland*.

While 99 percent of all auras are visual, they can also involve other sensory or autonomic changes (unusual smells, upset stomach, sweating, odd tastes), motor changes (focal weakness), problems with coordination, and even speech arrest (inability to speak, understand, or both), or altered consciousness like déjà vu, jamais vu, confusion, or unexpected emotion. These auras are unusual, but any sensory or motor event that seems to occur repeatedly in advance of a headache can reasonably be considered an aura.

During an aura, a cortical spreading depression (CSD) of nerve-firing moves across a section of the brain. In this case, "depression" has nothing to do with emotional depression, but refers to a depression of the electrical resting potential of the nerves. Previously, we thought this was associated with a decrease in oxygen due to local constriction of the blood vessels carrying oxygenated blood to that part of the brain, but recent work from Andrew Charles, M.D., at the University of California at Los Angeles, suggests that blood vessels actually dilate as the CSD advances. As with much of the science of headaches, we are just beginning to scratch the surface, and a clear story has yet to emerge.

One of the big questions among headache specialists is whether migraine with aura is a condition unique from migraine without aura. Certainly, patients who suffer both often feel that they are two distinct conditions. Yet convincing evidence suggests that all migraineurs experience the CSD—even migraineurs who do not experience an aura. These migraineurs' brains likely undergo the brain changes that the aura group experiences, but since most of the brain does not process vision or perform other "eloquent" functions, the CSD could occur in "silent" parts of the brain without symptoms, and these migraineurs would not notice the aura. This remains an unresolved question.

While there is not yet a definitive answer to the aura question, the laboratory offers some insight. We know that one of the underlying abnormalities that contributes to CSD is a variation in what is called the "slow calcium channel" or the "PQ channel." In support of this view, we have seen a variety of genetic mutations in rare migraine types, although we have yet to find these in common migraines. But interestingly, these cells with the abundant PQ channel are found in great numbers in the occipital cortex of the brain, the area that processes visual information, generates visual aura, and most often shows CSD.

Thus, migraine with aura may simply be a migraine that originates in the occipital or visual cortex, while migraine without aura might begin in another part of the brain. If this is so, the association between migraine with aura and other neurologic events, such as stroke, might merely reflect repeated damage to the neurovascular structures in this part of the brain. This is an overly simplified explanation, and this interpretation may have many problems. The reality is that at present we just don't know.

Interestingly, the aura phase of migraine is not always followed by headache pain. This is particularly true in older women, who often describe the visual changes without an attendant headache. So while aura and headache are associated with each other, they do not appear to be inextricably bound. By the same token, migraines in other individuals can be a prolonged, disabling event with weakness on one side of the body or inability to speak, every bit as depressing as the headache itself.

The relationship between aura and pain is presently a hot research topic. For headache sufferers who experience an aura, however, it is also useful in treatment, since the aura signals a coming migraine. These migraineurs can get a twenty- or thirty-minute jump before the onset of the headache, with the opportunity to take a rescue medicine, which can then often be more effective in avoiding or minimizing the pain phase. This is fortunate because migraine with aura is often a more severe, more painful headache than migraine without aura.

Understanding where you are in the progression of a headache provides a useful guide for selecting medication. If you think of migraine aura as a fire approaching your property, the triptans are effective in the same way that wetting down the property or clearing shrubbery is helpful in keeping the fire out of your house. When you feel the heat of the migraine coming on, go with the triptans. But once the house is on fire, hosing down the yard is not going to help. Instead, you need a fire retardant *in* the house.

The Headache Phase

Most of the world thinks the headache phase is the whole story. When we're in it, so do we. This is the phase when your head throbs, you might throw up, and you want to hide in a cool, quiet, dark hole. We know exactly what part of the brain causes nausea and vomiting; it is right next to the nucleus basalis caudalis, the area that becomes very active when the headache phase begins. Fully engaged in the process, the brain stem sends pain messages into the "higher" centers of the brain. The trigeminovascular system mediates headache pain through a complex of nerves that go both to the blood vessels around the brain and deep into the brain to connect with other nerves that spread to various other centers in the brain. Recent evidence even suggests that tiny branches cross the skull and send impulses to the muscles and other tissues outside the skull. The actual pain comes from throbbing blood vessels, but our awareness of the pain is made "louder" by sensitized nerves in the brain stem and thalamus, a "way station" between the brain stem and the higher parts of the brain. The picture gets more complicated when we add the fact that the brain becomes "sensitized" to these pain messages over time (hours) and may actually become self-stimulating in a vicious cycle. When this happens, breaking that cycle can be very difficult, and traditional rescue medicines become less effective.

Postdrome

Finally, the postdrome follows. This is the vaguely "out of it" feeling that most migraine sufferers experience after a headache. Often characterized by extreme fatigue, loss of appetite, scalp tenderness, altered mood, and foggy thinking, the postdrome can last hours to days.

Unfortunately, we know very little about why the brain reacts this way after a major headache, but we do know it is real. It is *not* your imagination, and you are *not* being a wimp. Of course, you know this, but I want to express it in black-and-white so you can show your spouse, employer, and colleagues.

Good-quality, well-controlled studies have shown that performance is impaired on cognitive and motor-skill tests, both during and after migraines. These deficits, though temporary, persist for a variable length of time, but the impairment *is* measurable.

Intuitively, this makes sense. Following a period of intense activity—whether physical, emotional, or cognitive—there is a necessary recovery period. We know that, during a migraine, a lot of activity takes place in the brain, and we can see this on PET scans (an imaging technique that demonstrates how much energy is being utilized by the brain). We also know that there is a wind-up process in which the responsiveness of nerves in the brain becomes increasingly altered. It takes time for these nerves to recover after the crisis is passed or the cycle is broken. This area of migraine treatment has not been explored to date but would hold significant appeal for headache sufferers.

To minimize the severity and duration of the migraine "hangover" phase, it helps to return to your regular schedule, especially for meals, sleep, and exercise. It is also important to rehydrate, since most people do not drink enough water during the increased sleep and general malaise of the headache phase. Remember, the postdrome is part of a headache crisis. If you try too hard to "get back to normal" and make up for lost time too soon, you will often end up frustrated at the very least and, at worst, may well have a headache recurrence.

Migraine's "Symptom Complex"

In migraine, many functions of the brain temporarily dysfunction. Not only do we see problems with pain, but also with all of the sensory systems and the autonomic nervous system, which regulates skin temperature, nasal congestion, sweating, and a variety of other functions. And migraine can adversely affect thinking and concentration, beyond what we would expect from head pain alone.

Vomiting

For some migraine sufferers, nausea and vomiting can be more disabling than the headache pain. It is probably not much comfort, but the association between migraine pain and nausea actually makes perfect sense—at least in terms of anatomy and evolution.

From an anatomical viewpoint, the nucleus basalis caudalis (often thought of as the migraine center) in the brain stem just happens to be located right next to the nucleus we associate with nausea and vomiting. So the nausea and vomiting may simply result from the physical proximity of the nausea/vomiting center in the brain stem to the headache center. In and around the "migraine center," other centers are involved with the sensations of dizziness and vertigo, which some migraineurs also experience. This lends credence to the notion that this is a local effect. When dizziness and vertigo accompany migraine, they tend to occur during the headache phase, not during the aura, so it is less likely that these symptoms come from higher in the brain, as the visual changes do. We have also seen strong associations between the neurotransmitters serotonin and dopamine, which are involved in migraine and nausea/vomiting. And interestingly, several of the drugs we use to treat nausea and vomiting also are effective in treating migraine.

From an evolutionary perspective, if we believe that migraines are a way for the brain to tell the body that it is in a hostile environment—and, sometimes, that hostile environment may include poisons or foods, as in the many food triggers some migraineurs suffer—it makes sense that one response to a hostile environment would be to empty the gut. So it follows that, hand in hand with migraine, we might experience nausea and vomiting, as well as diarrhea, which some migraineurs also suffer.

This should not be confused with the decrease in gut activity that occurs with migraine, called gastric stasis. It has been well reported that the processes of absorption across the gut is slow in migraineurs generally, and dramatically slowed during a migraine headache. One very real consequence of this is that medications taken orally will take longer to get into the blood and move on into the brain. There are no other symptoms. In the current teleology, we might think of this as part of the shift from vegetative/digestive activities to the "flight" response required to remove oneself from a hostile environment. The gut shuts down in a variety of threatening situations, as blood is shunted to the muscles and brain for quick action.

Throbbing

If you have ever smashed your finger with a hammer or cut yourself while chopping onions, you know that sickening, familiar throbbing. Many people who suffer from headaches are equally familiar with a pulsatile, relentless heartbeat in their head. We do not know the precise reason for this phenomenon, but it clearly is related to the way blood vessels, and the tiny nerves that cover them, respond to a "hostile" stimulus.

If we step back a little and look at how blood vessels work, this becomes clearer. The body's demand for blood varies depending on how much oxygen that part of the body needs, so the blood vessels need to be able to change their diameter to meet the need. If you've just had a big meal, you need more blood to go to your gut and less to your legs. On the other hand, if you are being chased by a large bear, you need lots of blood to the legs and not much to the digestive tract. So the blood vessels need to be able to dilate and constrict according to need. They do this with the help of tiny nerves wrapped around the walls of the vessels (which are actually specialized muscle tissue). These nerves cause the vessels to dilate or constrict. In the case of the smashed or cut finger, or a migraine headache, the normal regulation of blood vessel diameter stops and the blood vessel becomes a passive tube in that area. In a migraine, as the blood flows with the ebb and flow of your heart's pulsations, the nerves on the vessels pick up that pulsing signal and translate it into throbbing accents to your headache pain.

Photophobia

Sensitivity to bright lights so frequently accompanies migraine that it is included in the criteria that *define* the condition. Why is sensitivity to light more frequently associated with migraine than sensitivity to sound or smell or touch? In my experience, it is not.

During a headache, most migraineurs feel assaulted by bright lights, loud sounds, and strong smells (if they can smell at all). In fact, one or two hours into a headache, many migraineurs become extremely sensitive to touch, as well. Migraine begins as a hypersensitive response to some environmental stimulus and then the brain becomes hypersensitive to *all* stimuli. Over a short period of time, the brain becomes hypersensitive to its own stimuli, and no longer requires an external source. The headache begins to feed on itself. This is the phenomenon of central sensitization.

But remember, many migraineurs are also more sensitive to any sensory stimuli *between* headaches, and some migraineurs report that an excess of these stimuli will trigger a headache. The fundamental fact is that migraineurs are more sensitive to sensory input than people who do not experience migraines, and this is true even between headaches, when the migraineur feels fine. Well-designed controlled studies have demonstrated this.

Recent studies have also shown that headache sufferers have a very "reactive" brain. Both during a headache and over years of intermittent headaches, the migraineur's brain becomes increasingly more sensitized to input. This phenomenon, called "windup," is also seen in other pain syndromes, and is the main argument for early and consistent treatment to prevent or minimize this process.

Bright light in all its variations (flickering lights, strobe lights, full sunshine) can be a trigger, bringing on a headache in some people. Like any other trigger, this one can also worsen an existing headache. The eyes are very sensitive conduits directly to the brain, and not much input modulates visual stimuli, especially simple stimuli like light, so light may be the most common such trigger. But certainly, noxious smells and loud sounds can both trigger and worsen migraines in susceptible migraineurs.

Phonophobia

Often lumped together with photophobia, phonophobia, sometimes called sonophobia or sound sensitivity, is another common accompaniment of migraines. Most migraineurs will tell you that even when they are not in the midst of a migraine they are sensitive to loud sounds. In the midst of a migraine, *any* sound can be painful, including your own voice. This is often difficult for nonmigraineurs to understand, and is impossible to explain in the middle of a headache.

Touch Sensitivity

Until recently, we had no clue why some migraineurs experienced exquisite sensitivity to touch. In fact, when some migraineurs reported that their teeth hurt or that their skin was extremely sensitive during a headache, they were often greeted with a raised eyebrow. Finally, we understand this phenomenon, and it turns out to be a critically important piece of the migraine puzzle. Of course, being doctors and scientists, we cannot bring ourselves to call this symptom "hair pain." Instead, the technical term for increased sensitivity to touch is called cutaneous allodynia.

Logically, this symptom should come as no surprise. Migraines are all about hypersensitivity to environmental input. We are sensitive to lights, sounds, and smells that don't bother nonmigraineurs, so why not sensations like touch?

Cutaneous allodynia represents a hypersensitization of nerves within the brain, such that they become almost self-stimulating in the pain pathway. Generally, this occurs later in the headache phase, as most people say that cutaneous allodynia begins about two hours into the headache, not when a headache starts, but I have seen huge variability in this. And a percentage of migraine sufferers do not experience the phenomenon at all.

What is so interesting—and informative—about cutaneous allodynia is that once it occurs the triptans (some of which cost fifteen dollars per pill, or more) are no longer effective. Triptans, more effective early in the headache process, work on the first-order nerves in the migraine pathway, those carrying messages from the environment into the brain. So once cutaneous allodynia is present, your brain is on fire, and your hair hurts, medications that work on prostaglandins and inflammation may become more effective. It's time to switch to anti-inflammatories (naproxen or Toradol) or phenothiazines (Thorazine or Reglan, for example) or neuromodulatory rescues (Depacon).

Other Syndromes Associated with Migraines

Before the International Headache Society renamed headache types, migraines without aura were called common migraines, so named because they were the most common type of migraine. But other presentations of headaches have come under the rubric of migraine for many years. Whether these various syndromes are variants, or formes frustes, of migraines or distinct entities, we do not know with certainty. But the migraine "variants" have sufficient characteristics in common to make them easily organizable into groups. Some of these respond differently to preventive and rescue treatments, and others have associated symptoms that need to be addressed independently of the head pain. And perhaps more important, some of these syndromes place their patients at greater risk for stroke. For these reasons, it is useful to know about the more easily recognizable migraine variants.

Complicated Migraine

Complicated migraine is a much rarer form in which the headache is associated with a neurologic deficit during and, often, after the pain phase. Common deficits include difficulty speaking, difficulty using one side of the body, and alteration in sensation on one side. People with this kind of migraine may also be at greater risk for stroke than those with simple migraine. Complicated migraine differs from migraine with aura in that the neurologic deficits are present during the headache phase rather than in advance. Most headache specialists agree that patients with complicated migraine should be on a preventive medicine, often a calcium channel blocker. There is also disagreement as to whether it is safe to give these patients triptans due to the vasoconstrictive action of this class of drugs and their theoretical risk of stroke in patients at increased risk.

Hemiplegic Migraine

This is a specific kind of complicated migraine in which half the body becomes weak during the headache phase of the migraine. About half of hemiplegic migraineurs have a very strong family history of the condition, possibly with other neurologic problems as well. Recent research has confirmed that familial hemiplegic migraine has a genetic basis. Hemiplegic migraine is usually treated in the same way as complicated migraine.

Basilar Migraine

Basilar migraine describes a migraine-like syndrome that includes severe dizziness, balance problems, nausea, and vomiting. The time course (how long the attack lasts) is similar to that of migraine, though basilar migraine may or may not have head pain associated with it. Basilar migraine often requires treatment of other symptoms such as nausea and dizziness. Many people feel that basilar migraine is one of the most disabling migraines because of these associated symptoms.

Migraine and the Eyes

Eye pain and visual changes are a big part of migraine and of other primary and secondary headache disorders. The converse is also true: Many medical conditions of the eyes have pain as a symptom. Determining which is the cart and which is the horse is a job you should leave to your neurologist and ophthalmologist.

A few guidelines are useful. Typically, the visual changes associated with migraine take place in the visual processing area of the brain, not in one eye or the other. Therefore, you can perform a simple test: Close one eye at a time and check to see whether your vision is normal when you look through one eye or the other. If the visual changes are exclusively in one eye, it is likely *not* a migraine.

The exception to this is the apparently rare syndrome known as retinal migraine. Occurring in women of childbearing age, this sudden loss of vision *in one eye* is associated with headache, which typically lasts less than an hour. In some cases, however, the visual loss eventually becomes permanent. For this reason, and others, this is a serious concern, and it is important to discuss a true monocular visual loss, however brief, with your doctor as soon as possible.

Ophthalmoplegic migraine is another rare syndrome in which an eyelid droops, and the patient is unable to move the eye in one or more directions. These signs are associated with significant head pain. Usually the episodes are brief and self-limiting.

Sometimes, visual changes in the brain are not associated with pain. This is variously referred to as ocular or ophthalmic migraine, and often presents in older individuals who had typical migraines during their younger years. Usually, these syndromes do not require anything more than reassurance.

Late-Life Migrainous Accompaniments

A benign syndrome that we see in older patients who had migraines when they were younger, late-life migrainous accompaniments present with episodes in which a hand becomes numb and/or weak, then the sensation marches up the arm and to the head, sometimes with speech arrest or other deficits. This episode may or may not be followed by a headache before it eventually resolves. Certainly, a doctor should check a patient with such a presentation, but when this happens repeatedly in largely the same way a vascular event is unlikely, and late-life migrainous accompaniments is probable.

Acephalgic Migraine

Oddly, not all migraines hurt. Sometimes, migraines present with dramatic dizziness, nausea, or a focal neurologic deficit, but no pain. What they do have in common with other migraine syndromes is duration, typically four to seventy-two hours, as well as some of the other common features of migraines: sensitivity to light, motion, or sound. Again, this is not a diagnosis you want to make over the dinner table, but it is out there and is something a headache specialist may consider. Acephalgic migraine may not require any acute rescue, or it may require a symptomatic treatment for nausea or other symptoms. But if the symptoms are frequent, a preventive may be appropriate.

Mixed Headache

Patients can certainly have more than one type of headache, and mixed headache refers to the specific combination of a migraine with a tension-type headache. This is probably not as common as we previously thought, though good epidemiologic studies looking at this are not presently available. More typically, patients have migraines with neck tension as one of their prominent triggers. Pure tension-type headaches are less common headaches, at least in the United States.

More important, patients with migraines *can* get other kinds of headaches, and it is crucial to discover these while taking the patient's history. For example, as we get older, some people develop autoimmune conditions such as temporal arteritis, which can be superimposed on underlying migraines. When you perceive a change in your headache presentation, it is important to discuss it with your physician.

Hypnic Headache

This rare headache form occurs in people between the ages of forty and eighty. A unique headache, it occurs exclusively at night, typically at the same time each night, and lasts from fifteen to sixty minutes. The pain tends to be global, not just on one side, and is not associated with runny nose, tearing, or other autonomic features. This kind of headache does not typically respond to the usual headache medications, but other, specific treatments such as caffeine can be effective.

Inherited Syndromes Associated with Migraine

Michel Ferrari, M.D., Ph.D. (at the University of Leiden), and other headache scientists are identifying an increasing number of genetic diseases in which migraine plays a significant role. Many of these conditions have associated blood vessel abnormalities in the brain or the eyes, balance and coordination problems, or motor deficits. These conditions are present in only a small fraction of migraine sufferers but are of major importance in our study of the underlying causes of migraines. These conditions often run in families, providing an opportunity to study many individuals with similar DNA and similar medical conditions. To the research scientist, this promises major advances in our understanding of migraine in general.

Migraines That Require Special Handling

Even if headaches are your only issue, certain kinds of migraines and other headaches do require special treatment, and it helps if patients understand the best approaches for dealing with these headache situations. Chief among these is chronic daily headache (CDH), which can have specific causes that are important to uncover. Typical migraines are not daily, but migraine is often the headache underlying CDH. We have techniques for treating CDH without hospitalization, but these headaches are extremely difficult to treat, and often require hospitalization or intensive outpatient treatment.

"Progression of Disease"

For many years, headache specialists have witnessed the transformation of episodic headaches into CDH. They coined the term "transformed migraine" to describe this phenomenon. Recent scientific investigation increasingly suggests that this transformation may actually be the result of progression of the disease. This means that over years the disease gets worse. Most of the evidence for this comes from looking at the MRIs of people who have had migraines for a long time, and from comparing the health of older migraine sufferers with that of nonmigraineurs of similar age, gender, and so forth.

So, good evidence suggests that for many of us untreated migraine headaches will increase in frequency and severity as we age, but we really don't know the long-term consequences of this. Not every migraineur ends up with chronic daily headache. Why is that? When we look at those people who develop chronic daily headaches, we try to find elements that these headache sufferers have in common with one another but not with migraineurs whose headaches do not become daily. For example, we find that being overweight *is* a risk factor for chronic daily headache, but it is *not* a risk factor for migraine in general.

Supported by the growing body of scientific evidence, headache specialists have reached a general consensus that migraine is a progressive neurological disease. However, today, this is about all we know. For example, MRI scans of migraineurs' brains reveal small, bright areas. We don't know the significance of these lesions, but they are definitely there. We see similar lesions in some other chronic diseases, such as hypertension and diabetes. What does this mean for us migraineurs? We don't know if the changes we see in MRIs are important to the patients' overall health, if modification of lifestyle or regular use of medication influences these changes, or if there is actually an advantage to the changes that we see. Further, we do not yet have evidence that the frequency or severity of migraines has any correlation with the changes we see on migraine sufferers' MRIs. So far the new information about progression of disease does not have implications for treatment—beyond an intuitive sense that if we can reduce the frequency and severity of headaches, it should be a good thing. It makes sense that this is yet another reason to prevent and treat our headaches early, when we can.

Chronic Daily Headache (CDH)

It is not normal to have a headache every day. When a headache crosses the line from episodic to chronic, it is certainly time to get professional help. Often this means going to your primary care doctor and getting a referral to a neurologist. This is well worth the investment in time and co-pays. Increasing data suggest that chronification of headache is bad for you on many levels. While it is most likely due to overuse of medications, it is important to rule out the scary stuff, and this is best done by an expert.

CDH is the mother of all headaches. It is every migraineur's worst nightmare, and the patient with CDH is the one internists fear the most. The most common type of CDH is medication overuse headache (MOH), also known as rebound headache (see next section). Other

CDHs include hemicrania continua, *new* persistent daily headache, and possibly, transformed migraine (natural progression). Other, much scarier causes can be even more difficult to treat than medication overuse: a tumor, leaky aneurysm, inflammatory disease, or infection.

For research purposes, most headache specialists often classify patients as having CDH if they experience headaches more than fifteen days per month for three months or longer. But generally, CDH means just that: The headache is present every day, 24/7.

Medication Overuse Headache

Most migraineurs have experienced the phenomenon of a medicine becoming less effective over time. This is called tachyphylaxis. It means that the body gets used to the medicine. When this happens, patients take a stronger dose (more tablets at once) or increase the frequency (take it more often). When you do either of these, there is a change in the brain such that a headache develops when it is time for more medicine. In effect, pain is the way for the body to tell us it is time for more medicine. This is called medication overuse headache (MOH). Older literature and many doctors and patients refer to this headache as a "rebound headache," and it is very different from pain that is due to a primary cause. Often patients have both MOH and an underlying headache type, such as migraine without aura. One interesting question still waiting to be answered is whether people who are not migraineurs can get MOH if they take daily analgesics or other pain medicines.

Perhaps the most consistent finding among CDH sufferers (not 100 percent, but close to it) is daily or near-daily use of rescue medications, most often caffeine-containing compounds like Excedrin or butalbital (Fioricet, Fiorinal, Esgic) and narcotic compounds like Norco, Tylenol with codeine, and Vicodin.

Typically, the rebound headache is present on awakening. The pain is often global (as opposed to one-sided), and it does not respond to anything other than the rebound medicine. For example, if you have been taking butalbital/APAP on a daily basis and you get a rebound headache, a triptan will not help that headache. The only thing that will help is more butalbital/APAP. Bear in mind that you are not suddenly immune to the type of headache that got you into the mess, so you will probably still get migraines or other primary headaches superimposed on your rebound headache. And triptans may help *that* headache, further confusing the picture. I know, life isn't always fair.

In 1951, when the only medication for migraines was a class of drugs known as ergotamines, it was suggested that overuse of the drugs could increase rather than decrease headache frequency. Years later, Lee Kudrow, M.D., confirmed these observations with carefully controlled studies in his own patients. Today, there is strong evidence that daily or near-daily use of headache rescue medications will lead to chronic daily headache. While other factors can contribute to chronic daily headache, medication overuse is far and away the most common cause.

A more "scientific" explanation is tougher to come by. One theory holds that when the body is exposed to the same medicine over and over, it produces more receptors in response. Thus, it requires more medicine to elicit the same effect. There is increasing evidence that suggests that the brain has a common response to rescue medicines that is not specific to any one medication. In this model, taking *any* rescue medicine too often can result in MOH. There is science behind each of these theories, but the final answer has not been found. It is an area of intense ongoing research.

Interestingly, when it comes to rebound headaches, not all rescue medications are equal. By far, the most difficult medications to stop are opioids (narcotics), followed closely by barbiturates and butalbital-containing compounds. Triptans are relatively easy to come off. A wealth of literature describes how best to accomplish medication withdrawal, but essentially the only way out of rebound headaches is to stop taking the overused medication. Depending on the medication, stopping it can be a relatively easy undertaking or an extremely difficult one. For roughly one-third of patients, the simple awareness of the phenomenon is enough, but others will need the help of a neurologist or headache specialist.

Anyone who uses analgesics or narcotics daily for headaches should discuss a withdrawal plan with a physician who is experienced in rebound treatment. Often, patients need a structured outpatient program with withdrawal medications. Hospitalization is sometimes necessary to prevent seizures, blood pressure problems, and even withdrawal symptoms like nausea and chills. If a short inpatient stay is deemed appropriate, it should be under the direction of a headache specialist, not an addiction or pain management specialist, and generally, inpatient detox at a drug abuse facility is not appropriate. The same is true for outpatient regimens.

The bottom line is that coming off daily rescue medication is the necessary first step in getting headaches under control. The alternative is a very long and uncomfortable roller coaster ride of escalating medication use with all the attendant side effects; hassles with emergency room personnel, family, and doctors; and largely unrelenting pain. However, in my experience, coming off the medication is only the first battle in the war. Unless the patient and doctor address underlying headache patterns, triggers, and lifestyle issues, the rebound phenomenon will recur in a month or a year. Sooner or later.

A further complication of rebound headaches is that while the patient is in rebound, preventives are ineffective for chronic daily headaches, although they may in fact help with the underlying migraines. This means that any preventives the patient tries and rejects while in rebound need to be retried when the patient is out of rebound.

The majority of patients whose headaches have gone from episodic to daily are overusing rescue medicines, but this is not true of every patient with CDH. Therefore, the first task is to determine the cause of the chronic daily headache, something best undertaken by a headache specialist who starts with a detailed history.

Once such a headache has been characterized, the treatment plan will follow. The neurologist and primary care doctor will guide the plan, whether it is due to medication overuse or not. If it is a medication overuse issue, several treatment options are available. These include hospitalization with biobehavioral management and detox for medication overuse, and trials of drugs used for other indications.

Studies have compared the various approaches used to treat medication overuse. One study found that it was just as effective as inpatient detox programs to simply make patients aware that their daily use of analgesics for rescue was causing their daily headaches. To be sure, some patients just stop the offending medication when they become aware of the problem and their headaches go back to being episodic and responsive to prevention and rescue. In our experience, it depends on the patient, the medication being overused, the length of time on the medication, and many other factors. The best method needs to stop the daily rescue *and* provide a long-term plan to prevent relapse. In some studies, with certain patient groups, the relapse rate at one year approached 100 percent. But with careful selection of the most appropriate plan, relapse rates can be very low indeed.

We are learning more and more about CDH, and medication overuse headache in particular. Very recently, for example, we learned that starting patients on preventive medication while in rebound actually can have a significant benefit, even while the patients are taking daily rescue medicine. This is very different from what we thought before this research was published. As a result, most headache specialists start a preventive medication either before or simultaneous with commencement of drug withdrawal. This does not mean that you can see improvement in your headache by taking a preventive simultaneously with daily rescue medicine, but that starting a preventive while in rebound can make withdrawal smoother and show a benefit during and after withdrawing the offending medication. And it is still worthwhile to revisit preventives that "failed" while you were taking daily rescue medicine.

If you are taking the same rescue medication every day for daily headaches, you definitely need to see a headache specialist. Sudden withdrawal of certain rescue medicines can be dangerous, with side effects ranging from seizures to serious blood pressure problems and physical withdrawal symptoms.

Though some medications used for pain relief in migraines are narcotics, which can cause significant dependency, I don't think it is appropriate to refer to migraineurs who are overusing rescue medications as addicted. Aside from the obvious social overtones, this description is not accurate. This is *not* a drug abuse issue. If you are in this situation, do not let anyone make you feel like anything other than a patient trying to deal with your disease. You have used medications to combat pain. Medication overuse in migraines does not come from a desire to get high, "get off," escape reality, or be cool. It is most often a sincere, albeit somewhat desperate, effort to treat a real and debilitating disease. Moreover, it is most often accomplished with the complete knowledge and complicity of a treating physician.

For this reason, we prefer not to detox MOH patients in a facility for drug addiction, but to admit these patients, when necessary, to an acute care medical facility where we can treat the intractable headache condition, including withdrawing the offending medication. Whether a given patient is best served by inpatient or outpatient management of their MOH is a decision best left to patients and their doctors. There are many variables to consider, including but not limited to:

- the type of medication(s) being overused;
- any other active medical conditions;
- the level of support from family and friends;
- the medical and ancillary support services available in the community.

It is essential that patients accomplish medication withdrawal with the very active participation of medical specialists who know what they are doing. The specific medications and patient profile will determine the best approach for that individual.

OUTPATIENT STRATEGIES   The majority of patients experiencing MOH can be taken off their medications without being admitted to a hospital. But both the patient and the treating physician must be motivated, honest, and communicative, and the patient must have adequate support at home and in the medical community. Many studies show the need for this support after medication withdrawal if this treatment is to be successful. It is never enough to just stop the offending medicine without replacing it with lifestyle changes and appropriate medicinal strategies. Otherwise, most of these patients will be back on one drug or another—and overusing it—within a year. We can use either of two strategies to get many patients off their medications on an outpatient basis:

- **Cold-turkey withdrawal:** Some patients who use particular medications are able to simply stop the offending drugs without a tapering schedule, and this is fine. Cold-turkey withdrawal from the offending medicine requires supporting the patient with medications to handle withdrawal symptoms, as well as nonpharmacological therapies to shift the patient to a more successful management strategy.
- **Conversion:** In the case of narcotic or barbiturate overuse, patients can be converted to a less addictive medication, and their medicating is changed from "as needed" dosing to a set schedule, with a structured tapering schedule over several weeks or months to slowly wean the patient from the medication. This strategy usually involves preparing the patient for weaning by starting an appropriate set of medications designed to minimize withdrawal effects and establish a therapeutic level of an appropriate preventive medication. It is also important to implement nonpharmacologic support, lifestyle changes, and ancillary support services to help the patient maintain the treatment plan once the offending medication is stopped.

HOSPITALIZATION Under certain circumstances, such as when patients have complicated medical conditions, when they've been on multiple medications or particularly potent ones, or when the home environment is not conducive to outpatient strategies, we will recommend hospitalization to treat MOH. In the hospital, as we withdraw the offending medicine, we can use alternative medications to manage withdrawal symptoms and monitor pain while we watch for drug interactions, side effects, and other problems. Also, in the hospital, we are better able to initiate a biobehavioral plan, bringing any needed support services—like physical therapy, nutrition, and stress management counselors—to the bedside. At the Keeler Center, most hospitalizations take less than a week, followed by pretty intense outpatient management. Some other headache clinics use another model in which the hospitalization lasts several weeks or more.

Other Headaches

When headaches are the primary problem, not due to another disease or disorder, we call them primary headaches. The most common kinds of headaches—migraine and tension-type headaches—are examples of primary headaches. As complicated and variable as migraine is, headaches include plenty of other complications and variables. For some headache sufferers, these other issues might trigger migraines, exacerbate the headache pattern, or be the problem all by themselves.

Tension-Type Headaches

What is a tension-type headache? The International Headache Society set out specific criteria for tension-type headaches as frequent episodes of headaches lasting minutes to days. The pain is typically bilateral, pressing or tightening in quality, and of mild to moderate intensity, and it does not worsen with routine physical activity. There is no nausea, but photophobia or phonophobia may be present. Briefly, there are two types of tension headaches: episodic and chronic. Episodic tension headaches are usually bilateral (affecting both sides as well as front and back); are *not* associated with nausea, vomiting, or light sensitivity; usually improve with exercise, rather than worsening as migraines do; and occur less than fifteen days per month. Chronic tension-type headaches are similar but occur more than fifteen days per month.

After migraine, tension-type headaches are probably the most common headache type. Studies suggest that 40 percent of migraineurs may be misdiagnosed as suffering from tension-type headaches because, unfortunately, both headache types may include features that we commonly associate with the other. This happens because both headache types involve the trigeminal nerve system. The trigeminal nerve system dips down well into the cervical spinal cord, and in tension-type headaches it can irritate the nerves that travel to the neck muscles and the muscles that tense the forehead and temples. Almost anyone with a headache of any type is likely to tense the shoulder and neck muscles, so muscle tension is *not* a reliable indicator for headache type. While migraine and so-called tension-type headaches are two distinctly different things, most often we see migraines, perhaps *triggered* by tension.

This is a complicated picture, compounded by the fact that some people have what are known as mixed headaches, with both headache types or features of both types coexisting in the same head. When a patient has both tension-type and migraine headaches, one can transform or trigger the other, but this is distinctly less common than patients (and doctors) believe.

The complicated role of stress and tension in headaches is one of the most compelling reasons for discussing your headaches with a physician who has special training and experience in headache. It is important to make the correct distinction between tension-type headaches and a tension component in migraines, because the treatment is quite different for these two types of headaches. So, specifically, we need to sort out whether our headaches are tension-type or actually *migraines with tension as a prominent trigger.* Most often, the latter is the case; the bottom line then is to treat the headache (migraine) as well as the trigger (tension).

Stress is a very common trigger for for both migraines and tension-type headaches. Headache sufferers need to understand that it is a common misconception that a severe headache is a migraine and a wimpy headache is just tension. But it's not uncommon for people to describe tension headaches this way, and most people who suffer from tension-type headaches will bristle at having their pain referred to as "just tension." Their angst is justified. The fact is that the kind of headache does not necessarily tell you anything about the severity of the pain. I have seen mild migraines as well as tension headaches that will bring you to your knees. As a rule, tension headaches are not as severe as migraines, but some of my most challenging and disabled patients have suffered from pure, severe, tension-type headaches. The notion that they are less painful or less disabling than migraines is a myth. The International Headache Society spends hundreds of hours working out classification systems to help doctors determine what type of headache a given patient is experiencing, and severity is only *one* factor in that determination.

Patients with tension-type headaches can experience *almost all* migraine symptoms to varying degrees, and their headaches can last from hours to days. Tension-type headaches typically present with prominent, pressure-like pain in a hatband pattern around the head, as if a tight hat was putting pressure on the back of the neck and around the head to the temples and forehead. This pain is not usually restricted to one side of the head, as migraines often are. But a majority of all migraineurs also experience neck pain with their attacks. And some migraineurs, especially young ones, experience their headaches as frontal (across the forehead) or global (over the whole head), rather than one-sided. With all these common presentations, how can we possibly differentiate between migraine and tension-type headaches? The following clues help us make reliable distinctions between the two:

- Tension-type headaches do not have the aura phase that *some* migraineurs experience prior to headache pain; the presence of an aura certainly distinguishes a headache as a migraine.
- While bright lights or loud sounds can exacerbate a migraine, these *usually* do not exacerbate a tension-type headache.
- A migraine is often associated with nausea or vomiting, while a tension-type headache is *usually* not.
- Tension-type headaches might improve with mild to moderate exercise, while activity will typically *worsen* a migraine.

Patients who do have true tension-type headaches need to make this distinction in order to treat these headaches effectively. These headaches often respond to physical therapy, relaxation therapy, anti-inflammatories, or muscle relaxants. Like migraines, tension-type headaches are best managed through a combination of lifestyle modification, prevention, and rescue. However, the specifics vary depending on presentation. For example, muscle work and stress management may take a more prominent role in the treatment plan than medications.

We don't know what the relationship is between tension-type and migraine headaches. A wonderful neurologist and headache specialist, Roger Cady, M.D., suggested that both types of headache are part of a continuum between pain-free and severe headache. Another, equally bright headache specialist, Todd Rozen, M.D., proposed that each headache type has its own module and that such modules are linked in unique ways in each individual headache sufferer. Regardless of which of these models is correct, or if there is another model yet unsung, it is clear that these pain syndromes are rarely pure. Our task, as headache specialists and headache sufferers, is to identify the most disabling type of headache—and treat it.

Temporomandibular Joint (TMJ) Syndrome

The hinge between your upper and lower jaws, the temporomandibular joint, allows you to chew and clench and grind your teeth. It is named after the two bones involved—the temporal bone, which is part of the skull, and the mandible, the lower jaw. Several muscles are also involved in the complex movements of chewing, and these are active even when we are not eating. If they weren't, we would all wander around slack-jawed, swallowing all the flying insects that cross our paths. "Tone" is the term we use to describe how contracted these muscles are when they are at rest. One of the major muscles involved is the temporalis, which is around your temples.

When we are stressed, our muscle tone increases. This is true of all the muscles in our bodies, but perhaps more so for the jaw muscles. This is the basis for TMJ syndrome. For many people, this increased muscle tone results from simple clenching, often during sleep. Others also grind their teeth, in a left-right or, more rarely, front-back motion. Because most clenching and grinding occurs during the night, people who clench and grind often awaken with a headache, often with soreness in the jaw and a palpable click when they open and close their mouths.

TMJ syndrome can coexist with migraines or be a trigger for them. If TMJ is the only problem, then correcting it often eliminates the headaches completely. If it is a comorbid condition (as when the same person has two medical conditions) or a trigger for migraines, then correcting it can greatly reduce the frequency of the headaches. Bite guards, medication, biofeedback, and other modalities can be used to treat TMJ. Some headache specialists within the dental community work primarily with these issues and utilize a variety of invasive procedures (surgery, bite correction devices, etc.), as well as medical treatments. When jaw problems seem to coexist with headaches, it is often worthwhile to see a dentist skilled in orofacial pain.

Sleep Apnea

Like TMJ syndrome, sleep apnea and other sleep disorders can cause headaches upon awakening. But also like TMJ, a morning headache is not typically the only sign or symptom of sleep apnea. Typically, people with sleep apnea snore with prolonged pauses (lasting seconds, not minutes) in their breathing while they are asleep. Often, despite a full night's sleep, they awaken feeling exhausted because, during these pauses, their brain is not getting oxygen, so the quality of sleep is not restorative. People with sleep apnea can also have typical facial and body features. They tend to be overweight, have a thick neck, and have a hypognathic jaw, which is a jaw that is set back from the plane of the face (the opposite of a Dudley Do-Right jaw). Of course, not everyone with this appearance has sleep apnea. But when sleep apnea is a possibility, a physician can order a formal sleep study to monitor breathing and other parameters to make the diagnosis.

The relationship between sleep and headache is just beginning to be explored. Clearly, we "sleep off" migraines and, just as clearly, disrupted sleep contributes to worsening headaches. Whether the specific sleep disorders such as apnea, parasomnia, and insomnia cause unique headaches or whether these syndromes make migraineurs' headaches worse is not known. However, from a practical standpoint, it makes sense to improve the quality of sleep regardless of whether the sleep disorder is causing the headache or is merely contributing to it as a trigger.

Sinus Headache

Though actually quite rare, true sinus headaches *do* occur but *only* as a symptom of acute sinusitis—a sinus infection—which *will* respond to antibiotics. Sinus infections are caused by bacteria, and present with a disgusting greenish nasal discharge and fever along with the headache. While an acute infection or inflammation in the sinuses can cause head pain (sinus headache), that is a much rarer occurrence than an inflammation of the nerve causing sinus pain (migraine).

Many patients have used course after course of antibiotics to battle sinus headaches, but *unsuccessfully.* Why don't these antibiotics work? Current research indicates that many headache sufferers experience sinus pain, but this is because the trigeminal nerve, the nerve that becomes very sensitive in migraines, also handles sensation and carries pain messages from the sinuses. In migraines, when the trigeminal nerve is malfunctioning, pain is generated in all the parts of the head that are innervated by the trigeminal nerve—including the sinuses. Patients get the impression that the sinuses are making the head hurt when, actually, it is the other way around. A sinus headache is *usually* a migraine radiating pain to the sinuses. When we make this distinction, we can appropriately treat the headache (migraine) at its source, rather than treat a suspected problem downstream, in the sinuses.

In all fairness, the rare sinus headache and the very common migraine can share a number of features: both can be associated with changes in weather, pain or pressure over the sinuses, nasal congestion, and runny nose or watery eyes. Today, however, we know that all these symptoms result from activation of the parasympathetic nervous system; they are not specific for either sinus headache or migraine.

According the International Headache Society, the definition of sinus headache entails:

- "purulent nasal discharge" (greenish-yellow stuff coming out of the nose);
- imaging (X-ray, CT scan, MRI, or transillumination) that shows sinus disease;

- headache that begins at the same time as the sinus infection;
- point tenderness around the sinuses.

This seems straightforward enough. But in 1999, almost 40 percent of people whom doctors diagnosed with sinus headache actually met the criteria for migraine, *not* sinus headache. For billing purposes, about thirty million doctor visits each year are coded as sinusitis, and most of these people take antibiotics *and still have their headaches*. Searching for headache cures, well-intentioned doctors have even performed unnecessary sinus surgeries on innocent headache sufferers. It turns out that the "abnormal" mucosal thickening often evident on CT scans (leading doctors to diagnose sinusitis) is actually present in about half of the general population and about two-thirds of all headache sufferers. So, unfortunately, after sinus surgery, a migraineur will still be a migraineur. Even in the rare case that *does* warrant sinus surgery, it is extremely unlikely to eliminate the headaches, because the sinus problem was likely one of many migraine triggers.

Doctors aren't the only ones who make this mistake. Many patients, often with the help of vaguely misleading advertisements for over-the-counter pain relievers, conclude that because their pain is near the sinuses, it must be a sinus headache. But the fact is that more than 90 percent of migraineurs have at least one feature commonly associated with "sinus headache."

The consequences of this confusion are pretty dramatic. Obviously, treating a migraine with antibiotics won't work. Plus, overprescription of antibiotics can create significant stomach and gut problems, as well as foster antibiotic resistance and contribute to "super" infections. These are all reasons why both doctors and patients need to be aware of the symptom overlap between these two conditions. Remember, migraine is the most common kind of headache.

Other Nonmigraine "Primary" Headaches
Classified as trigeminal autonomic cephalalgias (TACs), cluster headaches, hemicrania continua, paroxysmal hemicrania, and SUNCT syndrome are not migraines, and they require special handling.

CLUSTER HEADACHE Contrary to popular belief, a cluster head-ache is not simply a collection of headaches that come in a bunch, but a distinct type of headache that belongs to a class of primary headaches called trigeminal autonomic cephalalgias. Compared with migraine, a cluster headache is relatively short-lived, lasting from twenty minutes to two hours. It is always one-sided and associated with symptoms such as a stuffy nose, tearing, an enlarged pupil, or a droopy eyelid on one side. By reputation, clusters are some of the most painful headaches imagin-able, and they tend to occur several times a day for days or weeks. Then they disappear, usually for weeks to months. Treatments for cluster headaches differ significantly from treatments for other headache types. Lithium, oxygen, and steroids are often effective in cluster headaches but less frequently in other headache types. At the same time, other treat-ments are common to both, such as triptan via injection and valproic acid in prevention. Since the pain is so severe, people who tend to get cluster headaches should have a treatment plan in place before a cluster headache begins.

HEMICRANIA CONTINUA A chronic headache, hemicrania con-tinua shares features with migraine and cluster headaches, and usually requires diagnosis by a neurologist or headache specialist. Typically one-sided and moderately severe, this headache tends to be constant with very short-lived, intermittent jolts of increased pain, usually with a stuffy nose, droopy eyelid, or tearing from the eye on the same side as the headache. Hemicrania continua is unique in that it will almost always respond to one specific medicine, indomethacin.

PAROXYSMAL HEMICRANIA This rare headache form can be epi-sodic or chronic. The pain is always on the same side, typically lasting from two to forty-five minutes. Usually there are five or more attacks per day. The attacks are typically associated with tearing, nasal fullness, a droopy eyelid, red eyes, or swollen eyes. These headaches usually respond rapidly and completely to indomethacin.

SUNCT SYNDROME   Probably one of the rarest headaches, SUNCT (Short-lasting, Unilateral Neuralgiform headache with Conjunctival injection and Tearing) consists of anywhere from three to one hundred very brief stabbing pains, typically lasting less than a minute. The pain is usually around one eye and is sometimes triggered by touching certain parts of the face or head. Anyone with SUNCT should be evaluated by a headache specialist or headache clinic.

"Secondary" Headaches Can Be Dangerous

Most headaches are migraines unless proven otherwise. As a migraineur, you should know how to differentiate migraines from some other headaches and be able to recognize when you have a new or ominous symptom that signifies a change in your headaches. The fact is that uncommon but potentially dangerous headaches do happen to all kinds of people—even migraineurs. Just because you suffer from chronic migraines does not mean you are immune to other headaches or complications.

More than one hundred conditions can include a headache. Secondary headaches, which are due to some other condition, are uncommon compared with primary headaches. It is rarer still for secondary headaches to present *only* with headache. In almost every case, when a physician carefully takes a history and performs a physical exam, other signs and symptoms will be evident. Still, brain tumors, ruptured blood vessels, and infections are both serious and scary.

In people who have had headaches before, a severe version of the usual headache is not likely to be a harbinger of something dangerous. Painful, to be sure, but not dangerous. In fact, headache is rarely a feature of stroke or brain tumor, and it is almost never the *only* symptom. This fact alone reassures the majority of patients who see me about their headaches. The brain itself is insensate (has no feeling), so a stroke or mass would have to be large enough to disrupt an artery or the lining of the brain before it could cause a perception of pain; usually, by the time a stroke or tumor has reached that size, there is plenty of other evidence that something is very wrong upstairs.

That said, as a chronic headache sufferer, you should have your doctor evaluate your headaches when you need help managing them and *again when you perceive a change in your headaches.* You should also be familiar with some danger signs so you know when a headache merits a trip to the emergency room. Here is a good rule of thumb: *If you are concerned and wonder if something else is going on, you should probably talk to your doctor or go to the emergency room.*

Most of us who suffer from headaches can recall the worst headache of our lives. But if you use that phrase in front of an emergency room doctor, you will probably guarantee yourself the (perhaps) once-in-a-lifetime experience of a spinal tap. Physicians have it drilled into their heads from the first day of medical school that a patient with "the worst headache of their life" may have a subarachnoid hemorrhage (SAH), which is life-threatening. In SAH, a blood vessel in the brain ruptures, either from trauma or a weakness in a blood vessel. This rupture often causes severe headache, stiff neck, and, sometimes, neurologic deficits as well. In a cruel twist of fate, even a chronic headache sufferer can suffer this relatively rare condition. So even though it is probably just a really bad migraine, this may not spare you from having a spinal tap to rule out the more dangerous diagnosis.

"Red flag" is a term doctors use to refer to warning signs or symptoms that don't fit the usual picture but may point to something potentially dangerous. For example, let's say a patient comes in complaining of a headache with aching muscles, especially a stiff neck. He says that he has felt this way before when he gets a headache, but the doctor notices that he also has a rash developing (a sign) and that his throat is sore (a symptom). Checking the patient's vital signs, the doctor also learns that the patient's temperature is elevated. This collection of signs and symptoms raises a red flag: this is more than the patient's typical headache. In fact, he may have spinal meningitis, an infection of the lining around the spinal cord and brain. The doctor would order tests to confirm or rule out this serious illness.

Obviously, it takes a medical education to know all of the elements of the diagnostician's decision-making process. However, several red flags cause a physician to look beyond the immediate problem the patient presents. Migraineurs should be aware of the most common headache red flags:

- **A first headache in a mature adult.** Not always, but usually, most benign headaches begin earlier in life. When someone gets their first headache after age forty or fifty, we worry about inflammatory disease or, rarely, cancer or bleeding problems in the brain.
- **Headache that starts abruptly or suddenly.** A sudden, severe headache raises concern about a ruptured blood vessel in the brain, called a subarachnoid hemorrhage (see pages 67, 69). If present, this is a big deal and requires immediate medical attention.
- **Headaches that increase steadily in frequency or severity.** While many things, most of which are not serious, can cause this picture, brain tumors and bleeding problems can present with this pattern, so further studies should be done.
- **Headaches with other signs and symptoms such as stiff neck, fever, body aches, and rash** raise concerns about infection, and can also suggest certain diseases of the connective tissues and blood vessels. When the other signs are more neurologic, such as **visual changes or numbness, tingling, or weakness on one side of the body**, we must consider the possibility of stroke, tumor, or other abnormalities in the brain. In particular, when your doctor looks at your eyes with an ophthalmoscope, he can detect evidence of increased intracranial pressure on the brain, a potentially life-threatening situation, often before symptoms beyond headaches begin to show up. Similarly, abnormal eye movements, reflexes, and behaviors can signal concern.
- **Headache after head trauma.** Whether the patient loses consciousness or not, a headache after head trauma needs to be evaluated for concussion, skull fracture, subdural and subarachnoid hemorrhage.
- **A new headache in someone with HIV, cancer, or other serious illness.** Often, very ill people have impaired immune

systems. Regardless of the cause of the impairment, these patients are more susceptible to both infection and certain kinds of cancer. Therefore, anyone in these categories who has a new headache needs further evaluation.

> Headache is rarely a feature of stroke or brain tumor.
> And it is almost never the *only* symptom.

Subarachnoid Hemorrhage

I was barely a teenager the first time I heard the term "subarachnoid hemorrhage," and my hero, Rod Serling, had just died from it. Neither of my parents could tell me what it was, and I was terrified of it. (I still am.)

Subarachnoid hemorrhage refers to a ruptured blood vessel that spills blood into the space between the brain and its lining. In general, there are two causes: trauma or a weakness in a blood vessel. In addition to a severe headache, this rupture is often accompanied by stiff neck and, sometimes, neurologic deficits. When there is even the slightest suspicion of subarachnoid hemorrhage, ER physicians will image the brain with a CT scan and possibly also check the spinal fluid with a spinal tap.

While subarachnoid hemorrhage is rare, skillful and experienced doctors, usually in the emergency room, can recognize the signs and symptoms of this very dangerous disorder. It is important also for the person with a headache to know when it is different or unusual, and bring it to medical attention. When subarachnoid hemorrhage is detected early, measures can be taken to minimize the damage and repair the blood vessel, if necessary. But even today, many such hemorrhages are devastating.

Spinal Meningitis and Encephalitis

The lining that covers the entire central nervous system—the brain and spinal cord—is called the meninges. Meningitis is inflammation and infection in the meninges. Fungi, bacteria, or viruses can cause such an infection and, depending on the infectious agent, it can range from a fairly benign condition to a fatal disease. Most meningitis in the United States is viral and is usually not dangerous. Doctors, often in the emergency room, suspect meningitis when certain signs and symptoms present: a whopper of a headache, fever, a very stiff neck (especially when flexed forward, "chin to chest"), and malaise (feeling sick). But people with bacterial or fungal meningitis are a lot sicker than those with viral meningitis. If a patient has the above symptoms plus a rash or neurological deficits, such as double vision, facial drooping, or facial numbness, it indicates a more serious meningitis.

While other things can cause these symptoms, meningitis is high on the list, and a doctor needs to rule it out, or in. The definitive test for meningitis is spinal fluid examination, so a lumbar puncture may be indicated. You cannot "diagnose" meningitis on your own. It requires medical evaluation, so if you have a headache with these symptoms, you need to see a doctor. While it may turn out to be the flu on top of your regular headache, you must allow a professional to make this determination.

Encephalitis refers to inflammation of the brain itself. While the brain's lining and blood vessels can convey pain messages to the brain, the brain itself does not feel pain. When the brain is inflamed, the patient experiences a loss of function, which can present with confusion, sleepiness, seizure, unresponsiveness, or agitation, as well as fever and other signs of infection. When this combination of symptoms and signs is present, it is a neurologic emergency, and a trip to the emergency room is appropriate. Diagnosis will typically involve imaging with a CAT scan and/or MRI, and spinal fluid examination as well as urgent treatment, possibly with antibiotics, antiviral agents, steroids, and intravenous pain management.

Headache After Head Trauma

Sure, if you hurt your head, your head is going to hurt. That is not uncommon. But it depends on the nature of the trauma. Axe blows and gunshots tend to be more painful than straightening up and whacking your head on the car's door frame—although that *really* hurts too. But it is a mistake to think that there is a correlation among the severity of the blow, the resulting headache, and the danger it poses, because, often, there is not. For example, often, after a car accident in which there was no specific head trauma but a lot of jostling, a nagging, persistent headache can develop. On the other hand, some patients with major open trauma to the head do not develop a headache that lasts beyond the healing of the external wounds. Sometimes a relatively minor blow can result in a tear of a vessel and an accumulation of blood between the skull and the brain. The effect of head trauma and the damage a head injury might inflict are determined by many factors, including the patient's age, general health, physical condition, nature of the injury (whether it is a "deceleration" injury or blunt-force trauma), and more. All of these factors will determine the diagnostic tests that need to be performed.

Whether the patient loses consciousness or not, a more serious and potentially fatal headache can result from a blow to the side of the head with cutting or tearing of arteries. The dura is a tough, rubbery lining inside the skull. If blood leaks between the dura and the skull, this is an epidural hemorrhage, one of the cardinal reasons for going to the emergency room after any significant head trauma. This is a true neurologic emergency. When the bleeding is between the dura and the brain, the blood has a bit more room and, in most cases, the patient has more time to fix the problem. But this is a determination best left to medical staff in the emergency room.

Another potentially serious consequence of head trauma—particularly in immune-compromised patients, the elderly, and alcoholics—is subdural hematoma, bleeding between the dura and the brain. This, too, can present with just a headache after trauma. If an emergency room doctor suspects a subdural hematoma in a patient who has a headache after trauma, he or she will request a CAT scan to make this diagnosis.

"Shear injury" refers to the jarring effect of trauma on the delicate latticework of nerves in the brain. The associated headache is less serious in a medical sense, though it is often debilitating. In almost all cases, this resolves over time, but it can be quite disconcerting, and often requires symptomatic treatment.

Headache is a common feature of concussion, and can persist for months following trauma. Patients may need medications, often tricyclics, to effectively treat such pain. Head pain at the site of a trauma (where the stitches are) is distinct from headache, and has its own pain management.

When there is headache after head trauma, it is very difficult for a nonphysician to distinguish the serious from the benign, so a medical professional should always evaluate trauma to the head.

Temporal Arteritis

Also called giant cell arteritis, temporal arteritis is due to a chronic inflammatory process in the arteries that causes episodic headaches. While much less common than migraines, temporal arteritis headaches are more common in someone whose headaches begin after middle age. Temporal arteritis can have serious consequences, so timely diagnosis is important. Therefore, a new or different headache in a person of appropriate age warrants a visit to the doctor.

A cardinal feature of the condition is a new headache, not in young people, but in those sixty and older. Temporal arteritis also has several unique signs and symptoms. It is typically a global headache, throbbing in nature, with tenderness over the temples, and possibly joint pains, sore jaw (particularly with movement), and intermittent visual impairment. Another common feature is a tender, swollen artery at the temples, though the disease is not limited to this location and can affect other arteries in the head. The joint pains tend to occur early in the disease and the visual problems late, but not every patient has every symptom.

Believed to be due to an autoimmune response, temporal arteritis is easily diagnosable with laboratory testing and a minor biopsy of an affected vessel. The blood test is called an erythrocyte sedimentation rate

(ESR, or sed rate). When the ESR is elevated to many times normal, the diagnosis is confirmed. Physicians also follow the ESR to monitor the patient's response to treatment. Temporal arteritis can threaten the patient's eyesight, and even result in blindness, if it is not diagnosed and treated appropriately with steroids, so it is very important that patients let their doctors diagnose any new or different headache.

Chapter 3

Why *You* Get Headaches

Nearly every new patient asks me why they get headaches. Implied in this question is a more primal concern: "What is wrong with me?" Sometimes, the essential, unspoken question is, "Do I have a brain tumor?" and sometimes, "Am I crazy?" It turns out that brain tumors are an *exceedingly* rare cause of headaches and are almost never the cause of headaches that have been around for years. And most people with major psychiatric disorders do not list headaches as their big problem.

There are a few things that migraineurs need to understand, to get through their heads. First, migraine is *not* all in your mind. Migraine is *real*—as real as diabetes, asthma, or congestive heart failure—and it is no more imaginary, psychological, emotional, or "mental" than these other diseases. So no one should blame you for your headaches, because they are not your fault. It is (usually) not your doctor's fault, either. Migraine is a genetic disease so, if you must blame someone, blame your parents. When you get a migraine, a trigger probably caused it. But since you cannot know, much less avoid, all the possible triggers out there (or in your own body), you are going to get headaches from time to time. So nothing—not even this book or the Keeler Method—is going to make your headaches disappear like magic.

Aside from not being careful enough when we selected our parents, we have all wondered what we did to "deserve" headaches in general, and *this* headache in particular. I have found it useful to turn this question around and ask patients, "Why do you care?" When I do this, I usually get a response that translates roughly to something like, "What are you, an idiot?" I am willing to endure that response because the answer is probably the most important realization a headache sufferer can make. And it is not obvious.

The question "Why do I get headaches?" is passive. It asks, "What's wrong with me?" If we have pain, it should be *from* something, but often we are frustrated because we cannot find the cause of a particular headache that just seems to come out of the blue, and we feel victimized by our malady. But when we ask, "Why is it important to know why you get headaches?" we can replace that passive attitude with the declarative, "I want to know why I get headaches so I can figure out what to do about them, how to prevent them, and how to live with them." Then we take the first step toward taking control of our headaches.

Nearly every new patient tells me that she has several different kinds of headaches, or that she is in some way different from me and all the other people on the planet who suffer with headaches. This is both true and not true. Every headache sufferer is unique in their constellation of triggers, their perception of pain, and their lifestyle. At the same time, human brains are, more or less, wired pretty similarly. It is likely that, at the most basic levels, our headaches have more in common than not.

Within families, similarities tend to occur in both the triggering patterns and treatment responses, so what hurts your mom's head is likely to hurt yours, and what helps your mom's head is likely to help yours. These are just probabilities and patterns we see. At present, we don't know for sure because we don't have blood tests or imaging modalities that can predict who will or will not suffer from migraines.

Any treatment plan must seek to identify the unique contributions of your lifestyle to your headaches. Unfortunately, despite the most inquisitive detective work into triggers, not every trigger is known and, even when we do know them, we can't control every element that might contribute to a headache. Even with the best plan, migraines will still happen, and we still need early and effective treatment when they do occur. That is why we need to enlist the support of doctors, families, and coworkers. But headaches start with triggers, so treatments that focus exclusively on pain do not work. By the time we're in pain, the proverbial horse has fled the barn. Of course, we need ways of catching the horse (not to beat a metaphor to death), but it would be a whole lot easier to just shut the barn door.

Triggers—Myth and Mystery

Triggers get a lot of press in the headache business. Careers (and fortunes) have been made by individuals claiming to have found *the* trigger or triggers for migraines.

What is a trigger? In the most basic sense, a trigger is anything that will result in a migraine headache when a susceptible individual is exposed to it—either alone or in concert with any other triggers. From there, it gets more complicated. Some triggers are absolute. They will *always* result in a headache. Others are *partial*, resulting in headache only under certain "predisposing" circumstances. There are a number of reasons why trigger identification is such a tricky business:

- Not everyone has the same triggers.
- Not all triggers always result in headache.
- Lists only work for the people who write them.
- The only way to identify your triggers is to pay attention to your life.

For most medical conditions, the set of causes is fairly consistent from patient to patient, as is the consequence, the disease state. Too little insulin results in diabetes, exposure to virus causes the flu, and so forth. Not so for migraines. The great challenge of migraines is this: *All migraineurs share a consequence (the headache), but each of us has a unique set of triggers.* For example, I could eat a case of Ding Dongs every day without getting a headache (not that I would), but a long day in the hot sun will *always* give me a headache (unless I pretreat with medication). Yet I have many patients for whom eating chocolate is like skydiving without a parachute. Some of them can't even walk by a candy counter without getting a headache. Still, our descriptions of the headache that results will be almost identical. This is an area of intense interest among headache scientists. But as headache sufferers, *each one of us must do our best to identify our own unique set of triggers.*

Food Lists and Food Triggers

About the only thing I clearly remember from the single-hour lecture in medical school on primary headache is that I was handed a list of foods that patients should avoid if they suffered from migraines. It was three pages, with a big X through most of my comfort foods. Though I was disconcerted, even then I thought, *Wait a second! I eat aged cheese all the time, and it never gives me a headache.* Later, I spent some time at a famous headache clinic in Chicago. It provided its patients with a special diet for headache sufferers, with a multipage list of foods known to trigger headaches. A dutiful and earnest young doctor, I immediately incorporated a similar list and diet into my headache practice and used it for a while.

"You know," a wise patient said to me one day, with a withering glare, "this list takes away the few things in my life that give me any respite from my headaches."

Of course, she had a great point. Why was I telling every patient to avoid wine or aged cheese or legumes or even chocolate, with no evidence that those things gave *that patient* a headache?

If you ask any well-informed person who does not suffer from headache what triggers headache, the number-one answer will probably be chocolate. Ask a roomful of migraine sufferers and you will get a roomful of answers. Ask your doctor and you may get anything from a sympathetic shrug to a prescription for allergy testing and an elimination diet. Obviously, it is hard to get a clear answer. There is a reason for that.

Amazingly, every book on headache (except this one) still includes comprehensive lists of possible headache triggers, and a recent best seller even endorsed a migraine diet, despite the total lack of scientific study supporting such an approach. Some doctors still give patients lists of foods to avoid, including all the things that ever gave anybody a headache. Other doctors put their patients through painful hours of allergy testing—again, without a trace of scientific evidence linking allergies to migraines. And a few even believe that headaches are all in your head. Don't even get me started on that one.

Of course, we could just follow the list, anyway. This would certainly be better than getting a headache. And aren't the odds in our favor that the list will include our triggers? The problem is, if following the list worked, you wouldn't need this book and I wouldn't need to write it. Successfully managing your headaches requires an environmental awareness that goes well beyond checklists, because the lists of possible triggers are just that: *possible* triggers. *There are way more triggers out there than there are items on any list*, and odds are that *every* list will have *many* items on it that have *no effect on your headaches*. Why should you deprive yourself of them? The answer is, you should not.

In the Keeler Method, we teach you how to look at your world with a critical eye so you can spot a potential trigger and avoid it, rather than forcing yourself to conform to one list or another. You should not let fear of a headache dominate your life and constrain your every decision, but rather become aware enough of yourself and your world to allow you to move through it, headache-free.

Every migraineur is different, and this is the basic reason why trigger lists aren't helpful. Among migraineurs, some triggers *are* more common than others. I have many patients who get a headache as sure as night follows day if they drink any alcohol at all. So should alcohol be on the list? One patient gets headaches after eating a hot dog (probably nitrites) and another can't eat peanuts. Should nitrites and peanuts be on the list? What about chocolate? Since just about anything can trigger a headache in *someone*, is it necessary to list everything? The answer is no. Nothing should be on the list because so far migraine scientists do not have good evidence that nuts, carbs, Chinese food with MSG, meat with nitrites, or anything else causes *your* migraines. These things *might* be among your triggers, but they might *not*, and what triggers a headache in you may not trigger a headache in me. Unless we are directly related, more likely than not, our triggers are quite different.

As a doctor, I do not want to forbid my patients to indulge in the things they enjoy if I have no valid reason to think it will help their headaches.

While there may be plenty of good reasons why you should avoid aspartame or hot dogs or chocolate Easter bunnies, you—and I—have no reason to think that doing so will help prevent our migraines—unless they do. The basic fact is that *everyone should have a personal list.*

As far as foods and food lists go, two things are clear:

- Foods definitely can trigger headaches in some people, often in combination with other factors such as a day in the sun, a change in sleep pattern, or a particular time of the month.
- Everyone's list of triggers is unique.

Anything Under the Sun Can Be a Trigger

The problem with lists is that they are woefully inadequate. And since every migraineur is different, the lists cause patients to exclude from their lives many things that give them pleasure, even though most of those things are not causing their headaches. Plus, in the search for triggers, we must keep our minds open to the fact that *absolutely anything* can be a migraine trigger for any given migraineur. Triggers can be environmental, dietary, hormonal, psychological, social, or related to sleep, medication, other medical conditions, or *anything else.* Once headache sufferers understand this basic fact of life, they can begin to evaluate the elements of their environment and begin the detective work of finding their own triggers, and will usually be rewarded with big results.

Patterns as Triggers

Migraineurs do best when their behavioral patterns remain fairly predictable. So, while food triggers get a lot of press, I've found that food *timing* is a much more common trigger. While it is not true for every migraineur, skipping meals can often trigger migraines. In some people, lack of sleep can trigger migraines, and so can sleeping in. Many patients get headaches when they don't exercise regularly, and others have more headaches when they overdo exercise. From patients who stay up late on

Friday and sleep in on Saturday to the weekend warrior who sits behind a desk all week and plays three hours of full-court basketball on Saturday, the patterns of our lives, when disrupted, can commonly lead to break-through headaches.

Certainly you could argue that three hours of basketball on Saturday is better than nothing. For migraineurs, however, it cannot be an either-or situation. If exercise is to be a priority in your life, in most cases, once a week is not going to work. A pattern must exist such that exercise does not shock the system. This means that a minimum of daily or near-daily exercise is necessary to temper the weekend marathon. If Friday night out with the girls is important and it can be only a once-a-week deal, you need to anticipate this and take measures to minimize the impact on the rest of your weekend.

Patterns, consistency, and planning are essential tools for the migraineur. There is just no way around it. But this does not mean you must be a boring shut-in. It just means you need to pay attention to your patterns, be reasonably consistent, and plan ahead for those situations where a break in the pattern is unavoidable—or too much fun to pass up.

Stress as a Trigger

We blame a lot on stress. We blame our bad moods, our eating habits, our ulcers, and our headaches all on stress. In my opinion, stress is get-ting a bad rap. To be sure, there is a lot of stress in the world and in our individual lives, but stress is as much a part of our world as the weather. Everybody has stress, and it isn't likely to go away any time soon. While we have (to a degree) some control over the *sources* of our stress, there will always be some measure of stress lurking out there. So, as with any trigger, the challenge is to avoid or manage the trigger of stress.

That's right. Stress is often a trigger for migraine. In fact, *it is probably the most common trigger for migraine.* Does that mean there is no such thing as a tension headache? Certainly not. But the consensus among headache specialists today is that tension-type headache is much less com-mon than previously thought, and much less common than migraine.

External Environmental Triggers

Again, anything can be a trigger. That does not mean that *everything* is a trigger. On the other hand, we do see some triggers more often than others. For example, I frequently hear, "My headaches are always worse during the allergy season," and "I know I get allergy headaches, because my sinuses kill me."

Clearly, the immune system (which manages the body's response to allergens, substances to which we are allergic) has a relationship with the pain pathways (which alert the brain to problems between the body and its environment). Recent research from the Harvard laboratory of Rami Burstein, Ph.D., and elsewhere, has begun to elucidate the relationship between the inflammatory response and migraines. When a stimulus activates the pain pathways in the brain and peripheral nervous system, an inflammatory response follows. While not particularly prominent at the onset of pain, this inflammatory response is typically in full force several hours into a headache. We've learned in our own laboratory and elsewhere that, in the course of a migraine, prostaglandins and other inflammatory molecules are released into the brain. Measurable in the spinal fluid, these molecules have been implicated in prolonging a headache for hours or days, which lends insight into why anti-inflammatory agents are often more effective later in a headache, while antimigraine medicines work better earlier in the process.

Given that headaches often develop in response to something hostile in the environment, it seems reasonable that allergens could be headache triggers. Headache sufferers usually reward such a statement with a big "Duh!" but it has taken the medical community a while to accept this notion. The fact is that many patients do experience a dramatic increase in the frequency and severity of their headaches in the spring and fall "allergy seasons."

But be careful here. While for some people an "allergy" could be a trigger, it depends on what you mean by *allergy*. Many people say, for example, that they are allergic to tobacco smoke because it gives them a headache. However, true allergy requires an immune response, and this has not yet been demonstrated in a migraine. Rather, in the same way that peanuts, stress, or too much sun can be triggers, allergens can be headache triggers for some people, too, *but the headache they cause is a migraine.* This is important because, when the headache occurs, we need to treat it as a migraine, not as an "allergy headache" or any other kind of headache. Obviously, it's important to address exposure to the trigger, but once the headache is there, it is a migraine and you need to treat it as such.

Similarly, many people believe that allergies lead to "sinus headaches," but this is generally not so. Sinus headaches do exist, but are actually quite rare. A sinus headache is one symptom of a sinus infection, caused by bacteria. It would be extremely unusual for a headache to be the *only* symptom of a sinus infection. Other symptoms typically include a disgusting greenish nasal discharge and fever. As a symptom of an infection, a true sinus headache should be treated with antibiotics, while allergy-triggered *migraines* should be treated with migraine medicines. If allergies cause congestion or itching or puffy eyes *and* they are a migraine trigger, then addressing the allergies through lifestyle modification or medication should help minimize allergies as a trigger, and that is good. But when you have a migraine, you need to treat the migraine, because treating the allergy after the headache has begun is like slamming the barn door after the horse has . . . well, you get the idea.

In most cases, if you can identify a trigger ahead of time, you can eliminate or control it before it starts a headache and, perhaps, avoid the headache altogether. In the case of allergies as triggers, if you can use an allergy medication to treat the allergies early on, you can prevent the migraine they might cause. But once a headache is going, it doesn't much matter what triggered it—whether it was allergies or something else. The headache is a migraine, and migraine medications will be the most effective treatment, so the important thing at that point is to abort the headache with the appropriate migraine rescue medicine.

A few years ago, a new class of medications, leukotriene receptor inhibitors, came on the market for allergies. The headache community was very excited, anticipating that these medicines represented a new treatment for headache pain. Unfortunately, it turned out that these medicines do not cross the blood–brain barrier, and while they are very effective in aborting allergy attacks, they are not much help once a headache is present.

Searching for headache cures, well-intentioned doctors have performed untold numbers of allergy tests and unnecessary sinus surgeries on innocent headache sufferers. Unfortunately, after sinus surgery or other extreme measures to clean out the sinuses, a migraineur will still be a migraineur. Even in cases when sinus surgery is warranted for other reasons, it is extremely unlikely to eliminate headaches. The important message here is that we should not confuse triggers with the headaches they cause. Allergies can be a trigger for headaches, but they are rarely a *major* trigger—and almost never the *only* trigger. Migraine remains the most common cause of headache, and while it is important to identify triggers, the hunt should never overshadow the diagnosis.

Internal Environmental Triggers

In addition to all the assaults from the outside world that can give us headaches, there is a whole "internal" world of hormones, neurotransmitters, and neuropeptides that can just as easily trigger headaches. And just like external triggers, these internal ones vary among individuals in their ability to cause a headache. The most common (or at least the most visible) of these triggers is estrogen, but a wide variety of other molecules in the body may contribute to headaches.

Unfortunately, if you get hormonally related migraines, there is a good chance that your daughter will get migraines when her periods start. Your son, too, may well become a migraineur when he hits puberty. We also find that menopausal patterns tend to run in families, so if your mom's headaches went away in her fifties, there is a good chance yours will as well.

Other Sensory Triggers

It is useful to distinguish between things that trigger or initiate a headache when none was present and those that make an existing headache worse. Often, the things that make your headaches worse can provide clues to the subtle triggers that initiate your headaches, so it is important to note those things that seem to worsen your headache. For example, many of us find that loud sounds make headaches worse. It may be less apparent (yet equally true) that spending hours in a noisy environment can help trigger a headache. The same can be said for overly bright or visually assaulting stimuli, like fluorescent lights or disco balls. Indeed, when we are in a susceptible state, *almost any sensory input may trigger a headache*—including odors, physical sensations (particularly heat), and even certain tastes.

The part of the brain responsible for perception of smell is called the olfactory cortex. Just above the nose near the front of the brain, it is only one short nerve away from the outside world (compared with touch, for instance, which has at least four nerves in the chain from the stimulus to the brain's perception of that stimulus). One of the most primitive inputs for environmental danger, smells are among the most potent stimuli to the brain. So it is not surprising that people who are very sensitive to environmental stimuli are sensitive to smells. That is why many migraineurs cite incense, perfume, cigarettes, and gasoline as triggers.

We now have good evidence that weather changes, particularly barometric pressure changes, can trigger headaches in some people. This comes as no surprise to those who experience this particular trigger. These migraineurs often get a headache a day or two before the weather actually changes, because the barometric pressure changes in advance of a weather front. This information can really help these patients. With a weather forecast, they can anticipate and avoid the headache by using a brief course of preventive medicine or, possibly, through a heightened willingness to treat at the first sign of pain rather than waiting to see if the headache becomes serious.

Some patients who are sensitive to weather changes are also sensitive to motion (as in car sickness or seasickness) and changes in altitude. Of course, these sensitivities can occur independently of weather changes, but often they go hand in hand. When these patients are aware of this predisposition, they can anticipate a headache and take preventive measures before they get into trouble.

It is also not surprising that one of the most common symptoms of altitude sickness is headache, described as throbbing and pounding. Sound familiar? If we assume that migraine is nature's way of telling us we are in a hostile environment and to move to more pleasant surroundings, then it should come as no surprise that the thin air at high altitude can be a powerful trigger. As we know, migraineurs are much more sensitive to environmental assaults than nonheadache sufferers.

Altitude sickness is usually an obvious issue when one moves from near sea level to ten thousand feet or more. But more practical questions arise. What about going from one thousand to five thousand feet? What about going from five thousand feet back down to sea level? What about going from sea level to forty thousand feet in the pressurized cabin of a passenger jet? For some people, almost any change of a couple thousand feet, perhaps just driving up to the local mountains, can trigger a headache. For many others, it takes a more dramatic change. Like all triggers, it is an individual question.

Most migraineurs experience severe pain when exposed to bright lights during a migraine. Photophobia, as we call it, is actually one of the criteria that define migraines. Studies have shown that certain wavelengths of light are better tolerated during headaches than others, but that standard fluorescent lighting seems to be almost universally problematic for headache sufferers. In addition to photophobia *during* a headache, in my clinical experience, bright or fluorescent lights can also be a big *trigger*, bringing on a headache in some people; in others, when these light sources are combined with another potential trigger, this is often enough to start a migraine. So it can be important to avoid bright or fluorescent lighting on a really hot day, in a stressful situation, or after a bad night's sleep, for example. I also encourage all light-sensitive patients to keep sunglasses with them at all times, and to do what they can to control the lighting in the places where they spend the most time, especially at home and work.

The primary principle to keep in mind about triggers is that anything and everything is suspect. For most of us, it can take some diligent detective work to identify our triggers. This requires a little bit of self-awareness. For example, an attorney came to see me. It was clearly his wife's idea. As far as he was concerned, he "gets headaches." He would just go to bed and eventually the headache would go away. I asked him if he had any idea what brought on a headache, what made it worse, or what helped it go away.

He stared at me blankly and shrugged. "It's a headache," he said. "What can I tell you?"

I prompted him a bit. "So you've never noticed anything that might give you a headache?"

"Like what?"

He seriously had no idea what I was talking about.

Bewildered, I offered a suggestion. "Like red wine?"

"Red wine?" he asked, surprised. "You think it's red wine? I can stop drinking red wine. No problem. Is white okay?"

The man was completely devoid of insight. (Perhaps that is what makes him such an effective lawyer.) It had never occurred to him that there might be a connection between his life and his headaches. With some coaching, however, he has done well, and we actually have become friends. He knows I am writing about him and will be flattered. What can I say? He's an attorney.

Partial Triggers

Some people *do* have very consistent and predictable triggers. We have one research patient who can reliably induce a severe migraine by drinking a light beer. We know this is true because she heroically volunteered to bring on a headache in order for us to study changes in her spinal fluid composition during the development of a migraine.

In general, however, our triggers are slightly less reliable. Most of us can recall the time we stayed up all night and didn't get a headache, or the time we drank that dreadful wine and actually felt fine the next day. For most of us, triggers *usually*, but don't always, bring on a headache.

Why is that?

As I've said, the brains of migraine sufferers are more susceptible to interpreting sensory input as painful. One way to think of this is that the brain sits in a delicate balance. Too much stimulus, or the wrong kind of stimulus, is enough to tip the scale toward a pain response—a headache. But unlike most scales, the brain has the ability to adjust its sensitivity so that, depending on the circumstances, a tiny disturbance may not tip the scale enough to throw off the balance. How sensitive the scale (your brain) is at any given moment depends on a lot of things, including how much sleep you got last night, your level of stress throughout the day, your hormonal status, what you ate for lunch, how much water you took in that day, and so forth. The brain must retain this ability to adjust its sensitivity in order for us to survive in the world. We cannot control every single variable that affects this sensitivity, so at least for headache sufferers, it's as if a given trigger affects a slightly different brain each time it is encountered.

Another way to think of this is to imagine that the brain is a fortress. Perhaps it can withstand the onslaught from one attack, but when there are two fronts—or three or four—the brain is more easily overwhelmed. In a practical sense, this might mean that skipping a meal won't cause a headache, unless you are premenstrual and your estrogen levels are trending downward. Or it might mean that perfume won't bother you unless you also didn't sleep well last night. Maybe you can get away with a night of drinking or pulling an all-nighter, but doing both on the same night is very likely to result in a headache. Or skipping a meal or spending a day in the hot sun may be okay, but together, the two are deadly.

Often, patients say that this or that sometimes gives them a headache. With a little digging, it often turns out that there is another trigger which, when combined with the "sometimes" trigger, is enough to start a migraine. Partial triggers are those that contribute to headaches when combined with another factor. Most common among these are changes in sleep pattern, stress, and alcohol. But of course, there are many others.

For example, I had a patient who often, but not always, would get a headache when she ate salted nuts. This was not a consistent trigger, but I felt it was significant that she brought up nuts at all. When we looked at this more closely, we were able to determine that the *combination* of salted nuts and its occasional companion, a nice cold beer, brought on the headache, but nuts in the absence of alcohol did not. The important lesson here is to follow your intuition—and for the doctors out there: *Listen to your patients.* If you sense there is something going on, investigate it until you are satisfied, either way.

Triggers don't exist in a vacuum, and most of us need to broaden our view of what circumstances will set us up for a headache. One important aspect of this is to discover your partial triggers, those things that contribute to causing a headache under the right (or wrong) circumstances but by themselves do not single-handedly bring on a headache. By careful observation and keeping a diligent headache diary, we can usually identify circumstances where several partial triggers conspired to take us down. Common examples of this are:

- staying up late *and* drinking alcohol;
- spending the day in the sun *and* not hydrating properly;
- skipping a meal *and* flying in a plane.

Personal experience says that if I take a partial trigger to the extreme, that trigger *alone* will give me a migraine. A slightly late night won't do it, but an all-nighter will. A glass of Pinot Grigio is okay, but three days in a row, probably not. So if a heavy dose of something will trigger a headache, this might indicate that a smaller amount *in combination with* a small amount of another partial trigger will produce a headache. We have not seen any studies to this effect, but it is logical that the information will help you understand your partial triggers.

As you get more familiar with your partial triggers and how potent each one is for you, you can devise modification strategies to minimize their triggering potential. I teach patients to rate the triggering potential of each of their partial triggers. Give each partial trigger a number of points on a scale of 1 to 10. You get ten points in a day, because ten points or greater means you'll get a migraine. One point of exposure is a very minor trigger, but if something is a 10, it is a trigger all by itself and will definitely cause a headache. For me, staying up late might be a 7 and red wine a 5, so if I do both, I'll be at twelve points and will almost surely get a headache. Similarly, if red wine is a 5 and aged cheese is also a 5, I'll get ten points of triggers and, again, I will probably be in trouble. But if jack cheese is a 2 and white wine is a 3, I can enjoy those and will probably be okay.

Maybe aged cheese is not a 5 for you, but a 3 or an 8. A hot afternoon might be a 6, loud noise a 4, and a late night a 7. If so, the midnight show at the Roxy would probably cause you trouble. If your premenstrual time of the month is an 8, it's a good idea to avoid every partial trigger you can. When you get an idea how strong each partial trigger is, you can avoid exposing yourself to additional triggers or modify your exposure to minimize the chance of getting a headache.

I can drink a really good red wine without a problem. Generally, I can stay up several hours later than my usual bedtime and not end up with a headache. However, if I stay up very late *and* drink red wine, it is a virtual guarantee that I will have a headache the following day. For me, wine and sleep changes are each partial triggers. Does this mean I never stay up late and drink a good Barolo? Of course not. But when I do, I know what I'm getting into and I take precautions before I go out. I have a patient who uses the same strategy before going out to dinner. She knows that having a fancy chocolate dessert after a meal that is heavy in carbohydrates will consistently give her a migraine, so she takes a long-acting triptan when she knows this is a likely scenario.

Of course, patients have many other examples, and this is one area where migraine management becomes art as much as science, for both patients and their doctors.

How to Organize Your Trigger Hunt

There are many ways to think about triggers. It is useful to classify them in some way in order to keep track, see associations, and manage them. For example, you can divide them into internal and external triggers; triggers you can avoid or modify and triggers you cannot; or complete and partial triggers. Because everyone's trigger lists will be different, no one classification scheme will work for everyone, but it *is* important to have a way to organize them into your *own* scheme.

It is true, in general, that paying attention to your life will help you identify your triggers, but it is always good to have a plan. When you first begin your search, it can be helpful to know where to look. For example, consider triggers that come from your external environment (barometric pressure changes, grapefruit, riding in a car) and triggers that come from your internal environment (your hormones, your sleep, your emotional responses). Later, when you have identified your major triggers and you are ready to do something about them, it is more helpful to organize them according to those you can avoid, those you can modify, and those you must simply protect yourself from, the best you can.

Many migraineurs develop long and convoluted theories about triggers, while others fly blindly through life in denial, constantly surprised and amazed when a headache strikes. Is there a middle course, a rational approach somewhere between making a career of searching for triggers and living the life oblivious? Yes, there is. It involves a little introspection and observation, and some rational behavior. But given the generally superior nature of the headache sufferer, it is well within our grasp.

FOUR STEPS TO TRIGGER IDENTIFICATION   The first step is to understand the realities of headache triggers and to dispel the myths. For example, it is a myth that all migraine sufferers should avoid chocolate— or peanuts, or anything else, for that matter. You need to develop a strategy to deal with that trigger only if you know from your own experience that any of these things gives you a headache. As we've discussed, we have other myths to dispel, as well. It is a myth that a headache around your eyes is triggered by sinus infection, that neck pain indicates a tension headache rather than a migraine, and that a headache that wakes you from sleep is always a sign of brain tumor.

The second step is to develop strategies for avoiding those triggers that are not particularly important to your quality of life. For example, if you know that incense always gives you a headache, it's not that hard to avoid places that burn incense. If you know that cheap beer is a reliable trigger, you can switch to good beer—or drink wine. And if you know that flashing lights will bring on a headache, you might convince your friends to get with the new millennium and hang out at a club that has retired the strobe lights.

The third step is to develop strategies to modify your exposure to those circumstances that you cannot avoid or, just as important, would *prefer* not to avoid. For example, if you know that skipped meals often trigger your headaches, but you frequently miss lunch, you can pack a couple of protein bars or a banana (or whatever you like) in your bag to eat at the appropriate time. If you know that a day at the beach can mean trouble, you can wear a hat, remember to drink a lot of water, take frequent breaks in the shade, and wear sunglasses.

The fourth and final step is to develop strategies to minimize the impact of those triggers that you cannot avoid or modify. The example is the unavoidable dinner party that will run late and have lots of alcohol—which are triggers for you. In these situations, you can work with your doctor to devise pretreatment strategies so you can get through the night headache-free, or at least with a less severe headache.

Identifying your own unique set of triggers can be difficult. I have seen many triggers—foods, barometric pressure changes, certain colors, noise pollution, harsh fluorescent lighting, poorly ventilated spaces, and particular times of the day, week, month, or season. One intriguing patient who complained of headaches only on the weekend turned out to have a car—which he drove only on the weekends—that had a leak in its exhaust system. One of my most difficult patients had daily headaches *except* when he went on vacation. For years, doctors (myself included, unfortunately) insisted that this must be due to work stress, and he tried every imaginable remedy. Only when he was forced to move from his home because of a mold problem were his headaches resolved. Tracking down triggers can take a bit of sleuthing, but it is always worth the effort when we finally find the offending stimulus. While these are extreme examples, it is important to remember that the environment, external and internal, is often the most likely place to begin the hunt for triggers.

False Triggers

One of the things we often contend with at the Keeler Center is what we call false triggers. One patient said, "I never listen to reggae music, because the first time I heard Bob Marley, I got the worst headache of my life." More commonly, I hear, "I can never eat broccoli," or "I can never ski," or "I never go to movies," or "I never take vitamins," and so forth. Patients eliminate such things because they associate them with migraines. But there is a world of difference between "The one time I did so-and-so it gave me a headache" and "*Every* time I do so-and-so it gives me a headache." If the purported trigger is not important to you, then avoiding it is no big deal. But if it is, then some additional investigation, to see if it really does contribute to your headaches, is well worth the effort.

From time to time, I get an e-mail from patients a day or two after I prescribe a new treatment reporting, "This treatment made my headaches worse." While this certainly could be the case, keep in mind that people wouldn't be trying a new treatment if they weren't getting headaches. Of course, it is hard to persuade people to try something a second time if the first time they associated it with an unpleasant outcome, but we have to be careful about this cause-and-effect business, and it is best to verify whether a substance or activity really is a trigger. This is best accomplished by tracking the suspect food (or activity) *over time* to see if it is consistently associated with headaches. At the Keeler Center, we use a headache diary to accomplish this. Some people maintain a food diary for a period of time, tracking the relationship between specific foods and their headaches. At the Keeler Center, we prefer a headache diary because for many people foods are not absolute triggers but rather partial triggers; a food diary won't reflect the combination of a particular food plus a nonfood as leading to a headache, while the headache diary will reveal these patterns.

Obviously, some migraineurs do have food triggers but for most of us our diets are not nearly as varied as we think. Keeping a headache diary for about a month will tell you a great deal about the connection between your headaches and your diet, as well as other potential triggers. This is a very important tool, because it keeps us from banning innocent foods and helps us pin down the nasty ones. It has been my experience, however, that when a patient has a food trigger, it is one of the first things they report when we start to talk about their headaches. It is the rare patient who has a significant food trigger that they had not discovered early on in their battles with headache.

Keep a Simple Headache Diary

The quickest way to become a careful observer of your life in order to identify triggers is to keep a headache diary, in which you write down everything you can think of surrounding each headache. The first month or two is a positively epiphanic time. Eventually, observation becomes second nature—and the appropriate measure to avoid a headache will also be obvious.

The headache diary is one of the few concepts that has survived intact from the early days of headache treatment—and with good reason. Even with today's designer medications and lifestyle coaches, the diary remains the best way to identify triggers, see patterns, and assess how well treatment strategies are working. Any diary in which you write down everything you can think of surrounding a given headache remains the best tool for identifying triggers and tracking your medication use and lifestyle changes. Using this simple tool, you will not have to avoid everything that has ever given any human being a headache, but can logically compare the circumstances of one headache with those of another to evaluate the validity of each potential trigger for *you*. A consistent trigger will show up again and again in your diary.

But why do we need to write it all down? Can't we just rely on our recollections to sort through our headache patterns? The answer is no. You need to keep a headache diary because:

- our memories are not that good, especially when it comes to remembering painful experiences;
- details about headaches are important, and the details that surround them (life events, medications, and so forth) can be equally or more important;
- when you record information about your headaches and show this to an expert, your clinician can actually detect patterns and triggers you might not see yourself.

Almost all of us who have headaches know that we do not think very clearly when a headache is building. Scientific studies confirm this.

Reaction times are slowed. Speech recognition, word finding, and abstract reasoning are impaired. Often, in the throes of a headache, we make just plain bad decisions—like not taking medication early or ignoring a worsening headache as long as possible. A good diary makes such decisions painfully obvious. Sometimes, diaries expose other headache patterns that are not readily obvious, such as headaches that build during the day or during the workweek.

In general, we migraineurs tend to underestimate the frequency of our headaches until they are dominating our lives. By then, it is usually much more difficult to reverse the trend. Ideally, we want to know that our headaches are worsening *before* we get to that point, so one purpose of the diary is to keep you informed about your current headache status. The simplest headache diary can help reveal an accurate headache pattern, most fundamentally how many headache days you really have in a given month. This is usually an eye-opening discovery.

In your headache diary, simply note any headaches, recording their severity (on a simple scale from 0 to 10) and anything else that might help you understand them. The nature of your entries depends on what information you want to get from your diary. For example, if you wish to know the relationship of your activities to your headaches, you will need to do more than simply record a number for headache severity at the end of each day. Rather, you'll need to log your head pain along with information about your activities. On the other hand, if your main concern is in decreasing the number of headache days per month, then a simpler daily log should suffice.

In the beginning, particularly if headaches are frequent or daily, keep the diary for at least thirty days, marking it several times per day on headache days. This should be enough time for patterns and triggers to emerge. Of course, this is not always the case. For example, if you are on an alternating day shift/night shift in three-week blocks, or if the month you are monitoring includes a trip to Greece, then you may need to rethink the time period. Just give your diary enough time so that most of the elements of your life emerge a couple of times. An effective diary does not need to be complicated. When you begin, every day that you have a headache, simply note:

- a number corresponding to your pain severity using the typical pain scale, in which 0 equals no headache and 10 is a day from hell, the worst pain you can imagine;
- any potential triggers—any external or internal disruptions that might have caused the headache (simple notes like "chocolate fondue with cheap red wine for dinner last night" or "up all night studying" or "started my period" can be extremely helpful);
- any medications you tried and how well they worked.

❖ The Pain Scale

The pain scale gives a reference point whenever you are evaluating whether your headaches are getting better—or not.

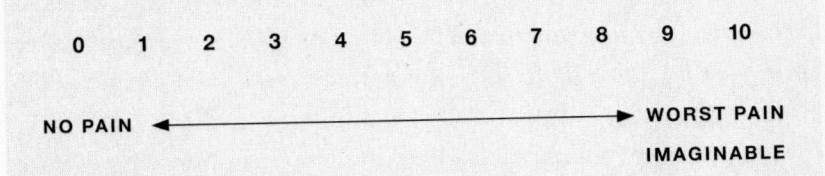

The pain scale provides important information, a relative measure of pain, so it does not matter whether your 6 is the same as my 6, or whether your 7 means the same thing to anyone else, even your doctor. Pain is, by definition, subjective. This means that you decide what number to assign to your pain, and you can never be wrong, argued with, or dismissed. It is *your* pain. *You* get to decide. If you feel like you need a little guidance on this to help you be consistent from one time to the next, the following guideline may help you:

0   **No pain**

1   **Faint pain**   I notice a twinge but don't think about it.

2   **Background**   I am aware of pain but can ignore it.

3   **Growing**   Pain interferes with my thoughts.

4   **Annoying**   Pain is bothersome but I can distract myself.

5   **Distracting**   I am hurting, and can't ignore the pain.

6   **Obtrusive**   Stronger pain interferes with my thoughts; I can function but don't want to.

7   **Difficult**   Pain is forceful; I will do only what I have to do.

8   **Disabling**   I feel consumed by pain, need help to care for myself.

9   **Misery**   Overwhelmed by pain, desperate, need someone to care for me.

10 **Worst pain imaginable**

While diaries are one of the most important tools we have for monitoring and evaluating your headaches, I caution you: *Do not make a career out of your headache diary.* This is not necessary or even desirable. The goal is *not* to major in migraine, but to minimize its effects on your life. All you need is a convenient way to record any environmental exposures or lifestyle disruptions that might contribute to your headaches. For most patients, a simple calendar does the job, or you can get forms on the Internet or from a doctor. At the Keeler Center, we have spent significant effort designing simple, effective, and efficient questionnaires, including the Keeler Headache Calendar.

Many of my patients have found that simply making headache notations part of their regular diary or blog has served them very well. There are many benefits to journaling, if you have a literary or introspective bent, but even if you don't, a few notes in the margin of your day planner or on the calendar hanging on the fridge can be just as useful. It doesn't matter what format you use. What matters is that you keep a diary, writing something down every day.

Any format will work. Our diary is very simple, but any calendar—a giveaway pocket calendar or a homemade grid—can work just as well. The key is convenience, which means keeping the diary where you will notice it and remember to write in it. Some people keep their diary in the bathroom, next to their toothbrush. That might make a diary hard to read, because of the water spots and toothpaste stains. Other people place it on the refrigerator, by the phone, near the front door, or in their nightstand. If one of these places—or another—works for you, then that is the answer.

Recently, more and more patients have found that using an electronic calendar is the easiest and most convenient way to go. One such program (the one I use) is part of Microsoft Office Outlook. It came with my computer, so the price was right, and I use it to manage my e-mail, which I check frequently during the day, so my calendar is always only a click away. To do this:

- Open Microsoft Office Outlook.
- See the first screen, which has a calendar option right next to the e-mail option.
- Click on the calendar option.
- At the top of the screen, click on "Month."
- Find the day and click on it.
- Type a number for how severe your headache was that day; add medications and known or suspected triggers, and any other pertinent information.

Playing with Outlook for about five minutes is all it takes to become a master. The advantage is convenience, especially if you already use this program for your e-mail. Also, it is easy to send the calendar to your doctor for review. Most patients simply paste it into the body of an e-mail, but some of my more savvy patients can export it to a data-processing program like Excel and create amazing and very informative graphs.

Over the years, I have used dozens of different headache diary forms,

Headache Calendar

MONTH:		HEADACHE PAIN 0–10 and time			RESCUE MEDICATION OR THERAPY	OTHER SYMPTOMS (e.g., nausea)	TREATMENT EFFECTIVE?	MENSTRUAL PERIODS	NOTES (triggers, exercise, etc.)
DAY:		A.M.	NOON	P.M.					
Monday									
Tuesday									
Wednesday									
Thursday									
Friday									
Saturday									
Sunday									
Monday									
Tuesday									
Wednesday									
Thursday									
Friday									
Saturday									
Sunday									
Monday									
Tuesday									
Wednesday									
Thursday									

Friday										
Saturday										
Sunday										
Monday										
Tuesday										
Wednesday										
Thursday										
Friday										
Saturday										
Sunday										
Monday										
Tuesday										
Wednesday										
Thursday										
Friday										
Saturday										
Sunday										

Pain Scale: 0 = no pain; 2 = discomfort; 4 = mild pain; 6 = moderate pain; 8 = severe pain; 10 = disabling pain, worst imaginable

Preventive Medication

RESCUE MEDICATION OR THERAPY
(e.g., ice, triptan, massage)

Number each medication or therapy
and put its number in the rescue column above.

(1) ——————— (6) ———————
(2) ——————— (7) ———————
(3) ——————— (8) ———————
(4) ——————— (9) ———————
(5) ——————— (10) ———————

but the *form* of the diary is not nearly as important as the *fact* of the diary. A good diary is a very important tool and well worth the effort.

Evaluate Your Diary

It is great to maintain the diary, but it is not enough. While the headache diary is the most important tool we have for monitoring headache frequency and severity, and for evaluating and improving the treatment plan, like most tools, it is only effective if it is used. Basically, it is a data set to which you can turn when you have questions. Ask any scientist. There is nothing like a good data set. Periodically, you need to review your diary. How often is periodically? That depends on where you are with your headaches. Certainly, if you are under a doctor's care, you want to show it to your doctor, every visit. On the other hand, if you are doing pretty well, it is useful to check it every month or so to make sure that your headache frequency is not creeping up or that you are not subtly increasing your medication use. Review your calendar for the last few months with these questions in mind:

- Are my headaches getting better or worse, or staying the same?
- How has my management plan impacted my headaches?
- Does my diary offer any insight into the timing, triggering, or management of my headaches?

One simple maintenance technique is to count up your total headache days each month and just note that number. This is an easy way to monitor the frequency of your headaches.

As patterns emerge, they will help you differentiate coincidences from actual triggers. Often people will come in and report that a new medicine made their headaches worse. Well, maybe. It is also possible that they got a headache and it had nothing to do with the new medicine, their sister's new cat, or the broccoli casserole. To determine that something is a trigger, it needs to be reproducible. The diary can help you make that determination, to help differentiate a coincidence from a true trigger—which can be the difference between a life without chocolate and a chocolate-rich, headache-free life. To discover important lifestyle patterns, evaluate your diary and ask such questions as:

- Are most of your headaches on workdays or weekends?
- Do they seem to build as the week wears on?
- Are your headaches most severe on awakening?
- Are they *never* present on awakening?
- Do they seem to come on a half-hour or so after you take a certain medicine?
- Do they fire up whenever you are preparing to go out to dinner with the Hendersons?
- Or only on the Saturdays when you go to your daughter's soccer games?
- Is there *any* relationship to your menstrual cycle?

Partial triggers may show up in association with other triggers. For example, I had a patient who got her most severe headaches when she had her nails done *during* her period but not at other times. It took her about four months of journaling to pick this up. When she changed salons to a place that didn't use heavy lacquers, she was fine.

Reviewing your Keeler Headache Diary on a regular basis should give you the tools to begin assessing your patterns and suggest questions to ask yourself and your doctor about your treatment plan. Whether you develop your diary with timed entries each day or a summary note at the end of the day, you will be able to harvest a wealth of information.

Tracking Triggers

Identifying triggers is tricky business. The Keeler Method offers many tools to help solve the important trigger riddle. The Keeler trigger questionnaires in this chapter will further help you identify patterns and potential triggers so you can better manage your headaches. We designed these quizzes to enable both patients and health care workers to more easily recognize patterns, and to break down lifestyle into the components that most often present triggers, then help identify potential problems in those areas. While we also look for *any* other triggers, the four main areas these questionnaires review are:

- sleep patterns and behaviors
- diet and eating patterns
- exercise and exercise timing
- stress and stress management

Using the Keeler trigger questionnaires, you will note environmental factors such as smells, barometric and atmospheric changes, toxic exposures, sounds, and so forth, then look for relationships with your headaches. By being a careful observer of your daily activities, you can consider various triggers and correlate each one with your headache diary and the frequency and severity of your headaches. Too often, we assume that a headache and an event are related when, in fact, they are coincidental. And conversely, some of our most routine and mundane daily activities are actually contributing to our headaches. The Trigger Tracker, along with a little common sense and scientific methodology, can tease out these relationships.

Usually, a Zen-like attention to your daily activities, ideally in conjunction with a headache diary, will give you all the information you need about your headaches, so you do not need to make your headaches a focus of attention. It is written: Pay attention to your life. If you find something that gives you a headache, work around it.

"Working around it" may mean avoiding it altogether, minimizing additional triggers at the same time, or taking preventive steps in anticipation of exposure to the trigger. There are several strategies we can employ to diminish the impact of triggers, but the key is to first identify them.

Anything that contributes to your headaches can be a trigger. *Anything.* Usually, if you have a major trigger, you don't need to buy a book to figure it out. You already know about it. But most of us have multiple triggers, some of which are obvious, others more subtle, some much more potent. But the lesser triggers can be the stuff of a monster headache—particularly when combined with several other minor triggers or just one big one.

This questionnaire helps you start your investigation, to consider the many things that might be triggers or partial triggers for your headaches.

Things You Consume

Have you associated any foods with your headaches?

_____

_____

Consider anything you eat, not just the common foods included on laundry lists of triggers. Remember, it is as important to rule out foods as it is to identify them as triggers.

Have you associated any drinks with your headaches?

_____

_____

Theoretically, even water could be a headache trigger, particularly since water is now supplemented and processed beyond recognition, so consider juices, milk, and all other beverages, not just alcohol. Keep in mind that dehydration (not enough water intake) is often the cause of a prolonged or intractable headache (one that just won't go away).

Do you take caffeine?

_____

_____

Consider coffee, sodas, energy drinks, chocolate, and other sources of caffeine.

Are there medications you take now or took in the past that you associate with headaches?

_____

_____

While headaches are listed as side effects for many, many medicines, not every medicine causes headaches in every person. It is useful to consult the diary and look for a correlation between starting a new medicine and a change in headache frequency.

Do you take any supplements now or did you take any in the past that seemed to worsen your headaches?

_____

_____

Not every medicine requires a prescription, and not everything in the health food store is safe and harmless. Remember, anything you put into your body is a potential trigger. Just because it is really expensive and comes in a dark bottle with a pastoral scene on it is no guarantee that it won't contribute to a headache.

Have you noticed an association between tobacco products or smoke and your headaches?

_____

_____

Aside from the fact that tobacco causes cancer, lung disease, heart attacks, and stroke, and smells really bad, it clearly makes many people's heads hurt.

Do any street drugs or other nontraditional substances seem to worsen your headaches?

_____

_____

Not all street drugs cause headaches. In fact, some (such as marijuana) help many people with headaches. It is important to be honest about the effect of anything that goes into your body, legal or otherwise.

Have any *combinations* of the above foods and substances ever seemed to contribute to your headaches?

_____

_____

Have you ever noticed that *stopping* something worsened your headaches?

_____

_____

Keep in mind that triggers often go hand in hand—as in "I only smoke when I have a drink" or "If I have caffeine in the evening, I don't sleep well." Patterned behavior is the central theme for migraineurs, and most migraineurs are at greater risk when they stray from their normal patterns of behavior. Keep an eye on this and see if it is true for you.

Your Internal Environment

What is your usual sleep schedule?

_____

_____

If you stray from your schedule, does this seem to trigger a headache?

_____

_____

We stress the importance of a regular sleep cycle over and over. But all people get a headache when they vary their sleep pattern. The best way to find out is to track your sleep against your headache diary.

What is your usual exercise pattern?

_____

_____

Does straying from this pattern affect your headaches?

_____

_____

It is important to understand the relationship between head-aches and your response to exercise. Exercise is best accomplished at the same time each day, and over time aerobic exercise raises our pain tolerance.

Have you noticed an effect from changes in hormone levels such as menstrual cycle, low testosterone, fasting, sleep deprivation, or thyroid illness?

_____

_____

This is not just about estrogen. When disrupted, many hormones likely influence headaches. Our sleep patterns affect cortisol, our eating cycle has an impact on a variety of hormones, and exercise, anxiety, and mental stimulation influence still others. While supplements or medicines can, in some cases, modulate these changes, they are generally best regulated by routine activity.

Have you noticed that headaches are more frequent during your workweek or during times of prolonged sitting, standing, or reaching/stretching?

_____

_____

There is an intimate relationship between the musculoskeletal system and the nervous system, particularly with respect to the neck and upper back. Most of us carry our stress in our neck and shoulders, and many of us sit at desks and computers for long hours each day. By becoming aware of this relationship and taking action to break the cycle, we can easily reduce or eliminate this trigger.

Does your headache frequency or severity increase during times of stress?

_____

_____

In one very real sense, headache is "all in your head." Stress and other strong emotions trigger the release of a variety of hormones and neurotransmitters that are active in pain pathways. Again, by recognizing these triggers and developing a strategy to dissipate or control them, we reduce their potency as triggers.

❖ External Exposures

Have you noticed a relationship between lighting and your headaches?

_____

_____

Try to distinguish between the effects of light on an existing headache (almost always painful) and sensitivity to light that seems to trigger a headache. Many migraineurs are sensitive to light in general. Consider sudden or prolonged exposure to bright light as well as flickering lights, and computer, television, and movie screens.

Does prolonged use of your eyes, even with proper lighting, elicit a headache?

_____

_____

Consider reading, as well as computer and video game use. It is important to note whether a headache is an immediate response or if it comes on after an hour or more of uninterrupted activity. Pain at the onset of reading often suggests that the problem is in the eyes themselves, rather than in the muscles that move the eyes, which is the case when pain comes on after prolonged use. Also, it is useful to note whether the effect is dependent upon the ambient lighting during the activity.

Does loud, persistent, or cacophonous sound bring on a headache?

_____

_____

Consider loud noises, straining to hear, sirens, and especially loud noise in conjunction with other triggers such as smoke, disco balls, and crowds. While sound might not trigger a headache when presented in isolation, many migraineurs are sensitive to sound in general, and sound is a common partial trigger.

Does strong scent, whether pleasant or noxious, trigger your headaches?

_____

_____

Note personal perfumes as well as environmental aromas such as air fresheners, incense, and candles; fumes; grass cuttings; smoke; and so forth. Smells, like sounds, are often partial triggers, not so much a problem on their own, but when combined with other triggers, they are often enough to push you over the edge.

Does extreme heat or cold trigger your headaches?

_____

_____

What is the effect of moving from a controlled (air-conditioned) environment into a natural environment?

_____

_____

Like many other triggers, for some migraineurs, it is not so much the warm or cool environment as it is the change from one extreme to the other that triggers the headache.

Observations and Associations

Typically, when you get a headache:

Are you alone or with others?

_____

_____

With certain people?

_____

_____

Where are you? At work? At home? Vacation? Driving? Alone?

_____

_____

What is the time of the day? Day of the week? Time of the month? Season?

_____

_____

What are you usually doing?

_____

_____

Do you associate any specific activities with headaches?

_____

_____

What do these activities have in common?

_____

_____

How do they differ from similar activities that do not lead to headaches?

_____

_____

Do you tend to avoid any situations (people, places, activities, or times) because you don't like them, for no good reason, though they don't consistently cause headaches?

_____

_____

Very often, these situations may include elements that you may associate as "partial triggers," elements that, alone, may not cause a headache but can, in combination with other elements, lead to a whopper.

Once you have identified some major, fairly consistent triggers, it helps to identify their essential elements. Then, it should be easier to predict other exposures that might also be triggers. This exercise is designed to help hone in on your triggers. If nothing comes to mind, that's fine. Skip the drill. But often it will turn out that it is a component of the trigger, not the whole entity, to which you're sensitive. For example, you may perceive exercise as a trigger when, in fact, it is only one *kind* of exercise (such as isometrics) or one *aspect* of exercise (such as improper breathing) that triggers your headaches. By refining your triggers, you can expand your activities *and* avoid the headaches.

Use your diary to list your known triggers here. Under each one, list three things that are similar to the trigger that do not give you a headache and three similar things that might. Make extra copies for more triggers.

TRIGGER:_____

Similar things that do NOT trigger   Similar things that MIGHT trigger

1. _____   1. _____

2. _____   2. _____

3. _____   3. _____

TRIGGER:_____

Similar things that do NOT trigger   Similar things that MIGHT trigger

1. _____   1. _____

2. _____   2. _____

3. _____   3. _____

TRIGGER:_____

Similar things that do NOT trigger   Similar things that MIGHT trigger

1. _____   1. _____

2. _____   2. _____

3. _____   3. _____

TRIGGER:_____

Similar things that do NOT trigger   Similar things that MIGHT trigger

1. _____   1. _____

2. _____   2. _____

3. _____   3. _____

TRIGGER:_____

Similar things that do NOT trigger   Similar things that MIGHT trigger

1. _____   1. _____

2. _____   2. _____

3. _____   3. _____

When you have identified a trigger, it helps to learn as much as you can about that trigger and its role in your headaches. Triggers change, as do our responses to them. By understanding the circumstances around the trigger and noting any ongoing correlative activity, we are better able to manage the trigger and thereby reduce its power over us.

> These questions will help you organize your observations about suspected triggers and other things that coincided with them, as well as information about the headaches that followed. (You may want to make enough copies of the list of questions for each suspected trigger.)

SUSPECTED TRIGGER:_____

Were you exposed to other triggers (suspected or definite) around the same time?

_____

_____

Were there any variations in your day? If so, list them.

_____

_____

Did you sleep well the night before?

_____

_____

Had you skipped a meal?

_____

_____

Had you been out in the sun?

_____

_____

Were you properly hydrated?

_____

_____

Had you been exercising more or less than normal that day?

_____

_____

Anything else?

_____

_____

Was the resulting headache typical for you?

_____

_____

If not, how was it different?

_____

_____

Did the headache respond to your usual rescue strategy?

_____

_____

Your Headache History

Probably one out of every three patients I see cannot tell me when their headaches first started, within three years. One in four cannot tell me if they have a first-degree relative who suffers from headaches, and probably half of my new patients cannot recall the things they have tried over the years to treat their headaches. This is not because years of headaches have damaged our brains—although mounting evidence reveals that migraines, left untreated over years, do take a toll on the brain. It is because most of us are not careful historians. As a headache specialist, I can tell you that *an accurate history is one of the most valuable tools I have in creating a successful treatment plan for my patients.*

At the Keeler Center, we use a computerized, structured, three-hour interview to tease out the details we need to understand your headaches. This book includes some essential components of this interview, to help you organize your headache history so you and your health care team can better understand your headaches and develop an effective treatment plan. Most of us take for granted that we know our own headache history, so using these forms may seem like a pointless exercise. But nothing could be further from the truth.

Do you need to bother with this if you are not working with a doctor? Absolutely. Should you be working with a doctor? Probably. If your headaches are bad enough for you to buy this book instead of some great work of fiction, then you probably need a physician's support to help you get your headaches under control. The rub, of course, is finding a physician who has the time, experience, and interest in getting a handle on your headache problem and devising a treatment strategy that will work for you. It takes a long time to clarify a headache history, and if the information you provide is organized and accurate, your doctor will be better able to fine-tune your treatment plan. So providing your health care practitioner with a concise, focused headache history helps facilitate a more efficient and effective appointment.

Of course, not every aspect of the history form is relevant for every patient and, sometimes, relevant information just isn't available. When you complete the Headache History (see Appendix 1), do the best you can.

Family History

Knowing your family headache history is important, but this is not simply a yes-or-no question. Beth, for example, is a seventeen-year-old high school senior with migraines and no clue about what triggers them. To my every suggestion of a possible trigger, her response was "maybe" or "sometimes." Reluctantly, she agreed to have her much older sister (with whom she did not get along) come in for an interview. The only thing they had in common was headaches. Her sister had a pretty clear idea of her own triggers and fairly good control over her headaches. Interestingly, it turned out that both sisters were sensitive to a similar list of triggers, and

❖ Family Headaches

Every blood relative who gets migraines—or used to get them—has a basic set of information that might help you deal with yours. Talk to your family and get all the information you can about the migraines that run in your family. Here are some important questions to ask:

How old were you when your headaches started?
How old were you when your headaches stopped?
How long did they usually last?
Did you have nausea and/or vomiting?
Were you sensitive to light or sound?
Did you know what your triggers were?
Did any preventive strategies work?
What were the most effective rescues?

responded well to the same preventive. Moral: Talk to other family members who have headaches.

Whenever possible, find out *what family members have done for their headaches* and *what their triggers are.* In fact, a good family history can be one of the most useful pieces of information you can bring to your physician because, often, what works for one family member will work for others, and triggers for one family member are often triggers for others, as well.

Your Current History

Headache is subject to so many variables that, in addition to your diary and trigger observations, we also need a broader perspective. Your diary is like a snapshot, a "day in the life," and your trigger observations provide clues to specific pieces of the puzzle. But your complete headache history provides the longer view, a comprehensive overview of your problem and the context for your immediate situation. As you develop, modify, and revisit your treatment plan, it is useful to understand your headaches from the ground up. This is why I ask all my patients to report their comprehensive headache history.

While a well-told story lends insight, some people just cannot tell a story. We have all had the experience of hearing the same story from two different people when, perhaps, one told it well and the other told it poorly. The same is true for a medical history. When a patient tells their history as a hodgepodge of anecdotes and impressions, I might not understand the problem any better than when we began. When a patient's story is well organized and logically presented, often the diagnosis and treatment plans seem to suggest themselves.

Since it can be a challenge to communicate your information in a manner that enables your health care team to understand your headaches, I have provided a Headache History at the back of this book (see Appendix 1). This form helps you organize and present your headache history in a way that makes it easy for your doctor to separate the important elements from extraneous information that might cloud the picture. Often, we are not sure what in our history is important and what is not. A good doctor can help with this, and so can this form. It also helps if your doctor understands your headaches in the context of your general health, your family and work situations, and your emotional life. This is an essential exercise for you, too. It will help you organize your information so you might observe the patterns that contribute to your migraines and better understand the nature of your headaches, even without the help of a trained professional. It also gives you a reference to which you can return. In other words: Do try this at home.

Plan Your Plan: The Three-Part Treatment Plan (Lifestyle, Prevention, and Rescue)

Once we have a good idea of the frequency, severity, and duration of a person's headaches, we can develop a treatment plan, starting with lifestyle and environmental changes. The best treatment plans also include prevention measures designed to avoid anticipated headaches, as well as a set of actions to use for rescue when a headache rears its ugly head.

Chapter 4

The Antimigraine Lifestyle: Recapturing the Good Life with Lifestyle Modification

xercise? I would love to exercise, but it makes my headaches worse."

"I decided not to take that trip because I didn't want to risk a migraine in a foreign country."

"A NASCAR race? You must be kidding! The noise alone would give me a migraine."

"No. I never fly. It gives me horrible headaches."

Besides sounding very familiar, what do each of these statements have in common? Each is an example of how headaches can control our lives.

Lifestyle has a huge impact on chronic diseases, and it takes practitioners a lot of time to learn enough about someone to tease out all the contributing factors. Sir William Osler, the father of modern medicine, taught that it is more important to know what sort of person has a disease than what sort of disease a person has.* Though this is especially true for patients with "chronic" diseases, unfortunately, many practitioners seem to have forgotten this approach. Doctors cannot cure these diseases with a pill, an operation, or a blast of radiation therapy. Treatment often involves little changes in many aspects of the patient's life. Most important, these conditions demand an open, accessible, interactive relationship between the patient and their doctor. These days, that is a rare commodity.

* William Osler, *Principles and Practice of Medicine*, 4th ed. (New York: D. Appleton, 1901).

Until we have a way to rewire the human brain to be less sensitive to environmental assaults, we will need to modify our environment to suit the brain we got. We don't have a magic pill for migraines, but once you do your detective work and identify your triggers, you can begin to establish your antimigraine lifestyle, which can *dramatically* reduce the number of headaches you get, and their severity. Understanding the theory behind this, however, is the first step toward a life with fewer, less severe headaches—a life in which *you* have control over your migraines, instead of letting *them* control *you*.

If someone were to ask me what is the single most important thing for headache sufferers to do, I would be stumped (but only for a moment). For any individual, there may be one thing he or she could do or change that would materially improve quality of life. But for the vast majority of headache sufferers, there is not one major thing; instead it is a whole collection of little things and medium-sized things that, taken together, end up dramatically improving their quality of life.

The fact is, of any treatment, **lifestyle modification has the greatest long-term impact on reducing the disability and pain of headaches**. Lifestyle modification is, at once, the most important aspect of the Keeler Method and the most neglected aspect of traditional and alternative headache treatments. This chapter is intended to help you tweak your lifestyle in subtle ways that will help you minimize, avoid, or modify your most troubling triggers.

The Antimigraine Lifestyle

We have all heard of adrenaline junkies, those guys who go bungee jumping in the morning, rob a bank at lunch, and skydive without a chute after dinner. These people are "wired" differently from how the rest of us are. Imaging studies of brain metabolism have shown that adrenaline junkies' brains respond to sensory input differently from how the brains of others do. There has even been a gene associated with "risk" behavior.

In a sense, and without making any value judgments, we migraineurs are just the opposite: we thrive on routine. This is not to say that we are boring or conservative. Anyone who knows a migraineur can attest that we are anything but. Any migraineur can tell you that as a group we are highly intelligent, remarkably productive people who just get a little carried away sometimes; we are among those who are euphemistically tagged type A. Still, the fact is that migraineurs do best when they are on fairly predictable schedules. We may not like it, but it is true. We do not handle change well, but do best (have fewer, less severe headaches) when our environment (internal as well as external) remains fairly routine, very *regular*.

Among the most common triggers for migraines are variations in sleep schedule, mealtimes, exercise, and hormones. And we migraineurs do best if our ratios of carbohydrate, fat, and protein remain fairly consistent from day to day.

Why is this? From fluctuating hormone levels to a shift in the weather, environmental change most often triggers migraines. It therefore stands to reason that the less change in the environment, the rarer the triggers and the fewer the headaches. Think for a moment what most of us do when we get a headache: we withdraw from the assaults of our environment and seek out a dark, cool, quiet room where we can lie still. We avoid the blowing air conditioner, the ringing phone, the aromatic food, and even the gentle stroking of our throbbing heads.

This doesn't mean that a migraineur can have no variety, no spice in life. It just means that as a rule we do better with regular hours, regular mealtimes, regular exercise. And it means that we need to be aware that, when we stray from our routines, we need to be vigilant in *monitoring* our environment, to watch for signs of an impending headache so we will be prepared to deal with it effectively.

My undergraduate degree was in philosophy, and as a result, I try to see problems in the broadest possible terms. This way, solutions tend to be applicable in many circumstances. Immanuel Kant used the term *Weltanschauung* to describe the way in which one views the world. I have found it a very useful concept in changing the way we, as migraineurs, approach our lives. A positive, proactive weltanschauung works much better than a laundry list of things to avoid, whether they are foods, social situations, or environments.

While migraine's "big picture" is important—and our weltanschauung guides us through unfamiliar situations—very often the little things are the ones that set us up for headaches. For some people, the occasional major carbohydrate load or chocolate binge or unlimited soda refills with dinner will do it. For others, a weekend construction project after a relatively inactive week sets them up. This is not to say that you *always* have to pass up a chocolate cruller, or that you can *never* take on a vigorous weekend hike, but it does mean that you need to be aware of the potential consequences of your actions and act responsibly. Often, this might be something as simple as taking an anti-inflammatory, hydrating well, and wearing sunglasses before you go out for a day in the hot sun, or thinking ahead about what you will take from the buffet, before you get to it.

Living an antimigraine lifestyle means bringing the proper attitude, or weltanschauung, to your daily activities, and being mindful of the little things that you have learned might set you up for a headache. Just as there is no wonder cure for migraines, neither is there one universal behavior that, when eliminated, will protect you from ever getting another migraine. At least, not yet.

The Elements of Lifestyle

What are the mysterious elements of lifestyle that protect us from headaches—or set us up for them? The bible for writers, a classic text called *The Elements of Style*, sets down in the clearest possible terms all the dos and don'ts of effective literary form. Just as *The Elements of Style* breaks down the written language into its components and provides guidelines for written communication, the Keeler Method's "Elements of Lifestyle" breaks down your interactions with the world.

Positive lifestyle patterns can certainly minimize headaches, and are the secret to an antimigraine life. Almost all migraineurs do much better when they live their lives with adherence to routines, especially around sleep, exercise, and meals. Good sleep patterns include practicing effective "sleep hygiene" habits, especially going to bed at the same time each night and waking at the same time every morning. Engaging in a regular, healthy exercise routine also contributes significantly to headache improvement. And following a consistently healthy diet with meals on a regular and predictable schedule completes the big three of a positive, antimigraine lifestyle.

In the broadest sense, we live in two worlds: an internal world of hormones, neurotransmitters, emotions, and drives, and an external world of environmental factors. Physiologist Claude Bernard described these two worlds 150 years ago, and it is just as useful today to understand them in order to address our place in the world. In an effort to gain control over our lives, it helps to further understand these two worlds. Our internal world, for example, runs on a schedule that is defined in broad strokes by our genetics, but we still have quite a bit of control over it. Unfortunately, modern culture allows us to stretch these schedules well beyond the limits of their natural rhythms. Consider that, in the temperate climates, it is dark for roughly one-third of the twenty-four-hour day, and for most of the last fifty thousand years or so, that's when human beings slept, getting their eight hours of sleep before rising with the sun. But thanks to the wonders of modern science and things like electricity, now we can stay up and do things all night if we wish, then nap on and off throughout the day, since we don't have to be out foraging for food or watching for predators.

What effect does this have on our internal environment? Our bodies still thrive on a roughly twenty-four-hour circadian cycle, particularly with respect to sleep and certain hormones. Cortisol, for example, fluctuates rhythmically with our sleep. When we mess with our biological clock, we disrupt our cortisol levels, which can trigger a migraine. This might explain why pulling an all-nighter or sleeping in on Saturdays often leads to a headache.

Cortisol is just one example of an internal cycle that we can disrupt. Throughout our daily cycles, our bodies also secrete a substance known as gastrin-releasing peptide (GRP), which links our digestive system to our daily rhythms. GRP may be involved in the well-known phenomenon of headache triggered by fasting; while this has yet to be demonstrated in a scientifically controlled study, it is at least as likely as the popular notion that low blood sugar leads to the fasting headache, which has been shown to be a myth. Most headache specialists believe the "fasting headache" is a migraine triggered by skipped meals. However, the relative roles of sugar, gastrin, insulin, grehlin, and other neuropeptides remain to be elucidated.

Hormonal changes associated with estrogen are perhaps the most obvious example of internal environmental changes that trigger headaches. The majority of female migraineurs can testify to the association between their headaches and fluctuations in their estrogen levels throughout the month.

Changes in our external environment likely trigger changes in our *internal* environment, whether they are hormonal or, more often, changes in our neurotransmitter responses, fatty acid metabolism, and inflammatory responses that in turn lead to headache. For practical purposes (and those things we can do something about), it is useful to be aware of the elements of our internal environment over which we have significant control. These include sleep, eating, and exercise patterns.

External elements often influence our lifestyle, simply in terms of the physical factors in our world, such as in our home, community, and workplace. But the *way* in which we interact with our environment—how we respond to stress, routines, and change—is another factor. Identifying those factors that cause our headaches is complicated, even for people who have been doing it for years, because we are not born knowing how to do it and because headaches do not come with an instruction manual. But if you look at the various elements of your lifestyle long enough and hard enough, patterns start to emerge, and trouble spots come to the surface.

We recently saw an accountant who came to us because her primary care physician was no longer comfortable providing her with a combination medicine generally known as Fioricet. She was upset because in her view she was doing fine, taking about ten of the pills a day. While she said her headaches were bearable and she was able to function with the medicine, she definitely could not function without it. Still, she did not think she had a problem. But her doctor did.

About three years earlier, she had started using Fioricet a couple of days per week, only when necessary. Within a year she was taking two tablets every morning, but that gradually increased. She awakened each day with a headache that she rated as a 5 on the pain scale, but she took two Fioricet every couple of hours while awake to keep the headache from escalating. When she came to us on this regimen, she was able to get through her days, pay her bills, and keep her family fed, but she found that ten tablets per day were not holding her. She wanted either more Fioricet or a second medication that "would work as well as Fioricet."

Despite her protestations to the contrary, her approach to migraine was not working. When we began to break down the elements of her lifestyle, she saw that her lifestyle patterns were not good. She was sleeping badly, constantly felt on edge, had neither the time nor the inclination for recreation and exercise, and so forth. We began by addressing *both* medication and lifestyle issues. She rearranged her priorities and started exercising, eating, and sleeping with a more deliberate rhythm to her day, and she formally set aside time for her family, her crafts, and herself. She also began using a preventive, which served as a mood stabilizer, and she began to taper off and eventually stop using Fioricet.

Like this accountant, most migraineurs do much better and minimize their headaches when they adhere to routines in terms of sleep, exercise, and meals. These are the primary elements of the antimigraine lifestyle, the secret to an antimigraine life.

Lifestyle Changes for Headache Sufferers

Many headache sufferers, bouncing from headache crises to catch-up days, lack a rhythm to their lives. The challenge is to create healthy, healing patterns with regularity in life, starting with these most basic ones— sleep, meals, and exercise.

In nearly twenty years caring for people with headaches (longer, if you count my years caring for my own headaches), I have *never* met a patient who could not benefit substantially from a careful examination of lifestyle for behaviors that contribute to headaches. In fact, with rare exceptions, a few minutes of careful questioning usually results in the patient's telling me exactly which things bring on or worsen headaches.

Not only does my clinical experience bear this out, but multiple studies on specific areas of lifestyle demonstrate the contribution of these factors to the frequency and severity of headaches. Of course, everyone is different. Some people find sensitivities where others do not. That is why you must always be suspicious of "quick fix" remedies (especially those with price tags attached). It is more useful to understand the components of lifestyle that often contribute to headaches, and then analyze *your* lifestyle to see where there may be areas to "redesign."

For example, if Friday night out with the girls (or boys) is both an important part of your lifestyle and a potent trigger for migraines, it makes more sense to develop a strategy that will allow you to continue this activity while minimizing the headache that follows, rather than dropping the activity or just suffering the whole next day. Lifestyle change does not mean joining a convent or monastery. It generally just means identifying your problem areas and tweaking them a little.

Sleep Routines

Solid scientific data and clinical evidence support the assertion that *good "sleep hygiene" is probably the most important element of lifestyle for most headache sufferers.* The fact is that for many migraineurs it is not enough to get the same *amount* of sleep; we also need to get our sleep at approximately the same part of the twenty-four-hour day. The body needs a sleep pattern it can rely on, so that your hormone levels are consistent and your body can coordinate the rejuvenating effects of sleep.

The body releases certain hormones on a diurnal (daily) basis. For example, cortisol fluctuates with our twenty-four-hour cycle, with the highest levels present in the early morning and the lowest levels present a few hours after we fall asleep. When we pull an all-nighter or sleep until noon, we change this internal cycle and disrupt our cortisol levels. In some people, this disruption is more than enough to trigger a migraine.

The whole idea behind sleep hygiene is to establish good habits that promote healthy, restorative sleep. As a major component of an antimigraine lifestyle, a few basic guidelines will help most migraineurs establish and maintain a healthy rhythm in their sleep cycles:

- Go to bed at more or less the same time each night. (If you have kids, go to bed an hour or two *after* they do.)
- Get up at the same time each morning, even on weekends, and regardless of how well you slept (or didn't sleep) the night before.
- If you are a napper, take your nap at the same time every day and for the same length of time.

Many migraineurs complain of weekend headaches that are often the result of sleep disruptions. Staying out late on Friday nights, sleeping in on Saturday mornings, and drinking less coffee while relaxing over the Sunday paper all upset the balance. Even if we stay up late and sleep late the next morning to get our eight hours of sleep, the problem is, they're not the *same* eight hours. When this triggers headaches, it creates many problems for migraineurs, particularly for shift workers, those who frequently travel across time zones, and those of us who would like to enjoy a Saturday night out on the town once in a while. And while it is important to live an antimigraine lifestyle, this is not to say that we can't live the life we want to live. When we choose to make an exception to any lifestyle routine, we might need to employ strategies to prevent the migraine that might result.

Dietary Habits

Not everyone has a problem with aged cheeses or chocolate or wine, but some migraineurs certainly do. In fact, not all migraineurs have a problem with *any* foods, but some do. So I urge all my patients to maintain a headache diary to uncover any specific foods that might be triggering their migraines. But that's not the end of the story.

Aside from the *what* of diet, other aspects are important. For example, meal timing is an essential part of most migraine treatment plans. Whether you eat three meals a day or five, most migraineurs seem to do best with a *regular* schedule of mealtimes.

Many headache specialists, myself included, feel that it is also beneficial to maintain the ratios of fat, carbohydrate, protein, and fiber from day to day. This does not mean you have to eat the same foods day after day, but that some attention to maintaining a relatively steady diet, whether it is high-protein, low-carbohydrate, low-fat, or whichever, seems to serve the migraineur well. Other areas currently under investigation (but not quite ready for prime time) include anti-inflammatory foods such as olive oil, walnuts, blueberries, and so forth.

Exercise

Exercise also influences our internal environment in many ways, and is very important for migraineurs. At the top of the list, it increases levels of the body's natural pain medication, proteins called endorphins, which affect our perception of pain and raise our pain threshold. If we had no endorphins, everything would hurt. But with unlimited endorphin levels, nothing would hurt and we would be dangerously immune to pain. So, through exercise, our bodies regulate how much endorphin is onboard. People who subject their bodies to lots of physical stress have very high endorphin levels and, as a result, have high pain thresholds.

For headache sufferers, this means that incorporating a regular exercise routine into an antimigraine lifestyle will (among other things) gradually raise endorphin levels. Higher endorphin levels will result in a higher pain threshold, so a 7 headache may feel like a 2, and a 10 may register as a 4. Like all lifestyle changes, this one does not come overnight, but clearly, it gives us an even greater incentive to exercise than the general population has.

For some headache sufferers, this may sound easier said than done, because for an unfortunate subset of migraineurs physical exercise can actually precipitate a migraine. While the benefits of exercising outweigh this downside, that doesn't mean you should exercise and just endure the headaches. The trick is to block exercise-induced headaches so you can enjoy the headache-reducing benefits of incorporating exercise into your lifestyle. We have strategies for managing such issues.

It is important for migraineurs to exercise on a regular basis rather than episodically. Twenty minutes every day or a half-hour three days a week is much better than four hours only on Saturdays. Regularity is fundamental to the antimigraine lifestyle.

Stress Management

Stress management does not "cure" migraines, but will often lead to fewer headaches and dramatic improvement. Besides, it's very good for you.

A good stress management plan requires that you recognize, anticipate, and, ideally, avoid your stressors (whatever is causing the stress), and when you can't avoid them you need a plan to dissipate or lessen their effect. It can be useful to break these plans into several parts: I use external, internal, and situational strategies.

External strategies involve adjusting your environment, for example, with calming music, comfortable furniture, soft lighting, and privacy so that you have more control over what comes at you, so to speak. Internal strategies include meditation, yoga, visualization, relaxation techniques, and prayer. Not everyone is comfortable with or suited to these approaches, but if they work for you they can be very helpful. Situational strategies are aimed at defusing situations that might cause stress to build. It is good to have a generous supply of these strategies on hand because stress tends to multiply and these tools can help minimize stressors before they explode into a headache. You might schedule breaks, plan downtime, write down things you are worried about, and offer to think about something before making a decision. These strategies should help you modify your lifestyle, reduce some of your stress, and minimize the effects of stress on your headaches.

Resolving Triggers

One of my great patients is a sixty-five-year-old teacher who has had headaches "since forever." The first time I saw her, she came in with her husband of forty-four years, and he sat in the chair next to hers with his arms crossed and an expression that was two parts boredom and one part disgust. When I came to the question that I always ask, "What do you think brings on your headaches?" she looked at me for just a moment too long and then slowly turned her head to glare at her husband. Some triggers are more problematic than others. For most of us, our triggers are not so readily identifiable. And parenthetically, neither were they for this patient. She and her husband actually had a delightful relationship, in a *Honeymooners* sort of way. But over time, we were able to identify and address several long-standing behaviors that dramatically reduced both the frequency and severity of her headaches.

If your headaches are triggered by peanuts, it is probably not a big deal to avoid them. But what if something that is essential to your health, family, or livelihood triggers your headaches? We cannot simply say, "Avoid your triggers." We need strategies that allow us to lead happy, productive lives in spite of our headaches. The key is to not let the headaches dictate or restrict your activities. At the same time, this does not mean that you just lower your eyes and run headlong into the wall. Denial is no better for your well-being than cowering in the corner. Once you have identified your triggers, you **value each one in terms of whether you can avoid the trigger, modify it, or prevent the headache**, and *then* integrate changes for a healthier, less headache-driven life. For some, it is merely a matter of avoiding chocolate, keeping regular hours, or taking some ibuprofen before exercising. For others, it may involve stress management, regular mealtimes, meditation training, a new line of work, or marriage counseling. Everyone is different, but everyone has triggers, and everyone can do better at managing them.

We have all heard the adage that if you approach life as a victim, you will be a victim. Certainly, our lives would be simpler and probably better without migraines. But for most of us, that is not a realistic option, and it is important to keep a constructive perspective on the whole migraine issue. The goal of the antimigraine lifestyle is to make migraines a footnote to your life rather than the focus. In other words, we want to live a life that is full and rich, not a life focused on fear, avoidance, and pain. Here are a few examples:

- I like to go out dancing, but the late nights, disco balls, loud music, and alcohol that go with it leave me with a horrible headache. A negative lifestyle choice would be to cite all of these reasons and avoid opportunities to go out dancing. Living an antimigraine lifestyle, I would employ a strategy that might include a preventive medicine, sunglasses, earplugs, and a flask of my favorite nonalcoholic beverage. Then I can dance the night away.

- A patient loves his job as a computer programmer, but by the end of the workday his head is pounding to the point that all he can do is go home and sleep. A negative lifestyle pattern would guide him to the state disability office. Instead, pursuing an antimigraine lifestyle, he would visit his human resources department and discuss the fluorescent lights, flickering CRTs, and excessive noise in the office, and he would make suggestions for simple, inexpensive changes so that he would not need to file a suit under the Americans with Disabilities Act. (Okay, a little extreme, but you get the idea.)

- A seventh-grader missed so many days of school because of his headaches that the school threatened to hold him back. Homeschooled for the last semester, he could sleep when his head hurt, study when it was not too painful, and play video games instead of exercising, because exercise gave him headaches. This child was miserable, isolated, and clearly living a negative lifestyle. A more positive approach would be to get back on a sleep schedule that corresponds to school, develop an exercise program that does not cause headaches, and take medications that allow a return to the social and academic environment appropriate for a twelve-year-old.

Obviously, if your antimigraine strategy involves prescription medication, you need to discuss this with your doctor and, if your primary care doctor is uncomfortable prescribing in this area, ask for a referral to a neurologist with experience in migraine management or go online (www.magnum.org, for example) to find a local headache specialist.

Regardless of whether you use prescription or over-the-counter medications, your physician should be involved in these decisions. Just because a medicine is available without a prescription, it is still a medicine, and if you have other health issues or use these medications inappropriately, you can get into a world of trouble.

The key to gaining control over migraine lies in gaining control over your lifestyle. This is twofold, as the triggers that cause headaches are embedded in our lives and, at the same time, an antimigraine lifestyle can be the biggest deterrent to frequent headaches. Before you begin to discuss medications and other therapies, take a long look at your lifestyle to identify those features that contribute to your headaches and those that help protect you from them. The former are our triggers, which are different for each migraineur. The features that tend to protect us from headaches are more often our routine behaviors—regularity in our sleep schedule, exercise regimen, dietary habits, and so forth.

Avoid, Modify, or Prevent

In my son's tae kwon do class, they teach the kids to walk away from a fight whenever possible. They also make sure the kids know exactly how to walk away *after* the fight, if it comes to that. It is much the same with headaches and their triggers. Once you know what your likely triggers are, you can make intelligent decisions about how to deal with them. Some you can easily walk away from without consequence. But others we would prefer not to avoid (like a really good rock concert or a fine Barolo). And others we would like to avoid but cannot or should not— like the horrible lighting in the IRS auditor's office, or the overheated, locker-room smell of the gym. These require a bit more finesse. Once you have identified your likely triggers, you *can* come up with intelligent strategies for dealing with them.

Sometimes, you can easily avoid a trigger without consequence, and that's great. If only it were all as easy as giving up okra. What about those triggers that we cannot or *should not* eliminate from our lives? The IRS office lighting might give you a headache, but if you avoid that particular trigger, headaches could be the least of your problems. Similarly, the stuffy, pungent air in the locker room may put your head into the danger zone, but you should not sacrifice the benefits of exercise to avoid a headache.

Another serious quandary arises when our triggers are things we *want* to keep in our lives—like that really good rock concert or wine, or Friday night out with the girls (or boys). Yes, we can live without these things, but we'd rather not. Even as a migraineur, you are entitled to enjoy a life that includes things you enjoy—the foods, drinks, and activities that make life fun, that make you feel like a "normal" person.

In the Keeler Method, lifestyle modification is not as simple as just avoiding all the triggers you identify, but includes an important middle step: *valuing your triggers*. Once you identify a trigger, you need to consider its value in your life. Ask yourself these questions about each trigger:

- Can you live without it, without regret?
- Would you miss it?
- Is it important to your life or to your loved ones?
- Do you have some degree of control over it?

If you can avoid the trigger without looking back, then the answer is easy: just avoid it. But if you would miss it, or if it is important to your life or to your loved ones, then it is worthwhile to tweak your life in order to minimize the associated headache. The idea is to develop commonsense strategies to work around the trigger and allow it to stay in your life while minimizing the impact it has on your headaches. If you have some degree of control over it, then you can likely make some modifications so you can keep the trigger without suffering from headaches. If you do not have any control, then you will need to take measures to protect yourself from the headache that the trigger will likely cause. So this step involves *evaluating* our triggers and classifying them according to their value in our lives:

- Avoid those triggers you can live without.
- Modify triggers over which you have some control.

- If you cannot or should not avoid or modify the trigger, prevent the headache.

Avoid the Trigger

Life would be a lot easier for migraineurs (and their doctors) if the only things that triggered our headaches were okra, Jerry Springer, and bad rap music. Then we could simply avoid all of our triggers and never look back. Unfortunately, it doesn't often work out that way.

Counseling patients to avoid things they love is hard. In fact, it is a little easier to tell a diabetic about the downside of sugar or a patient with sprue about the dangers of gluten than to tell a migraineur she can never eat nuts, cheeses, carbs, chocolate, red wine, Chinese food with MSG, meats with nitrites, and on and on. That's pretty harsh. Moreover, it is not necessarily true, at least not for every migraineur. That is why I want my patients to get good evidence that something is one of their triggers before they give it up.

Our triggers are often so trivial that a slight modification in behavior takes care of the problem. My favorite example of this is a patient who got a headache whenever he went to the mall with his family. His wife was convinced that he simply hated to shop, and he was half convinced of it himself. In collecting his history, he remembered that as a child he got headaches when he visited his grandparents. He said he could "still remember the smell," as his grandmother was overly fond of perfume. I asked him how they entered the mall and, as I suspected, they went through Nordstrom's and the gauntlet of the perfume counters. By simply changing where they entered the mall, he avoided the perfume counters (and the candle shop), and eliminated that particular trigger—along with a sticky family situation.

Examples of nonessential, easily avoidable triggers in your life should be obvious. These might include foods you hate, places where you need not go, and behaviors you wouldn't be caught dead participating in anyway.

"Partial triggers" might also offer options for easily avoiding headaches. Any one trigger taken alone might not give you a headache but a combination might be disastrous, so you can simply work to avoid the combination. Often, *one* of the partial triggers might be avoidable while the other is not. Fortunately, in this circumstance, avoiding the avoidable is often sufficient to prevent the headache.

Modify the Trigger

Triggers that are important to you, your health, and your joy in life are a bit more problematic. These might include exercise, business travel, and activities that are important to the people you care about, as well as foods or activities you just don't want to give up. And you shouldn't have to. Lifestyle modification often calls for a compromise. If you can anticipate that you will expose yourself to a known migraine trigger, your goal should be to minimize its migraine-producing potential. And you can do that.

One approach is to take care not to compound the anticipated trigger with others. For example, if you really want to go to a party at the beach but you know it could trigger a migraine, do everything you can to avoid *all* the other triggers that could contribute to a headache. Get a good night's sleep the night before. Drink and bring plenty of water. Buy an umbrella. Wear very dark sunglasses. Bring antimigraine drinks and snacks so you don't indulge in the cheap wine coolers and stale chocolate chip cookies that someone will inevitably offer you.

Every patient has many examples. Let's say you really want to go to a Metallica reunion concert. Really good earplugs may be counterproductive in this setting, but a pair of low-quality earplugs will mute the loud music and still allow you to experience the event. Do you want to go skiing in Aspen this year? Consider arriving a day or two early to allow time to adapt to the altitude before you launch into a day of rigorous skiing. (That's why they have base camps on Mount Everest.) If you want to fly across the country, take the redeye flight—and a sleep aid—to minimize the effects of a change in time zones. Or, if you want to go to Cape Town, try advancing your sleep schedule a few hours over the weeks leading up to the trip, to minimize the effects of the extensive time-zone change.

In most situations, an advance strategy and a slight change in plans can do a world of good in reducing the odds of getting a migraine. And when the trigger is a behavior, such as skipping meals or disrupting your sleep schedule, you can often avoid a headache with a little planning. Packing a lunch or rescheduling an activity, for example, can help you maintain your body's schedule and avoid the headache.

For the more type A among us, it is not a bad idea to actually prepare a migraine emergency kit to keep handy for those situations that unexpectedly barrage you with triggers. Such a kit might include a cereal bar, earplugs, sunglasses, a cooling pack, an anti-inflammatory medication, and your prescription rescue medications.

If You Can't Prevent the Trigger, Prevent the Headache

Many migraine sufferers are well aware that their headaches flare at certain times, under specific conditions, or when they encounter known triggers. Some of these are avoidable, but again, some are not. You simply cannot avoid or modify every headache trigger. In some circumstances, you need to *plan* for the headache so you can *prevent* it.

One common approach we use is to pretreat with an anti-inflammatory medication, usually a nonsteroidal anti-inflammatory drug (NSAID) such as naproxen or over-the-counter ibuprofen. Typically, NSAIDs can be very effective. In other cases, to prevent an expected headache, patients can use a long-acting triptan medication, such as frovatriptan (Frova) or naratriptan (Amerge). Over-the-counter medications can certainly work, but keep in mind that, just because you buy a medicine without a prescription at a drugstore or a health food store, it is still a medicine, and all the old rejoinders about checking with your physician before starting a new medicine apply. Obviously, you should discuss any such strategy with your doctor, particularly if your plan includes prescription medications.

With susceptible migraineurs, high heat or bright sunshine might be an automatic trigger but they might still have to work outdoors on summer afternoons, or want to take the kids to the beach once in a while. Before daring such a feat, they can take an anti-inflammatory agent, such as naproxen or Excedrin, or a long-acting triptan, such as frovatriptan, to avoid a heat- or sun-induced migraine. The same approach can be used in anticipation of most migraine-o-genic events, from vigorous exercise to a late night out on the town.

The trick of anticipating and pretreating is just that: anticipating. When we can anticipate our specific triggering conditions, we can take steps to prevent the headaches they cause. While this does require a flair for predicting your future, with minimal awareness and planning, it really will become easy—and automatic. I routinely take a couple of aspirin before I have a dinner involving wine. It is no big deal, but for me it will either prevent the headache altogether or, if it comes, it will not be as severe and I will be able to knock it out with my regular rescue medications.

PERIODIC HEADACHES Both men and women can experience hormonal changes that are potent migraine triggers. When we skip meals, sleep little, exercise too strenuously, or stress out all day, dramatic changes in our hormone levels occur. While this is a hot area for research just now, the current thinking is that when hormone levels fluctuate dramatically, they trigger migraines. Thus, it is not so much a question of "high" or "low" hormone levels, but a question of *change*—up *or* down. For this reason, when we see that hormones—estrogen, cortisol, or epinephrine (to name a few)—affect a patient's migraines, we try to develop strategies to level out or minimize these fluctuations.

In women, hormonal changes are an obvious and common example of a potent trigger you cannot avoid or modify. These include menstrual migraines and menstrually related migraines. In either case, the premenstrual days and the first few days of menstruation are guaranteed headache days for many women, while for others the midcycle days during ovulation are just as bad. In the past, doctors tried to modify this trigger through hysterectomy but today we know that hysterectomy will *not* improve migraines and can in fact make them *significantly* worse. Hysterectomy causes chaos in estrogen levels, estrogen receptors, and the chemicals that estrogen modifies. A migraineur's brain does *not* like chaos. It likes things nice and regular and predictable. Further, estrogen is not the cause of migraines, but the *changes* in estrogen levels have more to do with the association between migraines and menstruation. So women who experience hormonal migraines can use a number of strategies *other than hysterectomy* to prevent these headaches. For example, estrogen replacement strategies that maintain hormonal levels for long periods of time can be very effective.

Periodic headaches are those that are problems only at certain times, such as hormonal headaches and others with a known time frame of increased vulnerability, significant risk, or even the certainty of a migraine. (Hypnic headaches, which recur each night at a specific time, are periodic headaches, as are cluster headaches, which come, stay for a while, and then mysteriously disappear.) Such episodic headaches might come in groups, lasting a few days or a week or more, but they are often too seldom to warrant a daily medication, month after month. Learning about the specific features of various periodic headache syndromes will help you recognize them and develop strategies to preempt them.

We have a very valuable strategy for managing periodic headaches. Pulse prevention refers to a patient's taking a daily preventive medicine for a short period of time, before and during an at-risk period. Pulse therapy might last for the duration of your period, through a headache cluster, before a storm arrives, or just when your in-laws come to visit. Migraineurs who have trouble with travel can also employ this strategy, taking medication a few days or a week before and during travel involving significant altitude changes, flights, or multiple time zones. The trick is that this preventive therapy is not used permanently, day in and day out, but in bursts.

Along with menstruation, death, and taxes, we also cannot control the weather. Several recent studies have confirmed what many headache sufferers have known all along: Changes in weather and in barometric pressure before storm fronts move in can influence headaches. I also have patients who have found that their headaches are worse during allergy season, independent of any specific allergy. For reasons of biology or sociology, these triggers are unavoidable for some people, since we obviously can't change the weather. But we *can* employ strategies to help prevent headaches when the weather is likely to cause them.

Pulse prevention, using a migraine prevention medication during a season of increased headache risk, can be a very effective strategy. In addition to the triptans and NSAIDs, we also use steroids, D2 antagonists, and antiepileptic medications for pulse prevention. While medications are our main treatment for periodic headaches, massage, meditation, biofeedback training, and other options can be effective in some patients.

Some might need to use this strategy for a couple of months of increased vulnerability, or for a shorter term, say when the weatherman predicts a drastic change in the local weather. Starting a course of pulse therapy a few days beforehand will usually be effective in averting headaches. We can often anticipate and prevent episodic headaches and allow patients to successfully manage their migraines around their life, not the other way around.

Work It Out

We don't instantly go from suffering from chronic daily headaches to having no headaches at all. Improvement comes not in a straight line rocketing skyward, but in an undulating course, a wavy line trending toward overall improvement. This is partly because after a headache we tend to try to make up for lost time and end up overdoing it. Then the next day or two we pay for it. To create smoother waves, we need to learn to moderate our good days and not freak out over our bad days.

Since everyone is different and some people find sensitivities where others do not, migraineurs must always be suspicious of quick-fix remedies like "migraine diets" or "brain stimulators," especially when they come with a price tag attached. I have found it much more useful to understand the various elements of lifestyle that often contribute to headaches and then help patients analyze their lifestyle patterns to see where there may be areas to "redesign" without sacrificing control over their own lives.

KNOWN TRIGGERS *Think of all the triggers you currently recognize and note for each one whether you can avoid the trigger, can modify it to* *minimize its headache potential, or need strategies to anticipate and pre-vent headaches when you cannot or should not avoid the trigger.*

Trigger	Can avoid	Can modify	Pretreatment plan
_____	_____	_____	_____
_____	_____	_____	_____
_____	_____	_____	_____
_____	_____	_____	_____
_____	_____	_____	_____

Keep in mind that it is the rare patient who has one consistent trigger, avoids it, and has no more headaches. In watching for, identifying, and managing our triggers, the goal is to gain as much control as we can. We can never completely control our external and internal environments to the degree we might like, but we can go a long way toward managing them and thereby decreasing our headaches.

Chapter 5

Your Prevention Plan—Go the Distance

One of the big controversies among scientists and clinicians studying headache today is whether years and years of episodic migraine damages the brain. Magnetic resonance imaging (MRI) studies show that small lesions begin to accumulate in some migraineurs over time, suggesting that long-standing, untreated migraine can cause brain injury similar to that seen with long-standing hypertension or diabetes. While we do not yet know the significance of the changes seen on MRI, their very presence makes a compelling argument for preventing headaches early and aggressively—as if stopping the pain weren't enough. If many years of suffering from migraines *does* cause permanent damage to the brain, perhaps every migraine sufferer should be on a preventive medication, a neuroprotective agent to help minimize this damage. Many headache specialists feel that this alone is reason to use preventive medications in migraine, especially in migraine with aura. The jury is still out on this, but it is something we are working on.

Today, increasing scientific evidence also suggests that migraine is not just a chronic disease but also a *progressive* one. Like asthma or heart disease, if left untreated, migraine can become more frequent and more severe, and can last longer. Recent studies have even suggested that certain subgroups of women migraineurs are at greater risk for stroke as they age. The controversy centers on the increased risk of cerebrovascular disease (stroke) among people who have migraine with aura, complicated or hemiplegic migraine, or common migraine along with other risk factors such as estrogen supplementation or high cholesterol. At present, the connection is purely statistical: if you have these conditions, there is a slightly greater risk of stroke than is found in the general population. What is not known is how the two conditions are related: does one cause the other? Are the two conditions set up by a third abnormality in the brain or blood vessels? For now, we can only note the association and try to avoid making the situation worse by adding additional risk factors such as smoking or obesity. Because of this risk, a great debate is currently raging within the headache community regarding the advisability of placing certain migraineurs on preventive medication.

A more practical or immediate reason for prevention is to *avoid* or, if it is too late for that, to *correct* medication overuse headache (MOH). This headache results from the overuse of rescue medications, and is a daily or near-daily condition that is superimposed on the underlying headache syndrome. At present, prevention is our best defense against MOH. By decreasing the severity and frequency of headaches, prevention helps us avoid overuse of rescue medications and the resulting MOH. When you are already experiencing chronic daily headaches, initiating a preventive is an essential part of getting back to having episodic rather than daily headaches.

However, all preventives have side effects, and we don't want patients to take more medications than they need. And, as far as insurers are concerned, the cost considerations can be significant. It is often difficult to make insurers understand that short-term costs for preventives save them money in the long run by reducing the need for rescue medications and trips to the emergency room. For the patient, the problem can be compounded by the fact that many commonly used preventives are not FDA-approved for that purpose and, therefore, insurers are reluctant to cover their costs. On the other hand, if reducing headache frequency also reduces a patient's risk of brain damage or a life-threatening or life-altering stroke, a preventive medication seems a small price to pay. Right now, we just don't have enough information to make the call in most cases. But we're working on it. And as we learn more about the long-term effects of migraines, the neuroprotective aspects of prevention may change our approach yet again.

So Who Needs a Preventive Medication?

In the old days, we thought that any patient who experienced headaches more than four times per month was a candidate for preventive measures. Today, in the age of effective triptans, we prefer to interrupt and stop headaches with medication taken only four or five times a month, rather than put the patient on a daily medication to prevent such relatively infrequent headaches. But with the new scientific data about the possible dangers of ongoing headaches, headache specialists are rethinking this. For now, some patients need major renovation in certain aspects of their lifestyle (usually sleep hygiene, diet, stress management, and exercise), while others seem to have these elements well under control. *So those patients at risk for stroke and those with frequent headaches that persist despite lifestyle modification need a preventive medication.* And, in certain circumstances, preventive medication is mandatory. This includes patients whose headaches are associated with neurological deficits (such as weakness on one side of the body or the inability to speak), patients with frequent or debilitating headaches, and those whose headaches, while infrequent, are hugely disruptive to their professional or personal lives.

For most headache sufferers, this is my rule of thumb: *If headaches substantially interfere with life, the patient should be on a preventive.* When headaches are frequent or severe enough to disrupt daily activities, prevention is appropriate. If your headaches are disruptive enough for you to be seeing a doctor and your doctor is not suggesting a preventive, then you need to bring it up. Basically, every migraineur needs a prevention *plan*, but not every migraineur needs medication to be a part of that plan. However, most migraineurs who experience frequent or increasingly frequent headaches that substantially interfere with their lives will likely require a preventive medication as *part* of their prevention plan, at least initially.

But again, this requires the patient to make an honest assessment of how much their migraines impact their lives. This sounds simple enough, but we migraineurs tend to drastically underestimate both the frequency and severity of our headaches. This is why a diary (or a very observant companion) is so important to effective migraine management.

Medication Versus Nontraditional Remedies

Headache specialists generally agree that a preventive strategy is the most neglected aspect of headache management. Certainly this is true of the pharmaceutical component of migraine treatment. We have seen seven new medications to treat migraine pain and other symptoms since 1993, augmenting our arsenal of medications specifically for migraine rescue, but in that time, the pharmaceutical industry has added only *two* preventive medications. Neither one was developed specifically for migraine.

When daily preventive medication comes up, many patients want to consider alternative therapies, such as holistic or natural remedies. However, I don't make much distinction between natural and pharmaceutical, Eastern and Western, alternative and traditional. Headaches are so difficult, I like to use every tool in the box. I don't much care whether the FDA has classified a medication as pharmaceutical, neutraceutical, or something else. All treatments have their good and bad points, benefits and risks. So, for my money, the preventive that works best and does the least harm is the way to go. Not everyone sees it this way, but this has been my approach and it has served my patients well.

Although medication is considered the cornerstone of headache prevention, medications are just one aspect of a prevention program. A good prevention plan includes other measures to decrease the frequency of headaches, from traditional modalities (such as health maintenance, physical medicine, physical therapy, nutritional counseling, and stress management) to nontraditional therapies (such as biofeedback training, yoga, massage, acupuncture, and other techniques).

Some of us do really well with alternative treatments, while others do well with medication and physical medicine. Most of us find a middle ground, utilizing the best-fitting parts of headache treatments from around the world, based on personal preference, lifestyle, side effects, other medical concerns, and most important, what works.

Using the Keeler Method, patients learn how to select those treatments that will most likely bring the greatest benefit for them. For example:

- patients who find that one of their major migraine triggers comes from carrying a lot of stress in their neck and shoulders often do very well with physical medicine;
- people who feel a strong spiritual connection with their bodies often find craniosacral work and meditation to be very effective;
- "cerebral" types often have good results using biofeedback modalities.

Prevention Etiquette

Anyone who promises to cure your migraines is selling snake oil. We have no miracle cure or secret formula that works for everyone, so our goal is to make headaches infrequent and relatively painless, rather than a constant disabling focus of your life.

As you consider preventive treatment, keep in mind a few important points. First, no preventive works from Day One. It is important that patients give any preventive an adequate trial and a fair chance to provide lasting benefit. While some preventive strategies (such as massage, physical therapy, or meditation) may show benefit rather quickly, they must be incorporated into your lifestyle for a prolonged period in order to have a lasting benefit. Some of the prescription antiepileptic medications require a month or more to become effective, and many prescription medications and other substances like butterbur need about three months before benefit is evident. Also, *all* preventives, especially the medications but even the natural substances, have side effects that patients must consider.

Fortunately, not all side effects are bad. Like the surprise in the Cracker Jack box, some migraine preventives have beneficial side effects for certain patients, such as weight loss or gain. A medication with the side effect of sleepiness, for example, may be wonderful for someone with sleeping problems. So in the best circumstances, side effects will be beneficial. But in the worst, they can be dangerous or even disastrous, such as hair loss or numbness of the fingertips. Propranolol, for example, is one of the standard preventives frequently used to prevent migraines. It has been around for a long time, and we understand it pretty well. Propranolol might be great for a migraineur who has a rapid heartbeat, because it has the side effect of slowing the heart rate. However, it could be disastrous for an asthmatic migraineur because it can cause constriction of the airways in asthmatics. For this reason, doctors must *always* match the medication not just to the disease, but also to the patient, hoping to find a side-effect profile that is beneficial or at least fairly neutral.

I don't advocate a total reliance on preventive medications. The primary reason is that at present they are not 100 percent effective on their own. Second, because they need to get to the brain to work, and they modulate very complex neurochemical systems in ways we cannot entirely predict at present, they often have significantly bothersome side effects such as muddleheadedness, dizziness, increased appetite, and so forth. Most of these medications are also new and therefore pretty pricey, not covered by all insurance plans, and not well understood by some pharmacists. Still, medications remain an essential part of most prevention plans.

Prevention plans vary a great deal, as do their medication components. Some preventive medications are taken once, twice, or three times a day, depending on the medicine's particular characteristics, the patient's response to it, and other medications the patient is taking.

Rarely does a prevention plan become a static fixture in the life of a migraineur. We often prescribe a preventive medication for several months while the patient implements lifestyle changes to decrease her headaches or, in other circumstances, we will adjust preventives based on changes in the patient's lifestyle, headache pattern, or side-effect profile. To remain effective, prevention plans should be *actively* reassessed on a regular basis. As patients become pregnant, change jobs, acquire new tastes, enter menopause, change medications, or kick their children out of the house, their migraines will change. Prevention plans must be flexible and adaptive. You and your health care provider share the responsibility of reevaluating the plan every four to six months when things are going well and much more often when they are not.

It is useful to create reassessment time points, for example, intervals when a preventive medicine should kick in. Many patients are looking for a quick fix. And when your head is pounding, this is understandable. However, recent studies have shown that even the most common and effective preventive medicines may not reach their maximum effectiveness for *several months*. Of course, these are not absolute time points, but we humans find them comforting anyway and it is important and valuable to give a preventive therapy a good trial, so you know whether it is working. The other consideration when starting a new medication is side effects, as almost every medicine has some. The question is whether the side effects are worse than the condition you're treating. Often, side effects pass once the body becomes comfortable with the new medicine. In terms of headache etiquette at the Keeler Center, we ask that our patients:

- try a preventive for three months before deciding whether it is useful;
- try any medication for a week, if possible, before discontinuing it because of side effects.

Current Preventive Medicine Options

Nearly everyone has a sister, best friend, coworker, or Internet buddy who knows a guy who met a person whose brother had a friend who cured her migraines with a dab of this or a pound of that. In the science business, we call that anecdotal evidence, and it is considered the weakest form of support for a scientific statement. Unfortunately, patients who are not scientists often find it the most persuasive. Many fortunes have been made based entirely on anecdotal evidence that did not stand the light of day under scientific examination.

One product that is currently on the market does not even offer an explanation beyond "It works" when you rub it on your forehead. The substance is cool and soothing for a few moments, but that's only because it is nothing but scented alcohol. Still, it has sold millions. Most of these treatments are benign, and their only danger is to your wallet. But the reality is, we do not have a miracle treatment for migraines. If we did, all thirty million of us would know about it. Keep this in mind the next time someone tells you about anecdotal evidence from a friend of a friend of a friend.

Unfortunately, as I write this in 2008, we do not have great options for preventive medication. That is, we have no drugs that will reliably prevent migraines from occurring every time in every patient. It is best if doctors are up-front about this. Unrealistic expectations can't be met, and can undermine the very real good that preventives can do. Also, some of these medications work really well but have nasty side effects. Some are tolerated well but aren't very effective. Some are contraindicated with other common conditions (asthma, for example), and some can't be taken with certain other medications.

So when you evaluate preventive agents and strategies, remember, you are looking for *improvement*, sometimes dramatic improvement, but not cures. Also, virtually every medication that you put in your body— whether pharmaceutical or natural—will have a side-effect profile of some kind; you must balance these side effects with the benefits of the medication.

The science behind the various preventives is not overwhelming. Very recent work from the Harvard laboratories of Mike Moskowitz, M.D., Ph.D., has shown a direct effect on cortical spreading depression (CSD) with prolonged use of the FDA-approved preventives. We believe CSD is one of the very basic brain events that occurs when migraine begins. By raising the threshold for CSD, these preventives (which work by very different mechanisms) all have the end result of making the brain more resistant to the changes that lead to migraine.

Clinical studies (those done with patients, rather than in a laboratory) have shown benefit from all of the FDA-approved medications, as well as for butterbur and magnesium among the natural treatments, and mixed results for the others. Most work fairly well for about half the people who try them. But as we understand more about what these diverse agents have in common for the migraine brain, we can begin to home in on the essential properties they share, and begin to design drugs that are more specific and have fewer side effects.

A few years ago, before the class of antidepressants known as selective serotonin reuptake inhibitors (SSRIs) came out, the headache community was very excited that these might be effective preventives. By and large, this has not proven to be the case. While mixed evidence reports some of the SSRIs as being beneficial, many of them actually *worsen* headaches for some people. At the Keeler Center, we do use antidepressants, but primarily for coexisting headache and depression. We have had better success with the newer agents that increase brain levels of both serotonin and epinephrine (Effexor, Lexapro, Cymbalta). Remember, an older class of antidepressants, the heterocyclics (sometimes called tricyclics), remains a standard preventive for both migraine and tension-type headaches.

Selecting the right preventive can be tricky. At the present time, the FDA has approved only four medications for migraine prevention. Headache specialists actually use about twenty medications that are FDA-approved for other conditions but may also be helpful in preventing migraines. The list changes as we learn more about the mechanisms of migraines. Generally, in addition to a few natural agents listed later, we use five categories of medical preventives to treat migraines:

- **Neuromodulatory drugs:** valproic acid (Depakote, Depakene), topiramate (Topamax), pregabalin (Lyrica), levetiracetam (Keppra), lamotrigine (Lamictal)
- **Anti-inflammatory agents:** ketorolac (Toradol), indomethacin (Indocin), naproxen (Naprosyn, Aleve), ibuprofen (Motrin)
- **Vascular agents:** calcium channel blockers (diltiazem), beta-blockers (Inderal, Timolol) angiotensin-converting enzyme agents (Captopril, Lisinopril)
- **Antidepressants:** amitriptyline (Elavil), nortriptyline (Pamelor, Aventyl), protriptyline (Vivactil), duloxetine (Cymbalta), escitalopram (Lexapro), bupropion (Wellbutrin)
- **Serotonin/dopamine receptor antagonists:** olanzapine (Zyprexa), risperidone (Risperdal), quetiapine (Seroquel)

Side effects vary with each medication, and most patients do not experience any given side effect. Those that have been reported or that have been found during clinical trials are available on the Internet, from your physician, and from your pharmacy. I do not list them here for several reasons: first, it would take many, many pages to report all the side effects of these medicines, and second, I have found that people tend to focus on potential side effects (which are quite rare) to the exclusion of the benefits, which are not rare at all. The key is to notice if something doesn't feel right while taking a new medication.

For example, in some people on valproic acid, there is an increase in appetite and their hair becomes brittle. You won't wake up fat and bald the next morning, but over time, you may notice these things. If you do, it may be the medication and you should change it. Valproic acid can also be hard on the liver, so you should get periodic blood tests to make sure your liver function is okay. Finally, this medicine can be very dangerous if taken when you are pregnant and should not be used if pregnancy is a possibility.

Neuromodulatory Drugs

Sometimes called psychoactive medications, neuromodulatory drugs work directly on the way nerve cells in the brain fire, communicate, or regulate themselves. The neuromodulatory drug options that are FDA-approved for migraines include the so-called antiseizure medicines, valproic acid and topiramate, as well as pregabalin, memantine, gabapentin, levetiracetam, and several others that are FDA-approved for other conditions and are frequently given to migraine sufferers. As a class, these medications are probably the most widely utilized by headache specialists.

These medications seem to have the widest spectrum of effectiveness at present, and we feel that the benefits far outweigh the potential risks. This is a judgment every patient must make based on the information available, and if the fit is not right, alternative medications or approaches need to be considered.

Anti-inflammatories

Anti-inflammatories are an alternative in prevention as well as in rescue. Naproxen is one of the more common COX-1 inhibitors, and celecoxib is the most common COX-2 inhibitor. The COX-1 and COX-2 pathways are the primary ways in which our bodies mount an inflammatory response. By blocking one or the other, we can reduce this response and the pain that can follow. Indomethacin is the most potent nonsteroidal anti-inflammatory drug (NSAID), and we use it to prevent hemicrania continua and other less common headache types. It is a potent medication and can upset the stomach and thin the blood. Prednisone is a true steroid and also a very potent anti-inflammatory that we use to treat temporal arteritis and sometimes to break a particularly nasty migraine. When used often or regularly, steroids can have a host of potential side effects, including weakened bones, weakened immune system, cataracts, behavioral problems, and GI problems. Care must be taken with these medications. Anti-inflammatories can also be prescribed in pulse prevention of periodic headaches, often in conjunction with a long-acting triptan. The role of inflammation and other immune processes in headache is a hot area for research and, while the exact relationship is still not clear, anti-inflammatories seem to have a prominent role for migraine as well as several other primary headache types.

Vascular Agents

Vascular agents include beta-blockers (propranolol and timolol—the only FDA-approved vascular agents), calcium channel blockers (such as diltiazem), and ACE inhibitors (for example captopril) or modifiers (such as candesartan). The exact mechanism by which these medications work is not completely understood. Interestingly, a recent study showed that all FDA-approved preventives, regardless of purported mechanism of action, result in a decrease in cortical spreading depression in a rat model. This suggests there are several ways to create the same result in the brain. With respect to the vascular agents, it is presumed that by modulating the blood vessels' response to vasoactive agents such as calcitonin gene-related peptide (CGRP), substance P, and neurokinin A, these medications can reduce the throbbing response of the vessels—and their attendant pain. The vasoactive agents are part of a cascade of events involved in migraine and other kinds of pain. Released at nerve endings, they have a wide variety of actions. Scientists are very interested in blocking these agents from reaching their target receptor, or blocking those receptors, in order to prevent the pain process from continuing. In fact, it is likely that a CGRP blocking agent will be approved by the FDA as a migraine rescue medication in the near future.

Antidepressants

Amitriptyline (Elavil), nortriptyline (Pamelor, Aventyl), protriptyline (Vivactyl), duloxetine (Cymbalta), escitalopram (Lexapro), and bupropion (Wellbutrin) are in a class of medications that has been around for more than forty years, with new agents added all the time. Amitriptyline, one of the oldest, is often used as a headache preventive both for migraine and tension-type headaches. It is particularly useful when patients also have problems sleeping, as one of the main side effects is drowsiness. It is not recommended for use in the elderly, and can cause weight gain. At the other end of the spectrum is duloxetine, one of the newest antidepressants. It has been shown to have pain-modulating activity in addition to its antidepressant action. When antidepressants are used for headache prevention, the dosing is sometimes different than when they are prescribed for depression and, for this reason, it is important to discuss these medications with your headache doctor *and* your psychiatrist if you have concurrent depression.

Serotonin/Dopamine Receptor Antagonists

Olanzapine (Zyprexa), risperidone (Risperdal), and quetiapine (Seroquel), originally developed for use in schizophrenia and other psychiatric conditions, are powerful modulators of the dopamine system in the brain. Fortunately for headache sufferers, drugs don't know why they were developed or what they are supposed to treat. Because much of the pain pathway, and the associated nausea and vomiting, are mediated by dopamine, these agents have proven very useful for some patients. The hardest part usually involves reassuring these patients that we are not giving these medicines because we think they are crazy. Still, these are potent medications and can have significant side effects, including weight gain, diabetes, and sleepiness. These are not first-line preventives, but in the right patient, they can make a huge difference.

Other Preventive Medications

Because the menu of preventive medications changes often, it helps if you have tools to figure out if the medication your doctor suggests is right for you. Here are some questions to ask about any medication your doctor proposes:

1. What are the *most common* side effects of this medication? (The lists that you get from the pharmacist, in *Physicians' Desk Reference* [PDR], or online are written not by doctors, but by lawyers. For example, very few medicines in *PDR* don't list headache as a possible side effect.) Be sure to get the doctor's assurance that if you notice an odd symptom you can reach someone to run it by.
2. What is the dose range (the lowest and highest dose) for this medicine, and what are the signs of overdose or withdrawal?
3. What are the consequences of running out of this medicine, missing a dose, or doubling up by accident? And if you do forget a dose or double up, what should you do?
4. How often should you take this medicine? Should you take it on a full stomach or an empty stomach?
5. Does this medication interact with any other medications you are taking?
6. Inquire about any other specific areas that concern you. For example, if weight gain or loss is an issue, ask. Do the same if

mental clarity, sleep disturbance, hair loss, stomach upset, blurry vision, or dizziness is a problem for you.

But don't bother asking what the medicine is actually approved for. If you really must know, try not to put any stock in the information. Drug companies seek approval for an indication (a specific use for the drug) based upon where they are most likely to recover their development costs for a profit and where they can most easily and least expensively bring the drug to market. They know, as do most doctors, that once a medicine is FDA-approved, it will likely be used for any number of off-label purposes.

Hormonal Intervention

While some women's hormonal migraines respond to shorter, cyclical courses of preventive medication, this isn't true for everyone. We tend to introduce hormonal therapy when there is a clear association between menses or menopause and headache. For many women, fluctuations in estrogen levels strongly prime the migraine pump. By modulating these fluctuations with an estrogen supplement, we can minimize estrogen as a trigger. The most common approach is to supplement in such a way as to minimize fluctuation by avoiding the placebo period, which allows for menstruation. Current evidence suggests that there is no need for this break and that continuous estrogen replacement in appropriately selected patients is not harmful. Birth control pills, with their lower dosing, tend not to fully suppress the body's own estrogen production while the higher doses used for postmenopausal hormone replacement fully suppress estrogen production and may be more effective as a headache preventive. The downside, of course, is the concern over increased risk of stroke and ovarian cancer in susceptible patients. For this reason, women should discuss the issue of hormonal intervention with their doctors before making any decision.

Natural Preventive Agents

It has taken a long time, but Western medicine is finally waking up to the fact that it is not the only game in town. Some medicines out there do not require a prescription but actually work. In my opinion, the distinction between natural and pharmaceutical has more to do with marketing than with medicine. If you've ever seen a child in the emergency room after sampling the local plant life, or a cancer survivor jogging with her grandkids twenty years after chemotherapy, you know it is not simply a matter of natural = good and pharmaceutical = bad. You have to know as much as you possibly can about what you are dealing with.

In my practice, I take all the help I can get. Do the natural remedies work? For some patients, yes. Do the prescription drugs work? For some patients, yes. I have patients who go wholly holistic and other patients who want nothing but pharmaceutical grade. But the majority of my patients pick and choose among all the options, and together we come up with combinations that suit their needs.

While lavender and other topicals applied to the forehead are common natural preventives, there are presently only five natural substances available without a prescription that have been shown in rigorous scientific studies to be of benefit in headache prevention for headache sufferers. These are:

- feverfew
- butterbur
- vitamin B_2
- coenzyme Q10
- magnesium

Of the many, many products available over the counter for both headache rescue and prevention, only these five natural agents have undergone scientific testing comparable to the rigorous evaluation performed on prescription drugs. (Note that we are talking about prevention here;

no natural agents have been proven effective for rescue once a headache has begun.)

Feverfew

Feverfew and butterbur are often mentioned together for migraine prevention, but they are not related. Feverfew is a flower that has been purported to have fever-reducing properties. Its active ingredient, parthenolide, is a vasodilator (dilates arteries) and this is the mechanism that supporters maintain helps migraines. Unfortunately, many careful studies have shown this to be only marginally effective.

Most literature suggests that a strength of 3 to 5 percent is ideal, and it is probably most effective when used in conjunction with other natural preventives. Keep in mind that this herb has some blood-thinning properties and should be used with caution when taking other blood-thinning medications such as coumadin, aspirin, or anti-inflammatories.

Several commercially available preparations combine feverfew with butterbur in one capsule. The key to using these preparations is to remember that you need to give them at least three to six months before deciding whether the medicine is working. Some people see improvement more quickly, but as a rule herbs take a long time to effect change. Both are usually well tolerated, and side effects are minimal.

Butterbur

Butterbur (*Petastides hybridus*) is an herb that has been used as a folk remedy for centuries to treat headaches, allergies, and other ailments. The scientific literature supporting the use of butterbur is much stronger than that for feverfew. However, in 2004 a placebo-controlled study looked at two doses of butterbur as a preventive for headaches. In this study, 75 mg taken twice daily reduced headache frequency for half the patients in the study. The lower dose (50 mg twice daily) was no better than the placebo.

As with many "natural" treatments, it takes a bit longer to see results than with prescription medicine, often several months. Butterbur is usually well tolerated, with minimal side effects, but it is important to keep in mind that the herb in its raw form has some nasty toxins in it, which are removed during the processing of the product. Thus, home-brewed butterbur extract may not be the way to go. There are several products on the market that contain butterbur either alone or in combination with other nonprescription preventives. Several preparations combine butterbur with feverfew.

Riboflavin (Vitamin B$_2$)

Riboflavin (vitamin B$_2$) is essential for normal energy metabolism in the brain and elsewhere in the body. The scientific data suggest a major role for riboflavin in energy metabolism at the cellular level, and this is believed to be its role in migraine prevention. This vitamin is normally part of a daily diet. This is a good thing, since the body does not store riboflavin. The richest dietary sources include milk, yeast, cheese, oily fish, eggs, and dark green leafy vegetables. Other good sources include organ meats (liver, kidney, and heart) and certain plants such as almonds, mushrooms, soybeans, and whole grains. Also, flour and cereals are often enriched with riboflavin.

Riboflavin has been evaluated in both high doses (400 mg/day) and low doses (25 mg/day) for headache prevention. Unfortunately, it has not been studied in a controlled, blinded way that would yield definite results. However, one study, which compared low-dose riboflavin with a higher dose combined with magnesium and feverfew, found that the low dose was just as effective as the high dose served up in combination with other natural preventives. These kinds of studies are hard to interpret, but given the apparent "harmless" nature of B$_2$, and the potential benefit, this is a supplement that is often included in the nonprescription cocktails for headache prevention.

Coenzyme Q10

In the last five years, amid increasing interest in nonpharmacologic supplements for headache prevention, coenzyme Q10 (CoQ10) has been studied in controlled trials and has been found to be effective as a preventive. For example, a Swiss group looked at CoQ10 as a possible preventive treatment for migraines. While the study was small (fewer than thirty-five patients), researchers completed a double-blind, placebo-controlled assessment in which about one in three patients experienced a 50 percent reduction in the frequency of headaches over a three-month period. Though not a dramatic response, it is certainly statistically significant. The study needs to be repeated with a much larger group, of course, but given how well this medicine is tolerated, it is a reasonable part of a preventive program for many people who want non-prescription approaches to managing their headaches.

A molecule that is essential to mitochondrial metabolism, CoQ10 is found naturally in a variety of foods. The mitochondria have been heavily implicated in the pathophysiology (the disease condition) of migraine and many other neurological problems. One advantage of CoQ10 is that it has a very gentle side-effect profile including minor difficulty sleeping, mild irritability, and GI upset. It should also be used cautiously in people who are taking blood thinners. At the recommended dose of 150 mg/d of the gelcap form, it takes about three months of use before there is a demonstrable reduction in headache frequency.

Magnesium

An element that has significant benefit for many migraineurs is also a complicated one. More than ten years ago, the benefits of magnesium, for both prevention and rescue, were studied by two groups in New York. One gram of magnesium given intravenously in the emergency room offered a majority of migraineurs more than 50 percent relief. Four hundred milligrams daily showed a reduction in headache frequency after three months. But not all magnesium formulations are the same. Magnesium is not available in a "pure" form, but must be combined, and should be taken as magnesium gluconate, citrate, or a similar compound. Further, it should not be taken in combination with calcium compounds. Too much magnesium can cause problematic diarrhea, and too little can cause insomnia and even cardiac problems. Several small studies have suggested that 300 to 400 mg a day can be of benefit. But to further complicate this picture, the standard blood tests for magnesium reflect *total* magnesium, not the *free* magnesium that is available to the brain. A special blood test, looking for ionized magnesium, is necessary to determine whether you are actually magnesium deficient, for purposes of migraine treatment. Still, magnesium is generally a safe and effective medication—*when* an experienced headache specialist prescribes it. Some products on the market combine various over-the-counter preventives, such as butterbur, feverfew, vitamin B_2, and magnesium. While I think this is a reasonable approach, use caution when you purchase such products, since the guidelines for nutraceuticals are not nearly as rigorous as those imposed on prescription medicines.

A Word About Supplements

Patients often ask a broader question regarding whether a good-quality general vitamin or broad supplement will help headache sufferers. As far as I know, no studies have concluded that general supplements help in migraine prevention, but I think common sense suggests that promoting general good health could only be a good thing for headache sufferers, as for anyone else. Several recent studies, for example, have shown that being overweight or obese contributes to migraine headaches but not to nonmigraine headaches. Does this mean that only migraineurs need worry about their weight? Of course not. Keep in mind, however, that sporadic use of supplements, diets, and weight-loss programs may prove to be a problem for migraineurs, who should always aim to maintain routines and avoid sporadic modifications in activity levels.

Other Modalities

Several other modalities are also considered preventive, and medicine is not always the best way to treat medical conditions, particularly when the medical condition is a chronic disorder as opposed to an acute condition. Chronic conditions represent an ongoing problem in the normal functioning of an incredibly complex system—our bodies. Our bodies seek to maintain equilibrium, so when we throw something new into the mix the body responds with hundreds of thousands of complex chemical actions. Unfortunately, most of our drugs are a little too coarse to target the specific, subtle balance disturbances that cause the condition. As a result, medications often have effects beyond the one intended—side effects.

For this reason, a good prevention plan does not rely solely on medication, but also incorporates other modalities that have an effect that is easier on the body. At the same time, such strategies likely have longer-acting roles in treatment than we might expect from a single dose of medication. So the best treatment plans utilize all the tools in the toolbox—medication as well as physical medicine and spiritual and cognitive therapies.

Traditional Modalities

"Traditional modalities" refers to those approaches that most Western doctors (and insurers) recognize as appropriate treatments for illness. Personally, I find such distinctions artificial, divisive, and misleading. For example, the traditions of classical Chinese medicine predate even the antecedents of Western medicine by thousands of years. So who's to say what is traditional and what is alternative? Still, for purposes of organization and reference, if nothing else, it is useful to distinguish between the services that are routinely available through your doctor's office and those that are not.

HEALTH MAINTENANCE This catchall phrase gets bandied about a lot in health care circles and the popular press. The concept is quite simple: it means taking care of yourself and not doing stupid things to your body. Of course, this is easier said than done. In addition to the migraineur's responsibility to be self-aware, vigilant, and mindful of the things that can make headaches worse, health maintenance also simply means living a healthy life. Most headache sufferers report that their headaches get worse when they have the flu or some other chronic illness, but other, more subtle health issues, such as thyroid problems, vision problems, or chronic stress can also exacerbate headaches. Regular checkups with your primary care physician are important for this reason, if not others.

PHYSICAL MEDICINE "Physical medicine" refers to a collection of modalities, the best known and best established of which is physical therapy. But just as Western medicine is not the only kind of medicine, neither is physical therapy the only kind of physical medicine. At the Keeler Center, we frequently use physical therapy, to be sure, but we also rely heavily on alternative physical-medicine techniques such as craniosacral work, massage, yoga, and other hands-on treatments. We find that treating the whole body and, particularly, the head, neck and spine, has a dramatic impact on headaches in appropriately selected patients.

NUTRITIONAL COUNSELING What can I say? Garbage in, garbage out. While the food-trigger thing gets blown out of proportion, it is clear that diet strongly influences headache frequency and severity for most patients, and some gradually emerging principles appear to apply to all headache sufferers. Recent studies in our own laboratories, funded through an NIH grant, have indicated that certain fatty acids may promote headaches, while others may be protective. Other studies have found significant impact from magnesium levels, and less rigorous data have suggested roles for sugar and carbohydrates, protein, and even specific amino acids. While we don't have a specific migraine diet, several principles clearly do apply with regard to meal timing, overall diet composition, hydration, and so forth. When necessary, nutritional counseling can help address patient-specific questions.

Nutritional counseling can also help when someone is clueless about triggers but senses that food may be a problem. Strategies called elimination diets can help identify target foods. Rarely, to help guide a personal quest for the guilty foods, I will actually give patients some of the "potential food trigger lists" that have been generated over the years. But I always try to avoid blind rejection of foods without good evidence that they represent specific and personal triggers. In my case, I genuinely believe that the higher power felt bad about giving me migraines and therefore created chocolate without making it a trigger for me. I am grateful.

Keep in mind that nutritional counseling need not be limited to the specific foods we eat or avoid, but might also help with the timing of meals, portions, and the ratios of food groups to one another.

STRESS MANAGEMENT AND COUNSELING It can get pretty depressing running around with a headache all the time. In fact, depression is much more common among migraineurs than among the general population, as are many other medical conditions. Moreover, stress is probably the most common trigger for migraines. As smart as migraineurs are as a group, there are almost always things we can do to better manage our stress. A trained counselor, particularly one skilled in working with headache or chronic pain patients, can often provide insights and tips that significantly improve treatment outcomes.

Also, epidemiological studies show that migraines are more common among people who are depressed than among those who are not and that depression (as well as several other psychiatric conditions such as bipolar disease and obsessive-compulsive disorder) is more common among migraineurs. It would be wrong to assume that depression in a migraineur will automatically resolve when the headaches are under control. It might, but then again, it might not. It is best to address depression or any other mood disorder simultaneously with the headache.

Other Alternative Therapies

Western scientists have made major contributions to the field of migraine research, particularly in the last fifteen years or so. However, historical accounts of headache date back nearly five thousand years, and migraine is *still* a worldwide problem, as much in Asia as in America. Interestingly, the more we learn about the pathophysiology of the condition, the more likely it becomes that some "folk" remedies or "complementary" treatments have a sound basis. Moreover, the distinction between various therapies, particularly with respect to medicines, is largely political and artificial. When we put something into our bodies, whether it is fresh off the vine or synthesized in the laboratory, it is still a foreign substance and there will be consequences—some good, some bad. At the Keeler Center, we have seen positive responses to alternative therapies when none of the Western approaches have been satisfactory. Of course, the converse has been true, as well. Our best results come from a combination of the two.

YOGA   Many migraineurs do very well with yoga, particularly restorative yoga, which is what we use at the Keeler Center. Restorative yoga is nonjarring to the head, and the bodywork tends to be stretching as much as strengthening, which is good for people with lots of muscle tension. As a result, restorative yoga is better tolerated than some other modalities. Yoga also strongly emphasizes breathing techniques, which can be very helpful for headache sufferers. Since some migraineurs have problems with certain positions (such as inversions), it is good to work with a yoga instructor rather than exclusively from videotapes or group classes.

At the Keeler Center, we have weekly yoga classes and a yoga instructor on staff. While I can't think of a particular patient who credits yoga with a cure, neither can I think of a patient who has participated in our yoga program who does not feel that it contributed significantly to improvement.

ACUPUNCTURE   Acupuncture has many applications in pain management but in our experience at the Keeler Center it has not been as effective in migraines as some other modalities. One of the problems is that often you don't have a headache when you happen to have your acupuncture appointment, so it is difficult for the acupuncturist to know whether a given attempt has any effect. Several recent blinded, controlled studies looking at acupuncture and headaches have shown mixed results. Nonetheless, acupuncture is still a tool that should be available as an option.

At the Keeler Center, we use acupressure as a self-help technique. By applying steady pressure to the anatomic snuff box at the base of the thumb, then to the neck at the base of the skull, then the temple, many patients can often relieve a headache. This is a technique that must be demonstrated but it should be accessible through any traditional Chinese healer. An experienced practitioner can demonstrate the proper technique and you can find these points in books, such as *Acupressure Atlas* by Bernard C. Kolster, Astrid Waskowiak, and Nikolas Win Myint.

BIOFEEDBACK TRAINING Biofeedback is being used with good effect in selected patients. While definitive studies have not compared this technique with pharmacologic or other treatments, it certainly makes sense that biofeedback training would benefit certain headache sufferers.

There are several types of biofeedback training. The most common kind measures muscle tension, displaying—visually or aurally—the amount of electrical activity in the muscle so patients can become aware of the tension in their muscles and learn to relax them. Several quality studies have shown benefit from muscle biofeedback, particularly in helping prevent tension-related headaches.

Biofeedback can also measure minute changes in body temperature, skin surface moisture, and cardiac and brain wave activity. Using this technology, the therapist records objective information about the patient's physical responses to minor emotional or intellectual stressors, and displays this information for the patient. Patients can then learn relaxation techniques to minimize their physical responses to emotional stress.

Managing Your Treatment Plan

I spend a lot of time in Sedona, Arizona, a very mystical and spiritually charged place. While I was there, a young woman came to me for a second opinion. One of her advisers, an expert in the Chinese art of feng shui, had told her that to improve her headaches she would have to sell her home and move to another location, better situated among the various masculine and feminine vortices for which Sedona is famous. After taking her history myself, and visiting the allegedly ill-situated home, I concluded that she would be more likely to benefit headache-wise from a dramatic reduction in the number of pills she was taking on a daily basis. Her headaches did improve—significantly—and she was able to stay in her home.

In Ojai, we had a very complicated patient whose work required long, intense hours over a computer. His health was further complicated by bipolar illness, which could swing him from incredible highs to abysmal lows, often within twenty-four hours. Every medicine that helped one aspect of his health would throw others into chaos. When he worked with our craniosacral therapist, he began to settle for the first time in his life and, while he still wrestles with these twin demons, his overall quality of life is worlds better.

I consult with naturopathic doctors, herbalists, and other practitioners of complementary disciplines to arrive at the right treatment plan. This is one of the greatest advantages for patients in working with a knowledgeable headache specialist. Often, looking at an individual's lifestyle, other medical conditions, general health, diet, and more, we can predict which preventive regimens are likely to be of the most benefit and spare some of the trial-and-error routine that migraineurs can endure. Still, many of my patients have to try a few different preventives before they get satisfactory results.

Then patients frequently ask, "Will I need to take this medication or maintain this regimen forever?" Well, no. Some people do remain on preventives for many years. Others find that after six months or so their headaches have "cooled off" to the point that they can revisit management with rescue medications and lifestyle modification only. Still others find that over time one plan morphs into another, either because of decreasing effectiveness, changes in lifestyle, or the emergence of new options.

Unfortunately, only some of the triggers for migraines are under your control or within your sphere of influence. This means that for most of us, despite our best efforts, headaches will continue to happen. After all, we are still migraineurs.

Chapter 6

Your Rescue Plan—
When Disaster Strikes

I have a ninety-year-old patient, Bess, who has had headaches since she was thirteen. In the last fifteen years or so, her headaches have become a rare and minor annoyance for her, but when she was a girl in the 1930s, her doctor's advice was to "just leave her be until she comes out on her own." Her parents would set food and water inside the room but would not speak to her until she came out and apologized for her behavior. Sometimes she would stay in there for three days.

At first glance, this may seem cruel, uninformed, the product of ignorance. Actually, she remembers these episodes as what she called "unintended mercies," a most humane treatment. She was able to draw the curtains, avoid interactions, sibling noise, and kitchen smells, and retreat to the best respite available at the time. Rescue medications didn't exist, and the concept of trigger avoidance did not come until forty years later. Her doctor had the good sense to facilitate withdrawal from the hostile environment.

When I was a child (considerably more recently than the 1930s), I was once punished for making my mom pick me up at school after I threw up. Actually, I felt better after throwing up and wanted to go back to class, but my mom had already left work to pick me up from school, so we went off to the doctor, who confirmed that there was "nothing wrong with me." I remember a college girlfriend accusing me of using my headaches to get out of social functions. (Okay, this last may actually have held a grain of truth, but just a *grain*.) The fact is, no migraine sufferer would use a headache to get out of something; fear of divine retribution or bad karma would prohibit it. In twenty-plus years of headache care, I have never seen it happen.

When I was growing up with migraines, the medical community and the public at large knew so little about headaches that those of us who suffered them half believed the conventional wisdom of the time: that headaches were psychological, psychosomatic, or, at best, emotional. Too many people (including some doctors) still believe this, despite overwhelming scientific evidence that the opposite is true.

In my lifetime, we have come a long way in understanding and caring for headaches and, today, we have many more tools in our bag to treat an acute migraine attack. Still, not every tool works for every headache sufferer and, sometimes, peace and quiet—and a good night's sleep—are the best treatment we have. So things aren't all that different now than they were when Bess was a child suffering from migraines. In some ways, the treatment has not changed much from the old "Go to bed and call me in the morning." But we can do better than that.

We need to. Because even with excellent care, a brilliant treatment plan, and radical lifestyle modifications, sooner or later, every migraineur will get another headache. It is what makes us migraineurs. Too often, we see migraines as the enemy. Some books even describe migraine management as a war. That's a pretty intense approach. Migraines just *are*. When they happen, they're just something to get through. They aren't cancer, they aren't a psychotic break, and they aren't who we are.

Further, getting a headache does not mean your prevention plan failed. We still do not have a cure, and we cannot completely control our internal or external environments, so lifestyle changes and prevention plans are not usually enough to eliminate *all* of our headaches. No matter how careful we are, headaches break through now and then. The goal is to have fewer, shorter, less severe headaches. This might mean that you get one headache every few weeks instead of every week, or two times a week instead of every morning. It doesn't help to feel discouraged or frustrated when that infrequent headache shows up, despite fighting the good fight. And it does not mean the plan isn't working; it just means that you have a headache. And it means that *every migraineur needs a good rescue plan*, one with several layers.

Migraine Rescue

"Rescue" refers to any treatment aimed at breaking up a headache that has already started in any degree. For most people, medications work quickly, are well tolerated, and are the most effective, so they are the standard rescue strategy in the United States. But we do have nonpharmacologic treatments that will support your healing, whether you take medications or cannot tolerate them, or choose not to take them. Any of these strategies can help minimize your pain, and might include:

- environmental changes
- meditation, sleep, relaxation exercises, and biofeedback
- physical medicine techniques (physical therapy, massage, and yoga)

We don't have a one-size-fits-all fix for migraine rescue. *Each patient's first-line rescue should be the most effective remedy for that individual, both short-term and long.* In other words, the selected rescue medication needs to relieve the immediate pain without putting the patient at risk for dangerous side effects or more headaches down the road. Usually, that is a medication. While some patients will get relief from over-the-counter medications, first-line rescue medications will usually be in the class of drugs known as triptans, "designer" prescription drugs whose only indication is to stop a migraine before it really gets going. And we have many other rescue medications, including anti-inflammatories, antihistamines, and dopamine antagonists.

Abortive Medicines

"Abortive" medications interrupt or stop a headache that is already present. They are most effective when taken early in the headache, the earlier the better. Some of them are available over the counter, but the more potent and effective usually require a prescription. We have many options; the choice of abortive agents depends on a number of factors, particularly the frequency, severity, and duration of your headaches and also the other medications you take, finances, and a few other variables.

Popular nonprescription headache remedies include the combination of aspirin, acetaminophen, and caffeine, an excellent treatment for migraines that are relatively mild and infrequent. But these compounds have a tremendous potential for overuse that results in medication overuse headache (MOH). It doesn't say so on the label, but daily or near-daily use of this medication will make the medication less effective and *ultimately result in escalating headaches.*

While triptans are the current gold standard for migraine rescue, not every migraineur needs to be on triptans, which are expensive and can have some potentially nasty drug interactions. Moreover, not all triptans are equal. Some triptans take effect in as little as fifteen minutes, while others take up to an hour or longer. Some remain in the body four times longer than others. To make matters more complicated, depending on the deal your insurance company cuts with the manufacturer, some triptans will have lower co-pays than others, and some rescue medicines are not FDA-approved for migraines, so your insurer might not cover them at all.

Very recent information is out about a new rescue medication, a CGRP antagonist, which works very differently from the triptans. It *is* very different from the triptans. By the time this book is published, the medication will likely be on the market, radically improving our options for treating migraine. And there are other medications in the wings as well. As a result, what we know about migraine and how to treat it is constantly evolving.

Medication Plans Are Complicated Because of MOH

As we've expanded our arsenal of treatments, we've added risks and potential for complication. While medication side effects and drug-drug interactions could be anticipated, the use of rescue medications brought with it an unexpected consequence, one that has caused more problems than all the side effects combined: MOH, previously known as rebound headache. We don't know exactly why this happens, but it appears to be the result of a sensitization process in the brain whereby the very act of taking a rescue medication ramps up the pain pathways. It is also possible that MOH is actually a direct response to too-frequent an exposure to a particular medicine, making the brain less sensitive to its effect. This is an active area of research in migraine.

By definition, MOH is usually a daily headache resulting from the overuse of rescue medications. This is not to say that all chronic daily headaches are the result of medication overuse, but the majority of them certainly are. If you used to have episodic migraines, now have daily headaches, *and* are using rescue medicines on a daily or near-daily basis, there is little doubt that you are a member of the club. MOH can be recognized as a headache that is different from the underlying primary headache (usually a migraine). Typically, MOH is present upon awakening, and is a more global, constant headache that is resistant to the usual rescue medicines.

My patients in their eighties and nineties do not recall MOH ever being a problem, and I have not found any historical record of it before the latter part of the twentieth century. How can this be? The answer is simple: MOH is a product of modern technology—much like smog, radiation sickness, and reality television—and equally annoying. For many migraine sufferers, an awareness of MOH can be the difference between chronic daily headaches and occasional, easily treatable headaches.

Rescue medications are *not* meant to be used on a daily basis, but often nobody tells us this until it is way too late.

Most headache specialists feel that:

- *any* rescue medicine can lead to rebound headaches if used too frequently;
- some rescue medicines are clearly more likely to cause MOH than others;
- some rescue medicines are much harder to back off and cause "worse" MOH than others.

The risk of developing MOH is so great that we strictly limit each rescue medication to its rebound potential. For example, butalbital-containing compounds (such as Fioricet and Esgic) should be used only one day a week, and triptans limited to three days a week.

A first-line strategy for rescue is good, but not good enough. Unfortunately, the harsh reality is that until we change our lifestyles, identify our triggers, and find effective preventives, we may well be confronted with more frequent headaches. Consider:

- What if a patient has more headache days in a week than he has rescue medications?
- What if a patient maxes out on a medication's daily dose limit and still has a headache?
- What if a patient cannot take another dose for six hours but their headache is screaming again after just three hours?

Each patient, with their headache caregiver, needs to anticipate these and many other scenarios to create strategies *ahead of time* because, I promise you, making decisions about such complex issues when your head is pounding is difficult, to say the least.

You should take two or even three different *classes* of rescue medications, using each on a limited basis, no more than two days per week; rotating rescue medications in hopes of avoiding MOH is a temporary solution until the other elements of the treatment plan are working effectively. When you rotate, each rescue agent should work by a *mechanism different* from that of your primary rescue medication. For example, if a triptan is your primary rescue agent, something like tramadol or isometheptene might be your backup. At least in theory, this system should help prevent rebound headaches from overuse of a single rescue medication.

Your doctor can help you determine which medicines are in the same class, but here are some broad examples:

- Triptans: Imitrex, Maxalt, Frova, Zomig, Amerge, Relpax, Axert
- COX-1 inhibitors: Naprosyn, Aleve, Motrin, Dolobid, Toradol
- Muscle relaxants: Soma, Flexeril, Skelaxin, Baclofen
- Combination drugs: Treximet, Fioricet, Norgesic Forte

Honestly, no one knows yet whether taking three different kinds of rescue medicines two days each per week will avoid medication overuse headache. Some very smart headache specialists think it will. Others disagree. But we do know that taking *the same* rescue medication more than two days per week (in the case of triptans, more than three days a week) *will* result in more and more frequent headaches and MOH. The long-term solution is that you *must* pay more attention to preventive medication, lifestyle modification, and trigger identification to reduce your headache frequency below that two-day-per-week threshold.

Recent scientific literature has begun to link neuropeptides that regulate biorhythms to headaches. The most frequently discussed include orexin, grehlin, and adiponectin. There is mounting evidence that migraines are part of a much larger syndrome of biorhythmic dysregulation and that the orexins (produced primarily in the hypothalamus but with receptors all over the body) modulate a final common pathway of pain perception in the brain *regardless* of the mechanism of action of the rescue medicine. This is bad news. If it turns out to be true (and I suspect it will), it means that once a brain is amped up, *any* rescue medication will cause MOH, singly or in combination.

Timing Is Everything

For the majority of migraine sufferers, headaches are episodic, occurring fewer than three days per week and often only once or twice a month. For these patients, the most important factor in stopping a headache is early recognition and treatment. *The earlier you treat a headache, the more likely the treatment will work.* As soon as you think you are about to get a headache, you need to know what you are going to do about it—*and do it.* This first strike should be an automatic reflex act when you feel that first twinge. But the typical migraineur doesn't do this, for various reasons:

- **Denial.** "I can't believe I am going to get a headache today." For most of us, the prospect of losing another day to a migraine is so horrible, we just don't want to go there and, sometimes, we see taking the medication as acknowledgment of the wolf at the door.

- **Muddleheadedness.** Excellent studies show that as a migraine develops, our judgment becomes poor, our coordination fails, and our attention flags. As a result, we make poor decisions—and not just about whether to take medication or not. Studies of workers who "power through" their headaches demonstrate that efficiency is reduced by as much as 70 percent.

- **Cephalalgiaphobia.** One of my favorite words, this means "fear of headache." Plus, some of our rescue strategies include medications with nasty side effects or behaviors with unpleasant consequences (like telling the boss again that you need to go take a nap in the conference room). The consequence of cephalalgiaphobia is that we delay treatment because we are afraid of the headache (denial) and the side effects of the medication that has been prescribed.

- **Type A behavior.** It is more than a myth that the type A personality is overrepresented among migraineurs. One particularly troubling characteristic of this personality type is delayed gratification (or in this case, delayed self-care). We have a tendency to put off treatment until we are done doing whatever it is we are doing. Part of this poor decision making is the fear that if we stop to take care of our headache, we will not get done what we "need" to get done. Another factor is that when a migraine is building, we do not think clearly, make good decisions, or execute plans very well. A third element has to do with refusing to give in to something over which we seemingly have little control.

- **Rationing.** Knowing they are not supposed to use any rescue meds more than two days a week, but in the beginning stages of another headache, patients who don't have a backup plan won't take anything. As the hours go by, these headaches build, unabated, to misery. In desperation and with a migraine-addled brain, the patients eventually do something that is not part of the plan.

The best (and only) reasonable approach to managing an acute headache is to *take your best shot as soon as the notion of a headache enters your head.* I repeat: Take your best shot ASAP. If a triptan is the most effective medicine for your migraines, then take it and take it early. This works fine if you are having two or fewer headaches per week. But if you have more frequent headaches, you cannot take a triptan every time. Often, your physician will give you other rescue options for those times when a triptan is not an option. Which rescue to use when depends on the patient. Some patients find that a strict rotation is most effective. Determining when to use which medication can be the result of trial and error or of careful analysis with your headache specialist. We do not have a one-size-fits-all solution. In general, it is best to take your best medicine first; for migraineurs, this is usually a triptan. But over time, some patients find that a particular presentation of headache (such as a sore neck) may lend itself better to another rescue.

Too often, we try to play with our headaches by using cheaper, "safer," or better-tolerated medications first and saving our "big gun" for later, just in case the headache turns into a monster. Study after study has shown that this is a bad strategy. The most effective antimigraine medications, the triptans, are most effective when you take them early; many headache specialists (myself included) argue that they actually become ineffective once you are a few hours into the pain phase. And because your alternative medication is often less potent or less targeted, you end up taking more medicine overall than if you had taken your best shot first.

For example, Paul says he gets three kinds of headaches. One is his typical migraine, which comes on pretty quickly, and if he doesn't take his triptan, it will take him down for the day. His second headache is usually less intense and can build over an entire day. Sometimes he can just power through and eventually go to bed and sleep it off. This can turn into a migraine that is really hard to treat, even with a triptan. His third headache is a "sinus headache" that hits him right between the eyes and can last for days, often landing him in the emergency room. He gets these about twice a year. After investigating Paul's alleged sinus condition (not there) and his neck (really tight but no injury or illness), we suggested that he had only one headache type (migraine) with some different triggers. We also suggested that he should treat *all* his headaches early, and all with triptans. At the same time, we pushed hard for regular exercise and breaks during his day. Over time, Paul also found that using a muscle relaxant when his neck was tight saved him from using too many triptans.

It's very important to keep your medication close at hand, readily available. I keep mine at home, in my car, and in my office. I also have some in my briefcase and in my travel bag. You might need to keep yours in your medicine cabinet, purse, and gym bag. The important thing is to think this through when you're not sick, distribute your rescue meds according to your plan, and remember to replenish them after a headache.

Patients always ask, "What if I use up plan A and the headache never develops? Then I've wasted a valuable triptan day, burned one of my 'Get out of jail free' cards with my mom, canceled that meeting I'd been planning for three months, yadayadayada." This kind of reasoning makes both migraineurs and their doctors crazy. In the first place, how do you know that it wasn't the medicine that kept the headache from developing? You don't. And in a larger sense, who cares? Even at fifteen dollars, isn't one pill a small price to pay for a headache-free day? As for the other stuff, you can always call back, reschedule, enjoy a free day, or whatever. Sweating the small stuff can be a potent migraine trigger, and you should avoid it at all costs. With mounting evidence that increasingly frequent migraines can have long-term consequences in some people, beating a headache day—regardless of consequences to social and business calendars—has to be worth it. If you really don't think so, just have the headache. It is that simple.

Diary of a Mad Migraineur

10:30 a.m.   I become aware of the first hint of a headache, but I'm in the middle of three things, so I decide to keep an eye on it and see if it develops.

12:15 p.m.   Yes, I definitely am getting a migraine, but it isn't too bad. I've just got to finish a couple of things, then I will go to my car and get my medicine.

1:30 p.m.   My head is really starting to pound but I have time for lunch so maybe a triple-shot espresso latte along with my

	sandwich will knock it out. But I feel a little nauseated and can't eat half my sandwich. Ugh, I'll probably throw it up anyway.
2:40 p.m.	I am sweating, light-headed, and dizzy, and can barely focus on the ground under my feet. But I think I can make it to the bathroom to take my headache medicine, which I will probably promptly throw up.
3:10 p.m.	I'm blinded by light and pain, and ready to die. I decide to just lie down on my office floor for a minute, and then I'll feel well enough to go back to work.
4:00 p.m.	Mercifully, I drift off to a deep but unsatisfying sleep. God willing, I will awaken headache free, albeit out of it.

That was me. The *old* me.

Now I keep two of my medicines nearby at all times. They work well for me if I take them early in a headache, so I have them stashed in my glove compartment, my valise, my various desks and work areas, suitcases, you name it. I have an alert on my computer that reminds me every hour to stop whatever I'm doing, stretch my neck, and do a general assessment for a few minutes before I go back to work. And so on. My plan is no more elaborate than any of my patients' plans, but it is a plan that works for me.

In the middle of a headache, we don't make good decisions. Kendra, a thirty-one-year-old attorney, tells the story of sleeping badly the night before she had to litigate in front of a judge who "despised female attorneys." She did not take the sleep medicine we had given her, and remembers thinking in bed that she would probably get a headache the next day. When she awoke the next morning, she was aware that a hint of headache was looming in the background. She did not take anything but decided to see how she felt after breakfast. Kendra did not think of her headache again until she was stuck in traffic—without her medication. By the time she arrived at court, her head was pounding, but rather than have her office call the court and say she was sick, she decided to power through, and lost her motion rather badly.

How many bad decisions can you count in Kendra's story?

Of course, denial is part of this, but part of it is very real impaired reasoning and judgment that is a documented part of the migraine process. Good science backs this up. For this reason, we need to prepare for our headaches, so we don't have to make decisions when we feel one coming on. The plan should be in place, and all we need to do is follow it.

When Your Hair Hurts and Your Brain Is on Fire

In the last few years, two important theories about how a headache starts have emerged to greatly improve our understanding of what happens during a headache. The two theories seem to go hand in hand, but neither has been proven to be the seminal event in migraines. Central sensitization holds that once a headache has been present for a while, it no longer relies on external stimulation to keep it going but rather works on a feedback loop. Cutaneous allodynia is a condition in which normal stimulus to skin, hair, or other surfaces is perceived as painful. The two theories explain that once the head *aches*, the brain itself becomes sensitized, changing the nature of the headache from an external-stimulus response and altering the way we perceive pain.

While this may seem obvious to those of us who have laid in our beds, completely isolated from the world, and witnessed helplessly as our headache got worse, it has proven more difficult to demonstrate this phenomenon in the laboratory. Why is it important to reproduce this in the lab? Without a laboratory model, it is almost impossible to experiment with the system to locate and, we hope, correct the problem.

Using laboratory rats, we *have* been able to physically measure and track changes in the brain during these events. As a result, we have learned that once the brain has become sensitized during a headache, stimulus to the head (or even the paw) produces a pain response, even when the stimulus is as benign as a light touch. We have further found that this hypersensitivity can be prevented with a triptan early in the course of a headache, but not later on, and that the hypersensitivity *can* be blocked later on with an anti-inflammatory agent. A cause-and-effect relationship has yet to be demonstrated between the pain and the cutaneous allodynia. But it seems reasonable to assume that preventing central sensitization, either with early rescue, preventives, or both, is likely to have a positive effect on headache pain itself.

This is a wonderful example of how laboratory research can help us in the clinic, and observation in the clinic can help us understand basic pathophysiology as studied in the laboratory.

The Toolbox

Migraines are described in writings that are thousands of years old, and the Chinese identified headache treatments more than five thousand years ago. But the first medications designed specifically to treat migraines were only developed less than thirty years ago. Most migraine sufferers over the age of twenty-five remember the dark days before these migraine-specific drugs were introduced. With a severe headache, the best we could hope for was a dark, quiet room or a drug-induced dysphoria of narcotics or ergotamines, or a little relief from nonspecific medications designed for other uses, such as general pain, inflammation, or agitation.

Today, fortunately, we have these designer drugs, the triptans, that specifically target migraines. Unless there is a compelling reason to avoid the triptans, these are normally the big guns of migraine rescue. To complete your rescue plan, you will likely need to utilize various tools in our growing arsenal of migraine treatments, from other prescriptions to over-the-counter medications, natural remedies, and other modalities. Often these will include anti-inflammatories, antihistamines, dopamine antagonists, and other rescue strategies, such as nonprescription medications, meditation, sleep, and so forth. Our options *generally* include:

- Triptans: Imitrex, Maxalt, Zomig, Frova, Relpax, Axert, Amerge, Treximet
- NSAIDs: Motrin, Aleve, Indocin
- Muscle relaxants: Zanaflex, Soma, Flexeril, Skelaxin, baclofen, and Robaxin, as well as orphenadrine compounds
- Other prescription rescue medications: tramadol, butalbital, Midrin, Duradrin, and Amidrine; DHE, Migranal, Botox, and Myobloc; steroids, neuroleptics, Depacon
- Over-the-counter medicines: aspirin, Tylenol, caffeine, and the NSAIDs; diphenhydramine (Benadryl)
- Natural agents: cannibinoids (marijuana), butterbur, coenzyme Q10, riboflavin, magnesium
- Nonmedication rescues: breathing, meditation, physical therapy, acupressure

❖ Narcotic Rescue

Narcotics are never an appropriate rescue medication for someone with migraines or other primary headaches. In the short term, sure, narcotics will cover up your pain. But over time they will result in a lowered pain threshold, dependence, escalating doses, decreased effectiveness, nasty side effects, and MOH. So we are careful to avoid narcotics.

While there are reported cases of people who have used low-dose narcotics for many years without experiencing an increase in headache frequency or medication use, these cases are exceedingly rare. There is no reason to believe you are one of these rare cases. It is far more likely that you will become dependent on these medications, that side effects will become more of a problem (although you may not care), that you will need increasingly greater doses to achieve the same level of relief, and that your headaches will become more frequent and severe over time.

Solid science indicates that narcotics lower your pain threshold, making you less tolerant of pain, and that the effects of narcotics on the brain can last for many years beyond the point at which you stop. And then there is the problem of narcotics withdrawal, the difficulty of finding a doctor who will prescribe for your increasing need, and so forth. In short, narcotic use is a hard way to go. It is not that narcotics have no role in pain management. They clearly do—in cancer, postsurgical recovery, and so forth. They just don't have a role in the long-term management of migraines.

Triptans

Rob, in his mid-forties, had suffered with headaches as long as he could remember. Over the years, he had been given everything from Tylenol to Demerol. In 1993, for the first time, he was given a triptan, and found that his headaches could be treated effectively without significant side effects or difficulty. He continued to get headaches from time to time, and triptans remained effective for him. For Rob, like many, many migraine sufferers, triptans have made a huge difference in his life. Rob wrote this book. Today, we have seven migraine-specific "designer" drugs from which to choose. Known collectively as triptans, these drugs have become the standard of treatment for migraine rescue in the last dozen years. For the majority of migraineurs, they work well and have changed our world for the better.

Indicated only for the acute treatment of migraine headaches, the triptans are generally less effective once a headache gets rolling, so patients should take them as soon as possible.

The triptans all share action-specific receptors in the brain stem, in the walls of certain blood vessels in the lining that surrounds the brain (meninges), and elsewhere in the body. In general, the medicine is well tolerated, but there are receptors for the medication in the lungs and the heart (in much smaller numbers than in the head). As a class, these medications can be associated with a rare side effect, a tightening sensation in the chest, which is usually very brief. In addition, this class of medication is contraindicated for patients with unstable hypertension or active heart disease. Naturally, you should have a detailed discussion with your prescribing physician about the triptans or any new medication.

The first triptan was Imitrex (sumatriptan), which was followed in short order by Maxalt (rizatriptan) and Zomig (zolmitriptan). Today, the list has expanded to include Frova (frovatriptan), Relpax (eletriptan), Axert (almotriptan), and Amerge (naratriptan). All the triptans, however, are not created equal. They have significant differences. Some are administered as pills to be swallowed, others as rapid-melting tablets that dissolve on the tongue, nasal sprays, or injections. The triptans also differ in how quickly the medicine takes effect, how long it stays in your system, how it is broken down in the body, how it interacts with certain enzymes in the liver, and how they affect and are affected by other medications. So we can't say they are all the same, or that one is better than the others.

Several months ago, an internist approached me after a lecture and said, "I give my patients samples of several different triptans and just have them try some out." Cringing inwardly, I smiled politely and suggested that perhaps there is a better way, for the differences among the triptans can mean a world of difference to the patient. In selecting a triptan, it is important to match the characteristics of the medicine to the characteristics of both the headache and the patient.

How a particular patient's headaches present determines the selection of which triptan is most appropriate. For example, a triptan that comes on very quickly and wears off just as fast would not be much help with a headache that typically builds over several hours. Similarly, a triptan that reaches its maximum concentration in the blood in four hours is not going to be very effective against a headache that goes from a 0 to a 10 in twenty minutes. Some patients have monthly headaches (often associated with menses) that are present on awakening and last for days, while other patients have headaches that come on rapidly, knock them down for half a day, and then are gone. In selecting a triptan, I start out with two questions:

- What are your headaches like?
- What are you looking for in a headache medication?

Surprisingly, the answers to these two questions vary tremendously from patient to patient. For some patients, absence of side effects is paramount. For other patients, rapid relief is most important. Someone else might just want freedom from recurrence (the headache coming back when the medication wears off). The following guide to the various triptans provides a typical patient profile for someone who is likely to do well with each medication. Since all of the triptans are prescription medications, you will need to discuss these suggestions and your complete medical history with a doctor, and both of you will want to review the restrictions listed in the medication's package insert.

Rules for Triptans

Never exceed the daily recommended dose.

Never use triptans more than three days in the same week.

IMITREX INJECTABLE, NASAL, AND TABLETS Administered through an autoinjector just under the skin, Imitrex injectable has the fastest onset of action of any triptan presently on the market. It comes in both 6 mg and 4 mg prefilled syringes. Many migraineurs find that the 4 mg dose is sufficient to abort a headache. Since it is important to treat a headache as early as possible, this injectable is often ideal for patients whose headaches develop quickly. Imitrex injectable is also the ideal choice for patients with cluster headache. While it is used in some emergency rooms for acute treatment of migraine, in my experience, by the time you get to the treatment room in an ER, your headache is past the window of opportunity when triptans are most effective, and by then there are better alternatives. The downside with Imitrex injectable is that patients may experience more prominent side effects, including a brief sensation of tightness in the chest or throat. The injection itself is only slightly uncomfortable, and injection-site reaction is extremely rare.

Imitrex also comes in a nasal form, and many patients find that this formulation acts almost as fast as the injection, without having to give themselves a shot. For your first use, it is important to read the instructions ahead of time, as head position and other methods of use can be a little hard to process when you have a migraine. As with Imitrex injectable, the nasal formulation also has the advantage of portability, since it does not require a sip of water to wash down the medication, and this can be very convenient in certain situations.

Imitrex also comes in 25 mg, 50 mg, and 100 mg tablets and a recently reformulated 100 mg tablet that affords a response in about twenty minutes. All Imitrex formulations have a relatively short half-life of two to two and a half hours, which might be a problem for people whose headaches tend to recur after treatment, as this would require repeat dosing. When Imitrex is taken at the onset, which is ideal for any triptan, this is generally sufficient to knock out a migraine. However, some patients find that the headache will go away with the first dose, but then recurs later on. If you observe this pattern, you can take a second dose so long as you do not exceed 200 mg oral in a twenty-four-hour period. Sometimes, we recommend following up with a longer-acting triptan like frovatriptan or naratriptan, but mixing triptans is not recommended by the manufacturers (for obvious reasons). The recommended dose of oral Imitrex is actually 100 mg, not 50 mg or 25 mg. Rarely, patients find that they are successful with the lower doses, but we usually start with 100 mg and then go down, if possible.

AXERT   Effective for headaches that come on quickly, Axert is a good choice for people who are wary of the potential side effects of triptans because it is very well tolerated. In controlled trials, Axert had a side-effect profile that was identical to the placebo group, thus making it the most gentle of the triptans. We use Axert in patients who tend to be very sensitive to medications but whose headaches seem to require the power of a triptan. Its half-life ranges between three and four hours. Of course, Axert also has the same class contraindications of unstable hypertension and active heart disease, so always thoroughly discuss prescription medicines with your physician.

MAXALT   Maxalt wins the convenience award. Along with Zomig, Maxalt is one of two medicines available in a rapidly dissolving formulation that melts in your mouth. It is easy to take at the first sign of a headache, doesn't require you to find a drinking fountain or convenience store, and is easy to carry. Its onset of action is quite fast and, in my experience, since it has a half-life of more than four hours, recurrence is less of a problem. Maxalt is also available in tablet form in the same 5 mg and 10 mg doses, the latter being the standard dose in patients who are not also taking propranolol.

Rapidly dissolving formulations do not get into the bloodstream any more quickly than the tablet forms. The medicine is still absorbed across the gut rather than directly into the blood vessels in your mouth (the way true sublingual medicines, like nitroglycerin, are). The dissolving tablet is merely a convenience that allows the medicine to be swallowed along with your saliva. In addition to the convenience, the rapidly dissolving formulation is very useful in people who have prominent nausea with their headaches, when the prospect of drinking a glass of water to wash down a pill is just too horrible to contemplate.

ZOMIG   Similar in many ways to Maxalt, Zomig comes in two formulations, each available in two strengths. The rapidly dissolving formulation has an orange flavor that some patients prefer to the Maxalt, but this is a matter of personal taste (no pun intended). The main advantage of dissolving tablets is convenience, as it is easily carried and easily taken. Given the importance of early treatment with triptans, this is an important benefit. Zomig comes in 2.5 mg and 5.0 mg tablets, and the maximum dose is 10 mg in twenty-four hours. It is similar to Maxalt in terms of onset of action (about thirty minutes).

RELPAX The newest of the triptans, Relpax combines excellent tolerability, reasonable half-life (four hours), and good effect for relief of the nausea and light sensitivity associated with migraine. The standard starting dose is 40 mg, and the maximum daily dose in twenty-four hours is 80 mg. While I don't have a crystal ball, I suspect we will not see new triptans launched, and if this is the case, Relpax will be considered the "next generation" triptan. At this writing, it is the only triptan with head-to-head comparison data against other triptans and, in these studies, it came out ahead. As might be expected, the manufacturers of the triptans that did not measure up have criticisms of the studies. In my experience, Relpax is a very good drug, well tolerated and effective. Is it vastly superior to other oral formulations? No. In terms of treating migraines, these first five triptans do not have huge differences.

FROVA Frova is a unique triptan, used more often by headache specialists than by general physicians. It has a half-life of twenty-six hours, which means the medication remains in the body significantly longer than other triptans, and as a result, it boasts the lowest headache recurrence rate. It is also very well tolerated. On the downside, many patients report that Frova takes longer to kick in, which can be a problem if your headaches tend to build quickly.

At the Keeler Center, we often use Frova as a "chaser," following another triptan that comes on more quickly but wears off a bit too soon to prevent recurrence. Thus, when a patient reports that her headaches respond well to one of the "standard" triptans but then the headache comes back later in the day or the next morning, we recommend taking a Frova an hour or two after the first triptan. This approach is outside the recommendations approved by the FDA and is not listed in the prescribing insert that comes with the medication, so it is important to discuss such an approach with your physician.

Frova is also useful for "pulse" therapy during a brief period of frequent headaches, such as during menstruation. For example, suppose you are like many women who, month after month after month, reliably wake up with a headache on the day before (or after) your period begins. In this circumstance, it might be reasonable to take a medication the night before your menses begins and thereby avoid, or at least minimize, the inevitable headache. Obviously, a triptan that will be mostly gone by morning won't work, but one that has a long half-life will. We often recommend that these patients take the Frova for several days. Again, this is outside the usual prescribing practices, but sometimes you need to go outside the box. Frova comes in a 2.5 mg strength, but this does not mean it is less potent than, say, Relpax, which comes in 40 mg tablets. There is no correlation between the milligram strength and the potency of the drug.

AMERGE Amerge has a half-life of about six hours, which is longer than any triptan except Frova. It also has a very mellow side-effect profile, meaning it is pretty well tolerated. With this kind of intermediate profile, Amerge can be useful as a follow-up or chaser to one of the faster-acting triptans in patients whose headaches often recur after taking the first triptan. Another useful way to use Amerge is when you know you are heading into a situation that typically triggers a headache for you, such as a plane flight, a long drive on a winding mountain road, a party where you plan to have a drink or two, or an intense exercise session. We also use anti-inflammatories like naproxen in the same way and, sometimes, we combine the two. Amerge comes in 2.5 mg tablets, and the maximum daily dose is 5 mg. Like all triptans, it should not be used more than two days per week except in special circumstances and under the specific care of a headache specialist.

TREXIMET This addition to the triptan list is actually the first "combination" triptan. It is a mixture of 85 mg sumatriptan and 500 mg naproxen. The manufacturer's data indicate that combining a triptan and an NSAID is more effective in aborting a headache than taking either one alone. Whether combining the two medicines in one pill has any real advantage over taking the two separately and simultaneously, there is good evidence that combining members of these two groups (triptans and NSAIDs) is an excellent approach to aborting a headache.

NSAIDs

Nonsteroidal anti-inflammatory drugs (NSAIDs) include both over-the-counter options and prescription variations on the theme. These can be very effective in migraine rescue, but you also need to be very careful with these medications. Their greatest danger is overuse. When migraineurs take these medications too frequently, the risk of MOH is real and serious.

Ibuprofen and naproxen are the most common NSAIDs, though you probably know them by their brand names, Motrin and Aleve, respectively. Both are available in prescription formulations, which are higher doses of the same medicine.

As the name implies, this class of medicines is defined by their distinction from steroids. These medications work by blocking an inflammation pathway at various points along a chemical pathway. For example, aspirin blocks the pathway early in its course, while the COX-1 inhibitors like naproxen and ibuprofen only block one branch and COX-2 inhibitors like celecoxib block the other branch.

If your headaches are slow to build, an NSAID might be an effective first-line rescue *when* you can take it early enough. Some literature suggests that anti-inflammatories may also be more effective for a headache after it has been up and rolling for a while. The theory is that once a migraine is well established in the brain, significant inflammation is part of the problem, so triptans are increasingly less effective, and anti-inflammatory agents may, therefore, be more useful. In addition, we are learning more about cutaneous allodynia, a stage during migraines that about 80 percent of migraineurs experience an hour or two into a headache. During cutaneous allodynia, the migraine sufferer perceives normally benign sensory stimuli as pain, and the skin, particularly over the head including the scalp is painful to the touch. Once a migraine has reached this stage, triptans may not help much, but anti-inflammatories might.

Muscle Relaxants

Doctors often prescribe muscle relaxants for rescue and prevention. At the Keeler Center, we use muscle relaxants in patients who find that muscle tension, particularly in the neck and shoulders, is a potent trigger for their headaches. We tend to use these as rescue medications under the two-day-per-week rule. However, other headache specialists often use these in a preventive strategy either at night or several times per day. So far, no study has shown that the muscle relaxants result in rebound or medication overuse headaches, but I am very careful with these medicines. The major side effect in this class is sedation so, when sleep is an issue along with muscle tension, a nighttime dose can be very helpful. Medicines in this class include tizanidine (Zanaflex), Soma, Flexeril, Skelaxin, baclofen, and Robaxin.

Orphenadrine-containing compounds, such as Norgesic Forte and other trade name medications, combine orphenadrine, a muscle relaxant, with other ingredients, usually aspirin or Tylenol, plus caffeine. This is a very effective medication to give some relief in a headache that has been up and rolling for a few hours. The major downside is that it is very sedating. This is not a medication you can use while you work, drive, or even carry on an intelligent conversation. Still, there are circumstances where sleep is a welcome and practical alternative. You cannot take it more than three times a day and, again, not more than two days in a week.

Other Prescription Rescue Medications

TRAMADOL WITH ACETAMINOPHEN Tramadol is a prescription pain medicine that works at the mu receptor, which is the same site that accepts opioids. The difference is that tramadol does not bind irreversibly as opioids do. This makes it much easier on the body. It is not a narcotic. Neither is it a migraine-specific medication. It is a painkiller, but a relatively safe one, particularly if it is limited to two days per week. The usual dosing is one or two tablets, up to three times in one day. By taking acetaminophen with it (usually 250 mg to 500 mg), the pain-relieving effect can be significantly enhanced.

BUTALBITAL-CONTAINING COMPOUNDS These medications, which combine an analgesic like aspirin or acetaminophen with caffeine and butalbital, have been used for headaches for many years. Some of the popular trade names are Fioricet, Fiorinal, and Esgic. Let me say very clearly: *These are very dangerous drugs*. They are also pretty effective in ending a headache. This, of course, is a lethal combination for someone whose head hurts. How dangerous is this combination? It is dangerous enough that the German government has outlawed the medication and it is off the market in most of Europe. In our clinic, we find that people overusing these medications are far and away the most difficult to withdraw and have the highest relapse rate after coming off it. My best advice is to not get started with this medicine, even if your doctor offers it. There are other, better ways. If it is used, it must be strictly limited to no more than three pills in a day and *never* more than one day in seven.

ISOMETHEPTENE/DICHLORALPHENAZONE AND ACETAMINO-PHEN Commonly known by names such as Midrin, Duradrin, and Amidrine, this medicine combines a blood vessel constrictor (isometheptene) with a mild sedative and an analgesic. The usual dose is two pills at the onset of the headache and then one per hour as needed up to a maximum of five pills total in twenty-four hours and not more than two days per week. In my hands, this medication has been odd. Some people find that it works pretty well, others have found it totally ineffective. To date, I cannot identify a subgroup of patients who respond well to it. On the positive side, it is well tolerated and has few side effects. It is a medicine we often use in children or people who are very sensitive to medications.

ERGOT AGENTS Given intravenously over several days in an inpatient setting, dihydroergotamine (DHE) still remains a gold standard for breaking a migraine. Migranal is a prescription nasal formulation that many patients find effective. Unfortunately, it has some nasty side effects, including nausea, vomiting, diarrhea, and sweating. Overuse can cause constriction of blood vessels to the point where it can damage circulation. Again, patients must be careful to use ergotamines only according to their doctor's prescription and the package insert—and never more than two days per week.

BOTULINUM TOXIN AND OTHER INJECTIBLES Trade-named Botox or Myobloc, these medications have been used as rescue as well as preventive agents. At the time of this publication, the clinical benefit has not been established, but I suspect it will be, as my experience with this medication has been positive. At the Keeler Center, we have seen it work both as an acute rescue and as a preventive, lasting up to three months. There are two approaches. Using a tiny needle, we inject the medication into the patient's face, either in a standard array or following the pattern of the patient's pain.

Bupivacaine, either alone or in combination with a depot steroid such as triamcinolone (Kenalog), is also used as an acute treatment that can last for a prolonged period. These agents are injected, according to the location of the pain. If Kenalog is included in the preparation, we use a slightly larger needle. Such rescue treatments are, of course, not practical unless you live near a facility that is experienced and accessible. But an experienced health care provider can also apply botulinum toxin to the upper surface of the inside of the nose or around a focus of pain any-where on the head.

In some circumstances, a gel formulation of lidocaine can also be used on a Q-tip inserted on the upper surface inside the nose. This treatment is often used when the pain seems to localize between the eyes but has also been used for cluster headaches and migraines. The advantage is that the gel can be applied as often as needed. When it works, it works very well. But it is not for everyone. Again, this should be undertaken only with a health care provider experienced in the technique.

STEROIDS Steroids have had a checkered history in headache treatment. Even the current literature is mixed, with reports that IV steroids are not effective in breaking a migraine, and a large clinical experience (my own included) that indicates that they are. But it is clear that long-term use of steroids for headache control is not an acceptable alternative. The risks to bone density, vision, blood sugar, for example, far outweigh the benefits. However, short-term use, either over five to seven days or as briefly as a single dose following a failed triptan attempt, can be of tremendous benefit. Often prescribed orally in a tapering dose over days, steroids can effectively break a headache that has persisted for several days.

NEUROLEPTICS Neuroleptics are a relatively new player in head-ache prevention and rescue. Earlier generations these drugs had side effects that made them unwelcome outside the psychiatric arena, but the newer generation, known as D2 antagonists (the D stands for dopamine), is much better tolerated, although they can still, rarely, cause movement disorders, blood sugar problems, and increased appetite. By working at both the serotonin and dopamine receptors, these medications can often provide effective prevention when the more commonly used preventives have proven inadequate, and some headache specialists also use this class of drugs for rescue capacity at the onset of a headache.

DEPACON   Depacon is an IV formulation of the well-known preventive valproic acid (Depakote). It has been found effective as a way to break an acute migraine. Of course, it can only be administered in a medical setting, and therefore tends to be used rather late in a headache when more accessible rescues have failed. It has the advantage of bringing blood levels up into a therapeutic range quickly such that if Depakote is to be continued orally, no titration period is necessary. The problems of weight gain and hair loss that plague some patients with oral use do not seem to be a problem when the medication is used as a single rescue IV.

ANTINAUSEA AIDS   Ideally, in rescue, we want to treat the source of the pain. That is why recent work has focused on the triptans and current research has studied the vasoactive peptides, like calcitonin gene-related peptide (CGRP). However, a number of fellow travelers with migraines often need treatment because, when left untreated, their symptoms will worsen or prolong the headache. Prominent among these are nausea, vomiting, and subsequent dehydration. For this reason, acute treatment of headaches often involves medications for nausea—such as the phenothiazines Reglan, Compazine, or ondansetron—as well as hydration, electrolyte replacement, and other supplements, if necessary.

Rehydration is an important part of headache rescue. Whether you are dehydrated from vomiting or from simply not drinking water because your head is killing you, dehydration makes headaches much worse. It is critical to keep liquids onboard when you have a headache. We have seen cases where simple rehydration with an IV has ended a headache severe enough to bring someone to the emergency room. In these cases, the rescue meds may have failed because the patient was so dry.

Over-the-Counter Medicines

Many over-the-counter medicines (OTCs), and some of the NSAIDs, are available for people who get mild to moderate headaches relatively infrequently. Since you are reading this book, your headaches are probably more painful or more frequent—or both. So while aspirin and acetaminophen can be very effective and have their place in migraine rescue, you need to take them with a heavy dose of caution.

As with NSAIDs, the greatest danger is overuse. It is actually very easy for chronic pain patients to overdose on OTCs, damaging the heart, liver, and kidneys. As with any medication, follow package instructions on recommended dosing and daily maximums. And remember, from a headache management perspective, when migraineurs take these medications too frequently, the risk of MOH is real and serious. Also, to avoid exceeding the daily limits, be mindful of common ingredients in your prescription and nonprescription medications.

ASPIRIN In European emergency rooms, aspirin is given intravenously as a rescue, and it works very well, by all reports. This is not legal in the United States, but that is another story for another time. One report claimed that daily aspirin worked well as a migraine preventive, and there are many other indications for taking aspirin on a daily basis (such as prevention of heart disease and stroke). Further, no studies have shown that daily aspirin use results in rebound headaches.

But even though aspirin doesn't require a prescription, it is still serious medicine with side effects and drug-drug interactions. Keep two things in mind about aspirin. First, it is a blood thinner, and you need to be aware of that if you are taking other medications (like ibuprofen, warfarin, Coumadin, ginkgo biloba, and others). Second, many other headache medicines contain aspirin, so read the labels and make sure you do not take too much. Always discuss any medication, supplement, or over-the-counter health aid with your doctor to make sure you are as safe as can reasonably be expected.

ACETAMINOPHEN Commonly known as Tylenol, acetaminophen is a very effective analgesic. While there is no evidence that overuse of acetaminophen alone can result in rebound headaches, overuse of this medication can lead to problems in other organs of the body such as the liver and kidneys. A common ingredient in many other pain relievers, Tylenol overdose can be quite serious.

BENADRYL AND ANTIHISTAMINE Benadryl and antihistamine have both been used by some practitioners as migraine rescue medicines. Given orally or by injection, they offer relief to many patients. The scientific literature on this is mixed, and in our hands, we have found that Benadryl can be an effective rescue but can lead to nasty MOH if overused. Antihistamine is more problematic. A few prominent headache centers use it frequently as a twice-a-week preventive, but other centers (including ours) have not been able to reproduce their results.

CAFFEINE An ingredient in many migraine rescue medications, caffeine is a very controversial substance. Some headache specialists feel it has no place in migraine management and that it should be strictly excluded from every headache sufferer's diet and treatment plan. Many headache sufferers have experienced relief from a mild or early headache after drinking a caffeinated beverage and, clearly, a number of preparations include caffeine and provide relief. Our approach at the Keeler Center is that when headaches are out of control—too frequent, too severe—it is worth it to eliminate caffeine completely. When things are going a bit better, it is best to limit caffeine to a regular routine.

Needless to say, caffeine is a bad idea in the evening—unless you are suffering from a rare type of headache known as hypnic. This brief, painful headache occurs at the same time each night, wakes the patient from sleep, and is usually prevented by taking a small amount of caffeine just before bed. Curiously, in these patients, the caffeine does not appear to disrupt sleep. For the rest of us, a caffeine boost either in the morning or afternoon seems pretty harmless so long as headaches are under control. It is also good to keep in mind that "decaffeinated" does not mean "caffeine-free." Many so-called decaffeinated beverages contain more caffeine than a Dr Pepper.

On a scientific basis, caffeine is well recognized as an adjuvant. This means that it helps with the absorption of other medicines. This may be why it is included in several headache remedies. Why it seems to work in isolation (as in a Coke or Pepsi) to abort a headache, we don't really know. It has not been studied formally, but anecdotal evidence abounds.

MIGRAINE FORMULAS Over-the-counter migraine formulas often differ from their nonmigraine counterparts *only* in labeling and price. If you don't believe me, read the labels. Most "migraine formulas" are nothing more than a marketing ploy, admittedly a very successful one, designed to play on our need for headache relief. While many of these work well for the occasional headache, my feeling is that these packages should clearly state the risk for causing medication overuse headache. Of course, this would cut into their profits and, because they are over-the-counter, the FDA is not likely to interfere at this level. This is unfortunate because of the tremendous health care costs that result from the kidney damage and overutilization of emergency room resources as a result of analgesic overuse. Okay. I'm done. For now.

Natural Agents

I try to explore every option—from traditional medicine to New Age remedies. My only requirement is that they prove effective in rigorous scientific testing and objective evaluation. Little by little, natural remedies are meeting this standard. There is now credible data for cannabinoids (marijuana), magnesium, and several other preparations that were previously viewed as outside the realm of traditional headache treatment. Magnesium is used in an IV formulation as an acute rescue and orally as a preventive.

Curiously, many patients, in their desperate search for effective treatment, will forgo traditional modalities and medications out of hand, preferring to go natural. To me, this bias is no different than the bias some physicians have *against* medications and treatments that have not been vetted by the Food and Drug Administration. In the Keeler Method, we often combine traditional and complementary modalities in the same plan. Our only restriction is *Primum non nocere*: First do no harm.

MAGNESIUM　Magnesium has been linked to headache for many years, but only in the last several years has it been studied in an organized way. Part of the difficulty lies in the way most labs test for magnesium. The standard test measures "total" magnesium, which includes both bound and free magnesium, as well as magnesium that is bound to other molecules. It turns out that you can have normal total magnesium but low ionized magnesium. The test for ionized magnesium is hard to get and pretty expensive. It has been reported, however, that as many as one in three people has low ionized magnesium. It has also been reported that magnesium drops during a migraine attack. Often, we treat an acute attack with one gram of magnesium IV, which can be very effective, and oral magnesium is also used as a preventive. Keep in mind that there are several forms of magnesium compounds on the market and that the best compound for you may not be the best for me. It is a discussion that you should have with your physician.

MARIJUANA　Without going into the legal quagmire surrounding "medical marijuana," the substance has been promoted for headache relief for thousands of years. In fact, several controlled studies have shown significant benefit, particularly in patients with prominent nausea as part of their headache syndrome. Putting access issues aside, if you consider marijuana as an option, keep in mind that the damage done to the lungs from smoking is not limited to tobacco. Marinol, a pill form of marijuana, can avoid some of these dangers, but patients often report that it is not as effective as the inhaled form. The science is just beginning to catch up. Our lab has determined that enzymes that metabolize endocannabinoids are abnormal in the spinal fluid of migraineurs. These studies are very preliminary but point to a relationship between these substances and headache syndromes. We expect to know a lot more about this in the next couple of years.

OTHER PREPARATIONS　Several other preparations, available over the counter, have been proposed as headache rescues. The scientific evidence for their use ranges from thin to nonexistent. This does not mean that these preparations don't work, only that they have not been adequately vetted in the literature. Some patients find various balms applied to the forehead to be soothing, and there does not appear to be an obvious downside. However, these remedies should never take the place of a well-thought-out, well-executed plan.

Nonmedication Rescues

My experience dictates that when a migraineur needs a rescue nothing works quite as well as the right medicine in the proper environment, but this is not appropriate in some patients and some circumstances. For example, I have patients who are airline pilots, who are severely restricted in the medicines they can take and still keep their license. I have other patients who, for personal reasons, do not want to take any medications. And any one of us can find ourselves in a situation where medication and a quiet room are simply not available.

Many of these techniques are common sense. Some people get relief from a cold cloth on the forehead or the back of the neck. Some people also benefit from gentle massage of the neck or temples. However, an equal number find such stimulation almost unbearable. This may have something to do with the timing of these interventions, since the sensitization to stimuli comes on as the headache increases, and those measures that might feel good early on may be intolerable later in the headache. The same is true for some of the balms and lotions that are marketed for headache relief. For example, I have patients who swear by Tiger Balm, but I have other patients who say the scent worsens their nausea.

Rescue in the Keeler sense also includes many measures that help a great deal. At Keeler, we work very hard to provide rapid and *lasting* relief. Often this takes something more than medication alone.

PEACE AND QUIET—AND SLEEP When a headache is up and rolling, most headache sufferers long for sleep. Often, a headache will magically disappear once we fall asleep. *This is not an illusion.* For most people, sleep is a powerful tool in aborting a headache, especially if they can get to sleep early in the headache. The reason for this harks back to the reason we get migraines in the first place: migraines are the body's response to an excess of environmental stimuli. Not only do most of us structure our sleep environment to minimize light, sound, and movement, but the brain itself has the ability to decrease the "gain" on incoming stimuli during sleep, particularly in the deeper stages of sleep. So for most migraineurs, the best rescue in situations where medication is not an option is isolation from the environment—if possible, with sleep. Indeed, *this may be our best nonpharmacological rescue*, perhaps with other remedies such as balms, cool cloths, changes in environment, and so forth.

While we do not completely understand how sleep aborts a headache, we know that sleep dramatically modulates our sensory systems, decreasing our awareness of and sensitivity to environmental inputs. It may be as simple as that. But it probably isn't. Fortunately, this is a very active area of research, and we should know more in the near future. In our lab, we have determined that prostaglandins associated with sleep are abnormal in migraineurs, *even between headaches*, and they increase dramatically with a headache. Other studies have shown abnormal orexin levels in migraineurs. Orexins are neuropeptides intimately involved in the sleep/wake cycle.

All of this has important implications for structuring sleep when we have a headache. Much of it is common sense: Darken the room, turn off the TV or radio, and lie still. But some strategies are less obvious. For one, we should avoid common over-the-counter and prescription medicines that are often used to bring on sleep, because many of these actually *prevent* us from obtaining the natural sleep cycle that leads to migraine resolution. For example, Benadryl, phenobarbital, and benzodiazepines (Valium, Ativan, Xanax, etc.) disrupt the natural, restorative sleep we need. Whether the newer, prescription sleep aids have a role in the migraine/sleep continuum has not been studied. When appropriate, to help migraineurs fall asleep, I frequently use one of these newer medications, which seems to work well. But the jury is still out on whether this will become part of standard practice.

However, many patients say that going to sleep after taking a benzodiazepine *is* a good way to break a headache. But it is important to know what *kind* of headache you are treating. Aside from being addictive and disruptive to the natural sleep cycle, this class of medicines works as a potent muscle relaxant. If you are treating a headache that is primarily muscular—like a tension-type headache—then a muscle relaxer might be perfect, although we have other, safer alternatives than benzos. In fact, sleep rarely relieves a tension-type headache, because tension can actually *build* during sleep. In this case, the action of the medicine on the muscles, not the sleep, helps the headache, and other medications (tizanidine, for example) are safer alternatives than benzodiazepines.

MEDITATION   At the Keeler Center, we have found that various forms of meditation can help abort the onset of headaches, as can certain stretches, relaxation breathing exercises, and prayer, for example. We have found "minute meditations" (brief mantras that can be accomplished in almost any setting) to be particularly helpful. One book that we use frequently at the Keeler Center is *Flip the Switch*, by Eric Harrison. A variety of specific techniques in breathing and meditation may be appropriate for your treatment plan, but as with the other aspects of the plan, patients should explore these with a practitioner skilled and experienced in those disciplines.

ACUPRESSURE   Acupressure, a physical-medicine technique, can be useful to abort an existing headache. It is always advisable to have someone experienced in acupressure and Chinese medicine show you the proper technique.

Among many approaches, one that I have found effective is to apply constant pressure with a finger or the tip of the thumb at three specific points, on the *same* side as the headache—or both sides if the headache is global. You simply apply firm pressure to each spot for twenty seconds each. Major force is not necessary, just a firm pressure. You will know you are in the right place because the pressure point will be more tender (read: *painful*) than the area around it. The three points are along the same meridian, as follows:

- The first point is on the back of the hand at the base of the thumb in an indentation called the "anatomical snuff box." Looking at your thumb, flex the first joint and cock the second joint back toward your wrist and you will see the snuff box between the bones. It looks like a tiny triangle.
- The second point is on the back of the neck, just behind and below the ear. Feel behind the ear for the bone and then move slightly back and down until you find a tender point, just off the edge of the bone.
- The third point is on the temple at about eyebrow height. Again, this point will be tender to the touch. Interestingly, if you go straight to the temple without first applying pressure at the other two, the temple will be too painful to press.

Other Elements of a Good Plan

Throughout this discussion of rescue plans and backups, our plans also always include a component of escape. It is important that you consider, in advance, where you will go to find peace and quiet when you get a headache, and you need to think this through for all of the places where you spend a significant amount of your life.

Ample evidence shows that it is in a company's best interest, in terms of both productivity and compliance with the Americans with Disabilities Act, to provide a place of refuge for someone suffering from migraines. Most human resources departments can help you with this, if necessary. Of course, you can't accomplish this in every situation, but you should plan for it in the places where you spend significant time—at home and work.

Your refuge needs to be a place where you can quietly wait for relief, where—one hopes—noise, odor, or heat will not disturb you and invade your healing. Make arrangements for this place ahead of time so you can go there with a minimum of preparation or explanation, and so you don't need to set it up when you have a headache. Of course, the place can be your bedroom or a spare room, or it might be the factory infirmary or a spare office with a couch. If you spend significant time in your car, always keep a windshield sunscreen so you can park your car and quietly recline and rest.

If you are fortunate enough to have a gatekeeper (a spouse or maybe a secretary, coworker, or supervisor), you can plan a simple heads-up like "I need to lie down for a while." It's perfectly all right to request that your secretary hold your calls or that your spouse not check on you every five minutes. And by all means, the kids should know not to play basketball in the living room while they're waiting for you to get up and make dinner.

Of course, people who don't get headaches often don't get it. They are unaware of the way the flood of light stabs you when they open the door, or how "Are you okay?" sounds like the voice of Oz. Fortunately, in most cases, family, friends, and even coworkers can be educated and are often grateful for the opportunity to learn. So, as a chronic headache sufferer, you can gently educate the people around you about your headaches, and prepare them so they can accommodate—or at least, be aware of—your needs during a headache. The next chapter provides many more tips about how to help your support system help you most effectively.

Plan Your Plan

You might have noticed that in the midst of a headache you don't think too clearly. Not only is it hard to think through thunderous, glaring pain, but the brain actually undergoes changes during migraines that impair our ability to make decisions, focus on priorities, and even coordinate speech and movement. That's why it is important—in advance, during your precious, headache-free moments—to lay out your rescue plans and have them in place. Then, when you get that first sign of a headache, you are ready, almost reflexively, to begin early treatment.

A challenging question comes from patients who are on a complex drug regimen, with many different medications and a complex lifestyle on top of that. They can find no pattern to their headaches. This requires some very careful analysis. For example, let's say I have a patient who is on two preventive drugs, one with a half-life (how long it takes the body to burn half the dose) of twelve hours and a Tmax (how long it takes after ingestion to get to a peak in the body) of forty minutes, and another preventive with a half-life of twenty-eight hours and a Tmax of two hours. He takes the first drug twice a day and the second once a day. One night, he stays up two hours later than usual, thereby advancing his cortisol cycle such that it bottoms out two hours later than normal, and he wakes up with a headache. He then takes a rescue medication that has a half-life of six hours and a Tmax of thirty minutes. One hour after taking his medication, his headache is worse, so he takes a different rescue medication with a half-life of four hours and a Tmax of fifteen minutes. He would like to know why it is so hard for me to predict response to medication. If you think of this as a math problem, you can begin to see how difficult it would be to solve.

Picture wavelengths of different sizes to represent all the factors involved in headache triggering and treatment, and you can imagine that at times they will all come together as a node and cancel each other out (no headache). But there will also be times when the trigger wavelengths will add together, just when the treatment wavelengths cancel out or dip to their lowest ebb (really bad headache). Balancing all the factors such that headaches are completely predictable is not presently possible. But if we can simplify and routinize our schedules, it helps make this equation more predictable. By the way, the answer to the problem posed in the above paragraph is 7. (This is a little neuropharmacology humor.)

Using the Keeler Method, you and your headache specialist, neurologist, primary care doctor, or other caregiver should design the right rescue plans for your headache scenario and write them out in the clearest possible terms so that even when you have a pounding headache you will know and understand what to do. And if you don't, a loved one *will*. Of course, you will also need a medical practitioner to prescribe certain medications. Other than that, you can manage most of your plans yourself. These strategies include layers of contingencies for what to do if the first rescue plan is not effective.

If nothing else works, you need to know, in advance, where to go for help. At the Keeler Center, our patients have twenty-four-hour access by phone and e-mail to a doctor or nurse practitioner who knows them. If necessary, the last layer for our patients' rescue is *me*. As a migraineur, you need to have a good working relationship with your physician. This should include *access to a real, live person if you get to your wit's end*. This backup means everything.

Plan A

Your first step is to organize Plan A, a simple procedure for what you are going to do when a headache starts, including your first-line treatment and an activity, like lying down in a dark room or placing a cool cloth on your neck. Each plan should have three components:

- **Your "go to" treatment.** Your first-line rescue tool might be a medication, but not everyone wants to take medications, and not everyone can. Some people prefer a cold compress, Tiger Balm, meditation, and any of a number of rescue treatments. Whatever the strategy, it needs to be readily available and clearly identified as your first step.
- **Organized resources.** Prepare a list of phone numbers of people who are onboard with the plan and can help you with your treatment as well as the day's responsibilities.
- **Rescue environment.** Plan a place where you can go to rest undisturbed until you are ready to rejoin the world. It should be

a cool, quiet, and dark place where you can get water and help if you need it.

It may be useful to create time points when you (or your spouse or other family member) should assess progress during an acute headache. Of course, time points vary depending on the measures you use, but it is important and valuable to give a rescue therapy a fair trial for a predetermined period of time. At specific intervals, it is important to assess whether a rescue has begun to kick in, whether it is time to take a follow-up step, or whether it may be time for Plan B, if Plan A is not working at all.

Anticipating a time frame serves other purposes, too. If I know that in two hours I am going to do something specific, this relieves me of some anxiety (and we know that anxiety is not good for someone with a headache). It also spares us from incessant inquiries, such as "Are you all right?" and "Can I get you anything?" I can simply say, "I am going to sleep for two hours. Please come back then. If I am still sleeping, leave quietly, but if I am awake and in pain, give me the following.... It is all right here in my plan." Then you can let the paper fall dramatically to the floor from your outstretched hand as you lie on the bed. This is very effective and much easier on both you and your family. Even better, the paper would already be posted on the refrigerator, and everyone in the house would know what to do without all that drama.

During a migraine, it can be nearly impossible to *remember* the time, which makes it difficult to time follow-up medication. It is very helpful if you always keep a small notepad handy, in your nightstand or wherever you will go to rest—and use it. It also helps, then, to include reminders in your plan to record when you medicate so you know whether and when you can medicate again. A typical Plan A might look something like this:

- Take Maxalt and Naprosyn, and write down the time.
- Call Mom to pick up kids from school. Remind her to tell the kids that I have a headache and to play quietly when they get home.
- Call Bill to pick up dinner or take the kids out.

- Cancel any appointments.
- Go home, disconnect phone, close curtains, lie down, no TV.
- Assess in one to two hours. Take another Maxalt.

It can be that simple. Of course, your rescue meds may not be Maxalt and Naprosyn, and talking to your mom when you have a headache may be a bad idea, but the general concept works. You need to medicate, clear your schedule, and rest. In addition to those basics, you might include reminders for yourself, depending on your own habits. For example, while turning on the TV might seem like a good idea when you first get home, getting up to turn it off later, when your headache is really pounding, will be torture.

Multiple Plan B's

Sometimes, Plan A might not be effective, and your headache might still be raging after two hours. Even if your best plan has "always" been effective, it *can* occasionally fail. Maybe, for some reason, you couldn't treat your headache until it was in full bloom. Maybe you were exposed to a particularly nasty trigger—such as really old egg salad or some other noxious food. Maybe you were hit with multiple triggers at the same time. Perhaps you were dehydrated, didn't sleep well the night before, were very stressed about something you just couldn't put away, or are getting the flu. Whether we know why monster headaches happen or not, the fact of life is that they do. So if your "big gun" doesn't work, you need a clear backup plan for what to do in such situations. And you need it ahead of time because, if your first line doesn't work, you probably won't be in any shape to figure it out.

Suppose, for example, that a patient followed her Plan A to the letter but two hours later her headache is really pounding. She is lying in bed, contemplating her next move. Toilet? More medication? A different medication? Emergency room? A very sharp object inserted into one eye? It is hard to know what is right in this circumstance, because everything seems at once both reasonable and impossible.

Meanwhile, most rescue medicines have a daily dose limit, meaning you can take only so much in a twenty-four-hour period. If you max out your daily dose and still have a headache, you need a backup plan. If you cannot take the next dose for six hours but your headache is screaming again after three hours, you need a backup plan.

It is very helpful if you anticipate all of the different scenarios with your headache caregiver so you can create strategies ahead of time. I promise you, making decisions about these complex issues when your head is pounding is difficult, to say the least.

To make your rescue management even more complex, remember, *to avoid getting the dreaded medication overuse headache, you must limit your use of almost all rescue medications to two days per week.* This can be very complicated. What if you have a third headache day that week? You need contingency plans.

The Keeler Method calls for multiple contingency plans with "layers" of treatment in case you need a different medication or environment. To help you expect the unexpected and help you and your headache care team find the right elements for you, we provide several examples of backup plans. But remember, we have a lot of tools in the toolbox, and any rescue option might have a place in your plans.

In the most typical situation, Plan A didn't work. In this case, a basic Plan B might look like this:

1. If nauseated, take one Zofran and write down time.
2. If head still pounding, take Norgesic Forte and Vistaril. Write down time.
3. Try to drink two glasses of water—small sips if nauseated.
4. Ask Mom to keep the kids overnight (take their school stuff for tomorrow).
5. Call the office and tell them it's a bad one. Let them know who will cover your desk. (Identifying and prepping this person should be part of your prevention plan.)

Some migraineurs might need to anticipate circumstances in which they can't implement Plan A soon enough. For example, suppose you travel occasionally. What if you just boarded a plane to New Orleans, where you will meet five college roommates at a hotel overlooking St. Charles Street during Mardi Gras, and you're getting a migraine? (Actually, something similar once happened to me, but that's another story for another time.) This Plan B would anticipate measures you can take during a flight:

1. Take one Frova and one Sonata. Write down time.
2. Go to the bathroom.
3. Put on eye mask and noise-canceling headphones.
4. Ask attendant for a bottle of water.
5. Then ask attendant not to wake you until you land.

The specific medications and measures are less important than the fact of developing strategies when you don't have a headache that will make sense for your typical, individual situations and the circumstances of your life.

Fortunately, you can prepare as many Plan B's as you might need.

Plan C

Finally, unfortunately, you need Plan C. Plan C comes into play when you have exhausted your resources and need some outside help. You should *never* be in the position where you don't know what else to do. Plan C should involve a couple of other people: a support person and a medical caregiver. Your support person is a family member or close friend who is educated about your headaches. Your medical caregiver is a physician, headache specialist, or (as a last resort) the local emergency room doctor. The important thing is that you need to know where to go for another alternative when nothing works, and you need support from people who know you, know your medicines, and are available to you when you need them.

Needless to say, Plan C takes significant advance planning. It should begin with a discussion in your doctor's office, because you need to know how your doctor wants you to deal with a headache that seems out of control, despite his or her best advice for dealing with it at home.

I believe that as a part of Plan C *every migraineur needs to have access to a real, live person they can contact when they are at their wit's end.* Some doctors will give their migraine patients direct access via a pager or cell phone. Of course, you need to respect this added availability, but over the years I have found it extremely rare that patients abuse this accommodation. At the Keeler Center, our patients have twenty-four-hour access by phone and e-mail to a doctor or nurse practitioner who knows them, and the last layer for our patients' rescue is *me*. If your doctor shares an on-call schedule with other physicians or a nurse practitioner, it can't hurt to meet the on-call caregivers so that they have a sense of who you are when you are not in pain. Not all patients have 24/7 access to their doctor's office, however. Still, in these cases, you *must* know whom to call or where to go when you need help. It is important to have a relationship with your physician that includes access to a physician or other medical care when your rescue plans don't work. You hope such a time will never come, but knowing that you have backup means everything. In circumstances where this kind of relationship with your health care professional is not possible, you still need an ultimate backup plan. This may be a local ER or urgent care center where you can be known in advance, or a knowledgeable friend who can take control of the situation for you.

This is an important concept, because, if at all possible, you do *not* want your last resort to be an anonymous emergency room. Can you think of a more miserable environment for a migraineur? Just when you need peace and quiet, emergency rooms and urgent care facilities bombard your senses with bright fluorescent lights, loud noises, stiff uncomfortable chairs, and lots of activity. Not good. In fact, it is *exactly* the wrong kind of environment for someone with a headache.

Usually, the treatment is even worse. When migraineurs, in desperation, find themselves in an emergency room with no plan, the doctor will often turn to a cabinet full of narcotics, which is *never* the right plan.

The only time emergency room treatment *is* appropriate is when you and your doctor have included it in your plan. In these cases, the ER doctor knows your plan or has access to your doctor, perhaps via a letter that you bring with you, from your doctor. In these situations, your doctor might have requested that the emergency room physician administer a specific medication, since a number of fast-acting and effective treatments can be given only in a medical environment such as a clinic, ER, or hospital. This is the *only* circumstance in which a migraineur should go to the emergency room—unless, of course, you are having an actual emergency.

When Your Plan Takes You to the Emergency Room

If your treatment plan works, you should never need to go to the ER because of your migraines. And if your treatment plan and backup plans aren't effective, you should have a mechanism for working it out with your doctor so your headache does not take you to the ER. But in certain circumstances, you and your doctor might have included emergency room treatment in your plan. Sometimes, a rescue plan includes IV medications as one layer of treatment. A number of fast-acting and effective treatments can be administered only in the emergency room. Not everyone needs IV medication as part of a headache plan, but if your plan includes such a treatment, you need a mechanism in place that allows access twenty-four hours a day, seven days a week. As one of my patients always says, "Headaches don't punch the clock."

Some headache centers (like the Keeler Center) are set up to provide emergency treatment for their patients. But if you are not fortunate enough to live near such a center, your physician or headache specialist can arrange ahead of time with the local ER or urgent care center to provide such services, because the ER doctor needs to know your plan or have access to the doctor who does. If such facilities are part of your rescue plan, it is best to go armed with something more than a pained look on your face. Most ER doctors would be happy to follow an emergency plan set out by your doctor, but it really helps to have some kind of introduction to the facility, either a phone conversation between your primary doctor and the ER physician, or a letter—that you keep with you—from your primary headache doctor to the ER, providing treatment instructions. Also, always carry a list of your medications and drug allergies with you to reduce the amount of thinking and talking you will have to do when you arrive. It will make the ER doc's life a lot easier, as well.

By learning what nonnarcotic solutions are available in the emergency room, you can help direct treatment in the most productive way. While nobody (especially doctors) likes to be told what to do, the ER staff should receive constructive suggestions with a positive attitude. For example, you can go into an emergency room or urgent care facility and say, "I have a severe migraine and have been throwing up a lot. When this has happened before, some IV hydration and something for my nausea have really helped." In the ER, every patient and every circumstance is different. But several alternatives to narcotics have helped my patients at the Keeler Center, and you might ask your doctors or the ER physician to consider these alternatives in a crisis, especially if they are reaching for the narcotics:

- IV or IM Toradol
- IV DHE 45
- IV Depacon
- IV magnesium
- IV hydration
- IV steroids
- IV aspirin (not available in U.S.)
- IM Thorazine
- IV or IM Benadryl
- SQ sumatriptan
- Compazine or Reglan

Each of these rescues can be very successful in the right patient at the right time. The protocols for administering them (dosing, frequency, combinations) are available to every physician and ER.

Marta first came to the Keeler Center because her headaches were out of control. A thirty-one-year-old single mom with two kids and two jobs, she would use Excedrin Migraine, but when that failed she went to the ER. She was going to the ER for relief on almost a weekly basis. She had no primary care physician, and the ER was now balking at treating her, accusing her of drug-seeking behavior. She did not like Demerol, but didn't know there was any other option. As part of her treatment plan, she began carrying a letter from us explaining her condition, recommending an alternative IV rescue, and providing a phone number to call to confirm the legitimacy of the letter. This was an effective stopgap until her lifestyle and preventive measures began to work.

The *Only* Other Reason to Go to the ER: An Actual Emergency!

The emergency room is the ideal place to go when you have an *emergency*, because ER doctors and nurses are extremely skillful in treating emergencies such as broken bones, head trauma, heart attacks, and ruptured appendices. They are *not* trained as internists or general practitioners, and certainly not as neurologists or headache specialists.

Most ER doctors *are* trained to recognize secondary headaches, things like headaches due to subarachnoid hemorrhage, meningitis, brain tumor, or subdural/epidural hematoma following trauma. But a patient who has had headaches for ten or twenty years, and who is having a really bad day, does not rise to the level of "emergency" for most ER doctors. It is not that they lack compassion, but that emergency rooms and urgent-care facilities are not designed to manage chronic illness. Migraines are just *not* what they do, so you and your headache will be bumped to the back of the line to sit under the fluorescent lights for a couple of hours while life-threatening emergencies are triaged past you.

Is This Headache an Emergency?

When you suffer severe pain for hours on end, you might think going to the emergency room or urgent care center is a good idea. Ninety-nine times out of a hundred, it is not.

That means that about one percent of the time, it might be a good idea.

It is rare that a severe headache in someone who has had them before is a life-threatening emergency. For a given migraineur, headaches are pretty similar from one to another in *quality*, the main difference being in intensity. So when a migraineur's headache includes something new or unusual, the patient should consult a doctor to make sure it isn't a dangerous or life-threatening headache. "New or unusual" includes signs or symptoms like blindness in one eye, first-time weakness on one side of the body, or an unusually stiff neck, fever, or chills. Every migraine sufferer should be familiar with headache red flags (see page 68). When a chronic headache sufferer has a "different" headache or red flags, it warrants a call to the doctor. If you cannot reach your doctor, it warrants a trip to the ER. In such cases, be prepared to explain to the triage nurse what is different about this headache.

To use the emergency room more appropriately, migraineurs also need to know how to keep a headache from *becoming* an emergency. For example, migraineurs should be careful to avoid dehydration due to nausea and vomiting. This is best accomplished by drinking small sips over time. Sometimes this is not possible and an IV is the only alternative. Treating the nausea early can help facilitate taking in fluids. Using the Keeler Method, your rescue plans should include instructions for both nausea and hydration.

What Usually Happens in the ER

When a migraineur comes into the ER, the nurses and doctors quickly need to determine whether the headache is a life-threatening emergency, such as a subarachnoid hemorrhage, encephalomyelitis, impending herniation from a brain tumor, or some other *emergency*.

In most emergency rooms, a triage nurse will collect your basic information in order to determine how quickly you need to be evaluated by a doctor. That nurse may also check your vital signs (such as blood pressure, pulse, and temperature) for medical instability, and obtain an initial history, including medications, allergies, and other medical conditions. The nurse will give all of this information to the doctor before your consultation.

ER physicians approach medicine in a slightly different way from other doctors. Their main job—and skill—is in determining whether a patient is in imminent danger, in which case they are prepared to act, quickly. Focusing on the potentially dangerous headaches, most ER doctors will sort out the life-threatening from the serious but not life-threatening. Although pain itself can be an emergency, it is not usually life-threatening. The doctor who sees you will collect additional history and further information, and will perform a physical examination to look for any abnormalities that might point to a life-threatening condition. For example, when viewed through the ophthalmoscope, the eyes can have a typical appearance that raises concern over increased intracranial pressure, a potentially dangerous situation that must be further investigated. Similarly, abnormal eye movements, reflexes, and behaviors can signal concern, so when any of these signs or symptoms are present, the ER doctor will order additional tests. To determine whether a headache is a symptom of a more dangerous underlying disease or condition, the ER doctor might order a CT scan or MRI of the brain, a spinal tap, blood work, or other tests.

Once they know that you are not dying (even though your head is killing you), they pretty much need to get back to real emergencies and saving people's lives, so their work with you is mostly done. Of course, being physicians, they would like to ease your suffering, but they are not trained to manage chronic diseases such as migraine. So the ER doctor is concerned with making sure that the patient is medically stable, offering acute treatment, and making room for the next potentially life-threatening emergency by stopping your pain. And they can. They do know how to put you out of your misery—most often with narcotics. And while you may welcome this, narcotic pain relief is *never* appropriate treatment for a migraine.

At the same time, though, ER doctors don't want to be in the narcotic-dispensing business. For one thing, migraineurs are not the only people who come to the ER looking for pain relief on a recurrent basis. Even if you received narcotics for a headache last month, you will still need to convince the ER staff that you are not a drug seeker. This is not always easy to do, particularly when you have a splitting headache.

Narcotics in the ER

As a result, too often the ER staff will simply treat your pain, usually with a narcotic, and send you out with instructions to follow up with your regular doctor. Unfortunately, narcotics usually wear off before the headache resolves. Then you have to go back (looking like a drug seeker) or suffer for the duration, knowing that the narcotic lowered your pain threshold such that this and future headaches will likely hurt even more. Worse, the narcotic "primed" your pain perception to respond to more narcotics. It is a temporary fix that has serious, long-term, negative effects on migraine.

But unfortunately, there are still ERs out there where combined Demerol and Vistaril remains the cocktail of choice. You might get the Demerol or another narcotic pain reliever, which will probably make you feel better, and then go home. If the headache doesn't go away on its own, it will come back after a few hours, when the drugs wear off, since narcotics only cover up pain but do not treat the cause. Then you are confronted with the prospect of going back to the ER and starting the whole process over again, with the added burden of convincing them that you are not there for drugs but for headache *treatment*. Besides, narcotics are not an ideal rescue. These drugs prime the brain, changing its biochemistry in such a way that headaches become more frequent, more resistant to treatment, and more painful. They are not a good idea.

Some emergency room doctors are getting better at treating migraines. Many are becoming familiar with intravenous rescue options, and are learning that narcotics are counterproductive in migraine rescue.

Have a Plan, and Avoid the ER

Unfortunately, too often, migraineurs wait until a headache is so bad they can't see straight (literally), and then go to the ER, desperate for relief. In these cases, neither the patient nor the ER doctors have a plan, and so they resort to the cabinet full of narcotics. That is *never* the right plan. In addition, too many migraineurs use the emergency room instead of a personal physician; this is a very expensive, inefficient, and ultimately ineffective way to manage headaches. The emergency room *is* a valuable resource when all else fails or when you are very concerned, but it should never be your primary care facility, because ER staff are not in the business of developing treatment plans, generating differential diagnoses, or doing anything else beyond the immediate situation before them. For this reason alone, you should never rely on the emergency room to manage chronic conditions, including migraine. Instead, see your primary care physician, a neurologist, or a headache specialist for ongoing headache management.

Chapter 7

Build Your Support System

or most migraineurs, headaches are a fact of life. It doesn't help to get fed up with them. It doesn't help to deny that they exist. It doesn't help to blame yourself for being a bad person, or to blame anyone else. At best, you can fix partial blame on your parents, since migraines tend to run in families. Yet in our frustration and desperation, at one time or another, most of us do all of the above.

We live in denial. We blame our spouses, our doctors, our lives. But in the end, we still have our headaches.

One of the biggest problems we have is that we do not have a good time to deal with our headaches. When we have a headache, we are so befuddled and in such pain that it is difficult to put a sentence together, much less a treatment plan. And then, when we feel fine and normal and the headache is gone, the last thing we want to think about is what we will do next time our head hurts. So the essential question is: *When* is the time to develop a strategy for dealing with your headaches?

We have to remember that migraines are a chronic disease. In many respects, they are no different from diabetes, asthma, or depression. As with those disorders, we can manage migraines well or badly.

Patients are the best custodians of their own headaches. Of course, some migraineurs will need to consult a health professional—a physical therapist, a primary care physician, or even a headache specialist—but the better you understand your headaches, the better you can captain a team effectively and efficiently.

When it comes to dealing with headaches, doctors, family members, friends, and coworkers will all take their cues from you, the migraine sufferer. If you tell your doctor that everything is fine, odds are that the doctor will believe it. And if you report that medications aren't working, the doctor will likely go with that.

To manage well, migraine patients can employ some important tools to organize a support network to help with their headaches. Our Keeler questionnaires expedite this process. The detailed information you provide in these questionnaires will help you and your clinician analyze your headache history and current condition so you can promptly get on with the work of getting better.

Once you have your doctor onboard with your plan, it is important to also enlist the help of someone close to you, preferably someone with a soft voice, a steady hand, and a good measure of compassion. With a little education, you can engage a spouse, child, close friend, or coworker to help you when a headache begins. This on-call caregiver might tell you to take your medicine *now*, or take a walk, or lie down—whatever your rescue strategy calls for. This kind of support can make all the difference in improving your life.

It is hard to communicate when you have a headache, so you need someone who can speak for you, look for your sunglasses, or tell you that you are behaving irrationally. This is the person who would drive you to the ER or call your doctor and write down any instructions, put water by your bed or give you a shot of DHE-45, run to the pharmacy to pick up a prescription, or figure out how to block that sliver of light shining through the space between the window and the blind. It wouldn't hurt if this person had your medical power of attorney, but that is not essential. The Keeler Method includes more tips for educating family members about the dos and don'ts of caring for someone with headache.

A Migraine Personality?

As we approach the task of effectively managing our migraine strategy, it helps to understand a bit about who we are. The question often arises, *Is there a "migraine personality"?* To be sure, certain characteristics are more common among migraineurs. I like to cite depth of character, extraordinary grace and beauty, and boundless intelligence, though the scientific data on these are somewhat controversial. On the other hand, people often suggest the type A personality.

Beyond epidemiologic curiosity, I do not find these kinds of observations particularly helpful, since on an individual basis there is little we can do about such immutable characteristics. In managing migraines, it is much more helpful to identify patterns that either help protect us from headaches or seem to promote them. I have found that many patients tend to approach their lives with migraines in typical ways. Obviously, some of these approaches are better than others.

One way to judge how effectively you have integrated migraine management into your life is to look at the following "types" and ask yourself if there are elements of these admittedly exaggerated behaviors in yourself. Then consider how well they are working out for you.

- **The Professional Migraineur:** With the best of intentions, this patient has made a career out of their headaches, with every action aimed at reducing, avoiding, or understanding their headache syndrome. What is wrong with this? In substance, nothing. In degree, everything. These patients often have lost sight of the "big picture," which is to live as full and productive lives as they possibly can, given that they have a "condition." At some point, the professional migraineur needs to stop and say, "Okay. This is what I've learned. Now I am going to stop focusing on migraines and live my life." This is very hard to do, to be sure, but accomplishing this task is migraineurs' ultimate goal.

- **The Super Shopper:** There should be a pill out there that will take away headaches. I agree. There should be. Alas, there isn't. At least, there is not one pill for everyone. The Super Shopper keeps looking for the magic bullet, often going from doctor to doctor and from alternative therapy to alternative therapy, hoping that this will be the one thing that will put an end to the headaches. Unfortunately, very rarely do headache syndromes get "cured." For almost all of us, the solution will be an amalgamation of lots of little things and medium-sized things that ultimately result in fewer, less severe headaches.

- **The "Been There, Done That" Patient:** This subset of the Super Shopper group includes patients who look for instant results with each new treatment and, when the results are not dramatic, abandon it. There can be many reasons for a particular therapy's not working:
  - medication dosing problems;
  - duration of the trial (how long you give the treatment a chance to show an effect);
  - conflicting treatments that reduce the effectiveness of the trial;
  - bad timing (such as trying a new treatment the day you are served court papers or have your gallbladder removed).

  Treatments don't exist in a vacuum. We always need to look at the context of the trial and not give up too soon.

- **The Great Prioritizer:** Different from the Great Decider, Prioritizers are people who tend to put off addressing personal health problems (like migraines) in favor of taking care of business. The extreme case is outright denial: "I don't have time for headaches. I have too much to do." Of course, this doesn't work too well since a headache has its natural course. We try to encourage these patients to take time to try and identify the factors that may contribute to the headaches, map out a plan for what they will do when a headache strikes, and manage their headaches appropriately.

- **Fear Treaters:** Fear Treaters will do almost *anything* to avoid getting a headache. This often takes the form of daily medication, usually upon awakening. Sometimes, they say they "can't afford" to have a headache, but at other times the prospect of that horrible pain is motivation enough. The problem with this approach is that it often leads to medication overuse and chronic daily headache. A greater problem with this approach is that it puts the migraine in the driver's seat, while we are acting out of fear from a position of weakness, rather than from a position of knowledge and control.

Being the Boss: Four Qualities of an Excellent Headache Manager

To manage your life around your migraines, now and in the future, you will be more successful if you are a good headache manager. With a strong and healthy approach to living life as a migraineur, you can create healthy strategies for living with your headaches, rather than fighting them. To be an excellent migraine manager, you will do well to develop these four skills: openness, communication, consistency, and persistence.

Openness

As a disease entity, headaches have seen tremendous changes in recent years. Both the science and the care have gotten much better. As headache specialists, we have learned a lot from our patients, our research, and alternative and complementary approaches.

Everyone has a different threshold for trying new things. Some people prefer to wait until a treatment has been around for a while before trying it, while other patients want to try each new modality as soon as it is available. Ideally, with your physician, you can work your way through each new approach and determine whether it is legitimate, safe, and suitable for your situation.

Not every treatment is right for every patient, but every patient should have someone who is knowledgeable and who can educate you, answer your questions, and support your search for the best treatment. I have yet to meet the patient who couldn't teach me something about headaches, and I have yet to meet a patient who couldn't benefit from some time with the Keeler Method. It is important for chronic migraineurs to:

- consider both traditional and alternative treatments
- decide what fits your headaches best
- stay aware
- keep an open mind about contributing factors

Communication

Too often, headache sufferers tell me that their headaches are out of control but they won't see their doctor for another four months. On a larger scale, study after study has shown that the headache patients who do best are those who see their doctors on a regular basis, and whose doctors are actively involved in their headache management. As with any disease, when migraine is left unchecked, it is much, much harder to get back under control.

It is not always easy to engage a doctor who does not have a specific interest in headaches, but all doctors are sensitive to the patient in pain. (If not, they should consider a career in law.) Make sure your doctor hears you when you report how well or poorly you are doing. We see our patients weekly or more often when they are new to the clinic or not doing well. As things improve, we begin to spread out the visits, but even our shining stars come to see us for therapy or a follow-up visit at least monthly or every two months.

As the patient, it is important that you establish ground rules with your team, and ask yourself:

- Who is on your team?
- Will you work with and get headache medications from more than one doctor?
- Will others be involved (a pharmacist, chiropractor, yoga instructor, counselor)?
- Do the members of your team talk to each other?
- Do you present the same picture to each of your teammates?
- When do you decide whether your plan is working—or not?
- Whom do you call and under what circumstances?
- Is e-mail an option?
- How does your team feel about visits to the ER?

By establishing and respecting the lines of communication, your treatment plan can stay vital and organic, evolving with the inevitable changes of life. The old "Take two aspirin and call me in the morning" approach is outdated. To manage headaches in the best possible way, patients and their treatment team need to observe and discuss all aspects of the patient's migraine management—strategies for lifestyle monitoring, prevention, and rescue. To accomplish this, migraine patients need to:

- assemble a treatment team
- be an effective team leader
- help the physician understand their headaches
- strategize how to approach the treatment team with the plan
- guide the doctor to the best treatments

Consistency

Often, we decide, "To hell with it! I'm going to do what I want to do and if I get a headache, that's just too bad." The obverse is the person who says, "I'd love to do that, but forget it, I just can't handle the inevitable headache I'd get." Fortunately, with a little planning and some resourceful scheming, we can often do the things we want to do—without inviting disaster the next day.

Some evidence suggests that careful management of such things as diet, sleep habits, stress, and exercise can actually *increase your resistance to headaches*. Thus, triggers can recede, headache severity can lessen, and pleasure in life can improve. The key to this approach is in achieving consistency in these four important aspects of lifestyle.

For example, suppose salsa dancing is what makes your heart sing, but the smoke, noise, and alcohol that so often coexist with salsa palaces make such an evening out a sure bet for a migraine afterward. So, one migraineur might decide, "To hell with it. I'm going to have fun and deal with the headache later." Another might say, "I would love to go but I think I'll stay home and watch reruns of *Happy Days*, instead." But an alternative to either of these approaches is probably a better way to live. With a little modification, pretreatment, or restraint, you could enjoy the dancing without the headache. If you have the room, you can have the salsa dance at your home, where you can more or less control the environment—at least to outlaw smoking. Or, you can wear earplugs that do not completely eliminate sound but soften it so it is bearable. Or, you could dance but not drink. You could dance, but not until three a.m. You could be ultimately cool and wear sunglasses indoors, even late at night, to protect against the lights. (This last, however, may cross several lines.)

This example may be extreme, but the idea is not. When we anticipate triggers, we can usually find creative ways to avoid, modify, or protect against them with medication. These days, my headaches are not too frequent. I have the luxury of taking a triptan before going into a potentially triggering situation, and that is usually enough to allow me the freedom to live my life. When it doesn't work, a second triptan, usually with a nonsteroidal anti-inflammatory, does the trick.

Consistency does *not* mean life has to be tedium. It means that migraineurs try to maintain a consistent approach to the major areas—sleep, eating, stress, and exercise—so they can manage their headaches without making unconstructive decisions based on denial, fear, or fatalism.

Persistence

We don't have a perfect treatment. At best, a *good* plan will dramatically decrease the frequency, severity, and duration of headaches. So, when a patient goes three months or one month or even a week on a "new plan" and then gets a headache, it does not mean that the plan was ill conceived or even that they need a new plan. In fact, recent work from Michael Moskowitz, M.D., Ph.D., and others has shown that most preventives do not reach their maximum effect for up to three months. So we need to set realistic goals and then monitor (with a headache diary) to see if we're reaching those goals.

Suppose you decide you want to try the herbal preventive feverfew. Feverfew takes about three months to manifest benefits, so it does no good to take it for a week and then ask, "Now what?" Every treatment plan needs endpoints. This is the only way to systematically assess how well the plan is working—or not. Then it is important to stick with a plan until the results clearly indicate it is not for you. You may know within a day or two if a new medication has nasty side effects. Sometimes, a plan might be good enough to justify fine-tuning over several months, as is often the case with lifestyle modification, for example.

For better or worse, most of us developed and reinforced our behaviors over many years. When we set about changing these behaviors, it is unrealistic to expect changes to occur in days or weeks. It is the very rare headache patient who sees dramatic change immediately. Far more commonly, benefits from lifestyle modifications come gradually, over weeks and months of careful changes to our medicines, sleep rhythms, exercise patterns, eating habits, and stress levels.

Unfortunately, in most cases, we can't cure migraine. Even with the best plan and when the stars align just so, a headache can still come on. We can't control the stars, but we can manage and control many other triggers out there.

Use Your Resources to Your Advantage

Insurance and Employers

As a headache sufferer, you have many resources available to you.

If you have financial issues, remember that most pharmaceutical companies provide medications on a "compassionate" basis. You may need to jump through some hoops in terms of demonstrating need, but you can do this. Also, most companies that manufacture headache medications have a variety of patient services available via phone and on the Internet.

Insurance is a tricky business. Insurance companies don't exactly have the same priorities that you and your doctor have. Sometimes, it is necessary to explain to your insurer why it is in the company's best interest to allow you and your doctor to make your medical decisions. For example, some headache medications are expensive, as much as fifteen dollars or more for a single pill. To be sure, this is a lot of money, and some insurance companies limit the number of pills they will cover during a given period. This is *not* a medical decision, but an economic one. So telling them that you "need" more pills might not be a very persuasive argument. On the other hand, if you reason that without the doctor's recommended number of pills at fifteen dollars apiece they will likely have to pay more money because you will instead go to the emergency room, which will cost thousands of dollars, they may agree to cover the cost of the pills.

In general, when you provide adequate information to your insurer, you can get the coverage for what you need. To be sure, this is not always the case, but it is certainly worth the effort. It helps if you encourage your treating physicians to accurately document your history and treatment plan so that it will support any claim to your insurer.

Similarly, your employers do not always share your priorities, so it is important to present your needs in terms they will relate to. Start out nicely, and be constructive. You might point out the elements in the workplace that trigger or exacerbate your headaches, making you less productive. Many excellent studies prove this is so. If the flicker of the fluorescent lights hurts your head, then it is *in your employer's interest* to replace the bulbs with full-spectrum lighting. If wearing sunglasses allows you to remain at work, then the company's "no sunglasses indoors" policy may need rethinking, and so forth.

Unfortunately, sometimes "nice" doesn't work. That is why we have human resources departments and the Americans with Disabilities Act. These avenues are available *for people like us,* so do not hesitate to use them when you have to.

Enlisting a Doctor's Help

Several years ago, a new patient came to see me.

"I have had headaches for thirty years," she said. "I know I don't have a brain tumor, but I decided to come see you anyway."

Thank God, I thought, giving her my best look of concern. *You got here just in time!*

On the one hand, she was right: someone who has had headaches for years is not likely to have a brain tumor. On the other hand, what a tragedy that she waited thirty years to get help!

If migraineurs make one mistake related to seeking medical help for their headaches, it is in *not* seeking help early enough. Many migraineurs don't go to the doctor until their headaches have completely taken over their lives, and at this stage it is much harder to get the headaches under control than if the patient had sought medical attention earlier.

When you don't have a headache, you feel perfectly fine, and it seems silly to go to the doctor when you're fine. But in migraine management, we have a name for this: denial. It is very understandable. Headaches consume a lot of our time, and the last thing we want to do when we don't have one is work on our headaches. Yet it *is* important and worth doing. Migraine management requires strategic thinking and insight, which you do not exactly have when your brain hurts. Besides, a doctor can develop preventive strategies and be much more effective when you're well, with the luxury of time on your side. It is much harder to treat someone in crisis.

Except for a few very twisted individuals, people don't go to the doctor unless they have to. This is unfortunate, for a number of reasons. People often suffer longer than necessary, without the most effective treatment. And, without the best information, they can make decisions that actually *worsen* their condition.

So, if you wonder whether you need to see a doctor, you probably do.

The more complicated issue has to do with *what* doctor to see. We basically have three levels of medical help for headache care in this country. The front line is your primary care doctor—and everyone should have a primary care doctor. Some are very interested in headaches and skilled in their treatment, but others are not. If you find it difficult to get your doctor to focus on your headaches, it is fair to ask if your physician is interested and experienced in treating migraines. At any point, if you feel that you have exhausted your primary doctor's interest and/or expertise, it is time to get a referral to the next level of care.

The second level is a general neurologist. Most (but not all) neurologists have additional training and experience with headaches, and should be able to provide a more comprehensive treatment plan. Again, it is fair to ask neurologists about their interest and success in headache management.

The third level of headache care comes from headache specialists or headache centers. Often in private practice, headache specialists are usually neurologists with advanced training or long experience in headaches.

A headache center, on the other hand, is usually multidisciplinary, with ancillary resources for headache treatment, including physical medicine, counseling, inpatient treatment, and urgent care.

Prepare for Your Appointment

After you have decided to enlist the help of a physician, it's up to you to get ready for it. The first important thing you can do is schedule an appointment *specifically* to talk about your headaches. This establishes headaches as a health priority for you and, in your physician's mind, moves headaches way up on your problem list. It also ensures that the visit will be coded for headaches, and when your doctor submits the bill to your insurer, you will become a headache sufferer in the insurer's computer. This will, in turn, give you access to many medications that insurers will cover only if you carry that diagnosis, and should you request referral to a neurologist or headache specialist down the road, you will have a clear paper trail to support your petition. This is critical, especially for people with HMO-type insurance.

If possible, schedule enough time with your provider so you can adequately go through all of your headache issues. If they balk, you can honestly promise them that a little extra time this visit will result in fewer visits down the road, fewer late-night and weekend calls, and overall better care for your headaches.

It helps if you organize your headache history and your current situation so you can efficiently inform the physician about headache frequency, symptoms, triggers, medications, lifestyle issues, previous therapies, and so on. Either with the benefit of our questionnaires or through your own devices, it is extremely important to provide your headache doctor with complete and accurate information. When you come to your appointment well prepared, you will not only endear yourself to your doctor by saving huge amounts of time, but you will also improve the quality of the care you receive by focusing the history and exam through your excellent preparation.

One crucial part of this preparation is to know, and express, what you want and expect from the consultation with the doctor. If all you ask for is confirmation that your headaches are non-life-threatening, you may leave with that assurance and nothing else. If you ask for a cure, you may leave without anything at all. Be very clear in expressing your expectations, whether you need a prescription for a new preventive, a rescue strategy, a new lifestyle plan, nonpharmacological treatments, or referrals to specialists who can help you implement your treatment plan. Ask how you (and your doctor) will determine whether the plan is working or not. Ask if there is a backup plan. Ask if the physician uses e-mail for patients with episodic, recurrent conditions like migraines, or how else you can maintain contact. Ask about medications, concurrent illnesses, travel, physical activity, and other concerns. Ask! Ask, ask, ask!

During their training, most primary care doctors attend only a couple of hours of lectures on headaches. After that, they might learn more, but migraine competes against many other health conditions for each doctor's continuing education. Some doctors don't know much about headaches, beyond ordering a CAT scan or MRI to make sure you don't have a brain tumor. So it can be enormously helpful if you come to your appointment well prepared. I can't tell you how many times I have been met with a blank stare when I asked a new patient questions like:

- How old were you when your headaches started?
- About how many days per month do you have headaches?
- What things make your headaches worse or better?

Your carefully considered answers to such questions, combined with an appropriate neurological exam, can significantly help guide your clinician to the proper diagnosis. So if you work through the questionnaire in Appendix 1, you can arrive in your doctor's office prepared to answer these important questions. And, on the off chance that the doctor does not ask the right questions, you can provide a narrative of your headaches that will accomplish the same thing.

At the Keeler Center, on every physician contact, we have someone taking notes for the patient so that the patient can concentrate on listening. Most doctors' offices don't provide this luxury, so bring a pen and paper to your doctor visit. List your questions before the appointment and leave space to note the answers. There is nothing worse than waiting weeks or months for an appointment, then developing stage fright (or "white-coat panic") and rushing through the appointment only to find yourself sitting in the parking lot wondering what just happened.

After that, very often, there's a big gap between what *we* think we're doing, what our *doctors* think we're doing, and what we really *are* doing. These differences can result in overlooking or discarding potentially effective therapies—and worse. The questionnaire in Appendix 2 helps organize records of your medications to make sure that everyone is on the same page. If you don't overlook potentially effective therapies or trash something without giving it a fair trial, you and your doctor can assess the effectiveness of various therapies to find the most effective alternatives. These questionnaires will help you organize what you have already tried for your headaches so you won't end up repeating failed treatments, but will learn from them, and then be equipped to help your doctor design the most effective plan.

Interacting with Your Doctor

Most migraineurs get advice from many different sources, such as friends, various doctors, the Internet, direct-to-consumer advertisements, chiropractors, stylists, grocers, strangers on the subway… This is not necessarily a bad thing unless you have no way of validating the information you receive. Many times, patients' thirdhand stories have led me to interesting and unique solutions to the mysteries of headaches—Tiger Balm, jasmine tea, oxblood-red sunglasses, and the banana-peel cure, among many other tips. I turned over all sorts of odd explanations for why the banana peel might work, from transdermal absorption of potassium or other essential elements, to a cooling, patchouli-like effect from the skin. Finally, I learned that this miracle cure had come from a bogus letter to Ann Landers that was a complete spoof. Still, of course, the myth persists. Every so often, a patient still brings it up. In fact, if you go online and search "banana peel headache," you will get thousands of hits.

Another patient was admitted to the hospital with an incessant bloody nose. She had a somewhat rare headache type for which I had prescribed a powerful anti-inflammatory. But on her own, she had added the herbal medicine ginkgo biloba, which, unfortunately, thins the blood, as does the anti-inflammatory. She ended up in the hospital. Medicine is medicine, regardless of whether it requires a prescription.

It is important that you have someone who will oversee what you are taking and help you sort through the things you hear because, sometimes, the suggestions can be downright dangerous. One patient was told he needed "an adjustment" to get rid of his new headache, but he turned out to have a vertebral artery dissection. An "adjustment" would likely have paralyzed him, or worse. Ideally, you should talk to a doctor about these suggestions before you try them. This is an important function for health care professionals today, when information can be found everywhere. If your health care professional does not agree with me, you might look for another health care professional. That said, there are better and worse ways to bring these ideas to your doctor's attention.

Often, for various reasons, I am in the position of "recommending" a treatment to another physician who will write the prescription but who may not know as much about headaches as I do. I have found that it is better to educate and suggest rather than to order or demand. The same goes for the wily patient. When you hear about a new medicine or other treatment, before you talk to your doctor, do a little homework beyond what you heard at the water cooler. You may find out that it is not worth bringing up at all, or you may gain additional insight that will strengthen your case. Then you can enlist your doctor's participation in looking for possible solutions, such as the one you heard about. This may seem painfully obvious, but I can tell you from firsthand experience, it isn't. Consider these two scenarios:

- "Doctor Cowan, my stylist gets migraines, and she takes a medicine called Pixie Dust. How come you never prescribed that for me? I want you to write me a prescription for that." Several things go through my mind. If I have never heard of Pixie Dust, I am certainly not going to write a prescription for it, nor am I particularly thrilled about having to admit to my patient that I am ignorant. (I'm not saying I *won't* admit it;

I'm just not thrilled about it.) If I do know the drug and have ruled it out because it lowers the blood pressure and this patient already has low blood pressure, or because it causes hair loss and she's practically bald as is, or for some other reason, I am not thrilled about having to spend time defending my decision not to prescribe it. (Again, not that I won't, but it takes time that could be spent more productively.) Plus, nobody likes to be told what to do.

- "Doctor Cowan, have you ever heard of a medicine called Pixie Dust? I looked it up on the Internet and it says it can help headaches, but it's a blood pressure medicine and I already take a blood pressure medicine. What do you think?" Now, this is someone I can work with. She is open, has invested some time, and wants my opinion. I like that.

Doctors are human. We can feel threatened, overworked, intimidated, frustrated, all the things that other people feel. Sometimes, the white-coat thing can make patients (and doctors) forget that. But in general, if you approach your doctor with the same respect and openness that you expect in return, it will work out well. And again, if your doctor does not respond to this approach, you might want to find another doctor.

Fortunately, most (but sadly, not all) Americans do have access to a local health care provider. For the most part, these are bright, caring individuals who would love to help you get your headaches under control. Unfortunately, even the most well-meaning doctors are often overworked, undertrained (in headaches), and handcuffed by their employers and/or your insurance. What, then, do health care providers bring to the table? For starters, they can write prescriptions, and most people with headaches bad enough that they read this book are going to need a prescription, probably several. More than that, most health care professionals are also reasonably bright and have a more thorough understanding of human physiology, anatomy, and pharmacology than you do. So once you get them onboard, your health care providers can be a tremendously valuable resource.

Enlisting Your Loved Ones

In about 1992, I was involved in the clinical trial of a new migraine medication that had to be loaded into a complicated injecting device for delivery just under the skin. I had this "kit" placed prominently on the shelf in my bathroom, ready for launch at the first sign of a headache. About two weeks later, the headache came. Boy, did the headache come. It started around midday and, like an idiot (I really didn't know any better at the time), I decided to wait until the end of the day to try the new shot. Predictably, my day ended earlier than I had anticipated. By the time I got home, my head was pounding way too hard and the light in the bathroom was way too bright for me to read the seemingly complex instructions on loading and dispensing the medication. So I darkened the room and crawled into bed to wait.

When my wife got home an hour or so later, she came into the room, turned on the light, and asked if I was okay. I felt that I had been transported to an amphitheater's center stage. The forty-watt bulb seemed like a floodlight, my wife's gentle whisper the ring announcer's stentorian shout. The next fifteen minutes, while she figured out how to give me that medication, were some of the longest and most painful minutes of my life. Fifteen years later, it is still burned into my memory.

Fortunately, we have both gotten much better at managing my headaches. We have learned some painful lessons in how to deal with a severe headache—and how not to.

In families with migraines, we frequently see two approaches from significant others that result in bad outcomes. The first is the well-meaning person who wants to help but, not knowing what to do, turns to the headache sufferer for instruction. This problem is easily fixed with a conversation at another time, when the migraineur is well. This education can help the caregiver play an effective role, not just in migraine rescue, but in implementing lifestyle changes aimed at prevention as well.

The other type of person who can wreak havoc on a headache sufferer is the one who takes the headaches "personally." At some level, this person may feel that the headaches are his or her fault—or the migraineur's fault. These people might not understand why the migraine sufferer didn't get anything done all day, or why they couldn't do "the simplest thing." Often, they do not understand that migraine is a disease, as real as diabetes or asthma or heart failure. In my office, this person usually sits across from me, arms folded, leaning back in the chair with looks alternating between skepticism and contempt. These people do not help. In these cases, again, it is a matter of education. But it might be better if the education comes from the doctor, rather than from the migraineur. Until these "support" people understand the realities of headache, they will do more to worsen the situation than to improve it.

The people in your life should never think of your headaches as an excuse to avoid something unpleasant. If they do, they need some serious education. I hope this book will provide you with the tools to accomplish that education. With healthy support at home, this education can go both ways. You can learn a lot from your family. Your loved ones can often be very helpful in spotting triggers and behaviors that contribute to your headaches. The more they understand about your headaches, and headaches in general, the more helpful they can be, both during a headache and in preventing them.

Education

One day, my wife told me we had been invited to a cocktail party, and she immediately added that if I didn't want to go she would cover for me. Now, I am not exactly a party guy, and over the years, my wife and I have struggled with this, since she likes to socialize a lot more than I do. But in my defense, I have to say that I have made (what I consider) great strides in this area and, for example, no longer bring my electronic chess game to social events. So I protested, asserting that I would love to go to the cocktail party, couldn't wait to go, was *dying* to go. She reiterated that I didn't have to go, and we left it at that.

As luck (fate?) would have it, on the day of the party, I felt the beginnings of a migraine. Circumstances conspired such that I didn't treat it immediately and, by the time I got home, it was well on its way to becoming a monster. So I had a dilemma: my wife already expected me to wimp out on the party, to which I really did have every intention of going, and yet there I was with a migraine. Being a typical migraineur, I decided to macho through it, not say anything, and most of all, avoid that half-doubting look that every migraineur has seen in this situation.

Unfortunately, of course, the headache got worse. I couldn't cover it over. I needed a bathroom, a bed, and total quiet and darkness, doubting looks be damned. This particular melodrama actually played out fairly well. I medicated, slept, and, much to my wife's surprise, showed up at the party about two hours late, but I got there, nonetheless. My wife is a brilliant, compassionate person who genuinely loves me. Still, there are times when I sense she just doesn't "get" my migraines. And realistically, how could she? She doesn't get migraines.

We have all been through these complex emotional roller coasters filled with self-doubt and resentment, neediness and desperation. In retrospect, our stories can be funny, but at the time, they are painful, painful, painful. No matter how much scientific evidence and just plain common sense is focused on the subject, there is still no way for someone who does not get migraines to understand how we feel. At some level, nonmigraineurs often see migraines as things that are somehow under our conscious control, things that we can bring out at will for a convenient excuse, or roll back out of sight when it suits us. This "Not tonight, honey" view of migraine is a source of much tension and anxiety in many relationships. Thus, the impact of migraine goes well beyond the hell inside your head. It can stretch its nasty tentacles into the very fiber of your existence. Treating migraine is not just a matter of finding the right pain pill. Treating migraine means treating the lives of those affected by the condition, giving control back to the migraineur, and wresting it away from the migraine—as much as possible. On a regular basis, husbands, wives, parents, children, and friends ask me how they can help loved ones with their headaches. People who don't get headaches don't really "get" those of us who do. It isn't that they don't care or don't believe us. They just don't understand what it is like to have a monster headache. It is very hard for someone who has never had a migraine to understand how painful and disabling it can be. What's more, the timing of migraines can be incredibly inconvenient, often crashing in on social events, weekends, or routine responsibilities, like making dinner. Unless someone understands the condition, migraines can seem like an annoyance, an inconvenience, or even a ploy. So a big part of living with a headache sufferer is education.

At least usually, migraines are not used as an excuse to get out of exercise, vacations, outings, or travel. While we often hear of the "convenient" headache that seems to come up when it is time to visit the in-laws or go to the company Christmas party, anyone with migraines will tell you there is no such thing as a *convenient* headache. This is one of the most pernicious myths associated with migraines. If I could get one message out to the non-headache-suffering world, this would be it: No sane person chooses a headache over anything short of a firing squad, and some of us *would* choose the firing squad in the midst of a bad headache. It is extremely unusual (and probably really bad karma) to use a headache as an excuse to avoid anything. Often, however, the stress and anxiety associated with putting yourself in a vulnerable position (one that may lead to a headache) may in fact trigger a headache. But that is a far cry from fabricating a migraine. Still, the waters can get muddy.

When I speak on migraine, I often show a slide of a PET scan in which the part of the brain where migraines are generated lights up bright red. Even well-educated people are astonished to see this physical evidence of migraine. Of course, those of us with migraines say, "Duh!" But in fact, most of the conditions that we once thought of as "psychological" have proven to have very clear *physical* underpinnings, and functional imaging studies actually allow us to observe how the brain works in many of these conditions. Abnormalities are often obvious.

Those of us with headaches, and those of us who study those of us with headaches, know *without a doubt* that headaches have a clear biological basis. As a case in point, the newest class of drugs for migraine treatment, the triptans, effectively eliminates the pain for most patients—but is useless for other pains such as broken arms, back injuries, or post-surgical pain.

Unfortunately, even today, spouses, parents, and children of migraineurs frequently ask whether headaches are psychological, and even migraineurs themselves occasionally question whether their headaches are their own "fault." One problem is that migraine has no obvious outward sign, no easily obtainable blood test or X-ray, and no objective measure for the disease or its pain. Since headaches seem to come out of the blue and disappear just as mysteriously, it can be very hard for people who don't get headaches to understand them.

It is important for loved ones to discuss these issues at a headache-free time, because it is impossible to do so when a headache strikes, and no one wants to talk about a headache after it is over. Booklets and videos are fine, but nothing works as well as a family discussion about headaches and what to do when someone in the family gets one. The Keeler Method includes some tips and talking points for such a discussion.

Especially if migraines are chronic or poorly controlled, they do take a toll on relationships, not so much in the acute headache as in the cumulative effect on the family. If migraines become disruptive to the point where the person cannot actively and regularly participate in the relationship, it is important to start breaking down the relationship to look for triggers. You need to explore whether the relationship is an innocent casualty of other triggers, or if stress in the relationship *is* the trigger. It is tough, but do not shy away from looking at the relationship itself. Finances, responsibilities, sex, social obligations, and extended family can frequently be problematic. Sometimes, it is the kids, and you have to address this head-on as well. Remember, stress is the most common trigger for migraine. Your task is to identify the source of the stress, even if it is within the family relationship.

Very often, loved ones feel helpless, defensive, and even angry in the face of a migraine. This is especially so when the sufferer is the main character in the family, responsible for significant responsibilities, and depended upon for routine care and feeding. In these situations and many others, it helps when family members understand what a migraine is, how it affects the migraineur, and how it affects the rest of the family. Just as we educate loved ones about a family member's diabetes or asthma, we should also educate about migraines. The more your family knows about the disease in general and your headaches in particular, the better they can help you prevent headaches and manage them when they occur.

The Family "Headache Meeting"

It is important to sit down and discuss the issue, but how do you do this? Assuming you are at least slightly acquainted with the person whom you are hoping to educate, you have a better sense than I do of the best way to approach the subject. So I can't help you there. But I do have some advice regarding *when* to bring it up, as well as some talking points you should cover in this discussion.

Timing is important. I know, you do not want to talk about your headaches during your precious, pain-free moments. But it is really important to do this. Do not start to have this discussion when you are in pain, or when a headache is coming on or just resolving.

At a time when you are well, discuss with your loved one exactly what you would like them to do to help you, to care for you. In a given person, most headaches do not vary from one to another except in severity. Each headache is pretty much like the next, so you likely know what will help during your headaches, and you need to share this information with family members, and perhaps friends, coworkers, and others. Tell your support people what your headache feels like and what you would like from them. If you don't tell them, they probably will not have any idea what you go through and what you want or need.

You might explain something like this: "When I have a migraine, I need you to leave me alone in the bedroom. Do not just shut the door. Please leave a cool washcloth in a bowl on my nightstand, with a glass of ice water. It helps a lot if you make sure the TV doesn't blare in the next room, and if the kids don't shout conversations in the hallway. Please do not come in every ten minutes and ask me how I am, but if you could refresh my water every hour or so, that would be great. Just don't ask me any questions about household stuff. And, when you come into bed, please be as quiet as you possibly can."

Most headache sufferers experience a phase during the headache when *any* stimulus is painful. This may be right from the beginning or an hour or two into the headache, and it will help your family be sensitive if you tell them about this. A minority of migraineurs find that gentle stroking of the head or neck is soothing, but most do not want any stimulus, so if you just need cool water, medication, and maybe a damp washcloth, explain this clearly. Then your caregiver can quietly set them by the side of the bed—without announcing this small kindness.

It is best if you have your comprehensive meeting with your doctor *before* your loved ones get too involved. Until doctor and patient have a headache management plan in place, you cannot have a very detailed discussion with the family. However, sometimes, the first and most important thing family members can do will be to convince you that it is time to seek medical help. If your loved ones raise this with you, you should probably listen.

Taking your migraines for granted, you might not realize their impact on your life (and the lives of the people around you) until things are seriously disrupted. Sometimes, it helps if family members keep notes, maybe record how many headaches you have over a month or two, how many days you've lost, events you've missed, and appointments you've rescheduled.

When you have an appointment with your doctor to discuss your treatment plan, this is an ideal opportunity for your "primary caregiver," usually the spouse, parent, or child, to come along. Some doctors will be happy to discuss the loved one's role in headache care, while others will prefer that you work these things out on your own time.

Then, your family discussion should try to define what role the support person should play in headache care. This topic is well worth the effort, and helps eliminate a lot of stress on everyone's part. One migraineur might want their loved one to assume all the care and feeding responsibilities, give medications, and call their employer, while another might only want their caregiver to close the door behind them on their way out. Every headache sufferer has different needs. With a little effort, everyone can understand those needs during a headache, and the rest of the time, too.

Lifestyle Support

A good headache management plan has three parts—lifestyle modification, prevention, and rescue. The latter two might mostly be medications, so other than reminding a headache sufferer to take his or her medicine, loved ones cannot do much about those. But friends and family can have a *huge* role in lifestyle modification, and might even have a very positive impact on the migraineur's health. Lifestyle modifications include two categories: avoiding triggers, and maintaining healthy routines around sleep, exercise, and diet.

Every migraineur has a different set of triggers. The more the people close to you know about which activities are likely to set off a headache, the better able they will be to help and support your efforts to avoid or prepare for them.

Interestingly, migraineurs do get food cravings. It is not clear whether the cravings are simply a warning that a headache is on the way, or whether they're a more sinister symptom, like a trigger.

In any case, suppose your daughter gets a migraine when she eats chocolate. You might remind her that the chocolate in the cabinet is not good for her because it can give her a headache, and that when others are eating chocolate cake for dessert, she should not have any. Helpful? Not really. How about if you find alternative treats and desserts to keep around, and don't keep chocolate in the house? That would be a much more constructive approach. Is this fair to the rest of the family? Probably not. But that's not the question. After all, if you had a diabetic child, you probably wouldn't keep a pantry full of sugar.

Healthy routines are an extremely important part of migraine prevention, and it helps if the family understands this. Yes, adjustments can be difficult, particularly for younger people, but the return is considerable, and can make the difference between a fun, active life and many miserable days. All of this is most feasible when loved ones really understand the individual migraineur's headache situation.

While everyone requires regular exercise, it is especially helpful for migraineurs, but the key word is "regular." Exercise should be *routine*. When loved ones support and facilitate a regular exercise program, it helps a lot. However, if exercise can bring on your headaches, it's important that the family knows this. They can even remind you to hydrate aggressively, possibly take an anti-inflammatory, wear your sunglasses, and so forth. Gentle reminders of such precautions can be the difference between a great day and a day in bed.

What to Tell the Kids

Kids, even really young ones, are incredibly perceptive when it comes to reading their parents. They know when we are in pain, when we are scared, and when we are trying to fool them. Kids are also scared by the unknown. Kids, especially young ones, need to understand that Mommy or Daddy is not dying. We have found that it is best to explain migraines to the kids when you are headache-free. Assure them that your headaches are not dangerous, that when a headache is over you will be fine again, and that it helps a lot if certain things happen when you get a headache.

Try to focus this conversation on the positive, pointing out things the child can do to help, rather than emphasizing the negatives. At an appropriate level, kids can understand the importance of quiet and isolation. You can explain that when you have a headache you don't feel well, and disturbing you makes your head hurt more, so they should take questions, requests, or other interruptions to the other parent or caregiver. And rather than visit you, kids can engage in care from a distance, playing quietly in another room, helping keep the house quiet, and making drawings to help you feel better. Kids can also help prepare the house by closing blinds and curtains and turning off the TV.

Contingency Plans for Headache Days

For most of us, no matter how good our treatment plan, we will have headache days. When a treatment plan works, headache days should be few and far between, but they will come, so we need to have contingency plans in place for those times. It is important that employers, coworkers, family, and friends understand that you suffer from migraines. In my experience, people prefer not to be blindsided by an unexpected absence, but are grateful for the opportunity to help in such a circumstance. Education is important, because headaches don't often come with much advance warning.

At home or work, if someone will cover for you during a headache and they expect "payback" for your downtime, spell this out up front so that no one feels taken advantage of in the end. The more people know about headaches in general and your headaches in particular, the less disruption and stress you will experience during your headaches.

It is enormously helpful, both to the migraineur and to the rest of the family, if you all have a plan in place to pick up the slack when a migraine hits. It is almost impossible to change complicated plans when your head is pounding, so it is better for everyone if the simple announcement "I have a headache" shifts everyone's gears. In this case, your child might know to go into the bedroom, unplug the phone, put some water by the bed, and shut the curtains. Your spouse or significant other can take the lead during a headache, and assume the responsibilities of child care and other duties. For example, a husband can pick up another child after baseball practice, grab something for dinner, and "migraine-proof" the house, moving the kids away from the bedroom. Better yet, he might take the kids out to dinner or to a neighbor's house. In any event, no one will use the garage door as a tennis backboard, and the dog will not be barking outside. Without such family support, a moderate 5 migraine can easily escalate to a 10.

Creating a Migraine-Safe Haven

Every migraineur needs a place where they can go when they have a headache: the darker, quieter, and more odor-free, the better. If a headache hits on the hottest day of the year and you happen to be in the middle of Disneyland, this can be a problem. But when you are at home, or can get home, it should not. For most of us, the bedroom is our haven, but if the bedroom is also a family gathering place, the migraine-safe retreat may be the spare bedroom, the den, or wherever. The room should have a bathroom nearby and be furnished with light-occluding blinds or curtains—the darker the better. The important thing is to identify a place and make sure everyone in the family knows about it. In a big family, it doesn't hurt to put a sign on the door.

A primary caregiver can help implement the migraineur's treatment plan when a headache happens, but only if they are aware of every aspect of the plan. This means that this support person should be familiar with triggers, medications, and fallback plans. These can be most helpful when a caregiver needs to handle complex situations. At a minimum, a caregiver needs to know about rescue medications, other medicines the migraineur takes, triggers, doctor contact information, and when to get urgent care.

How to Help During the Headache

All you really need during a headache is a quiet, cool, dark, odor-free place and a cool glass of water. This may seem obvious, or even minor, but it is not. I have seen migraineurs guided to the family room, where the kids are watching the tube, and I have seen a mom voluntarily go to the couch rather than the bedroom to lie down. Instead, ideally, you have established a migraine-safe haven and, as a headache comes on, your family can quickly migraine-proof this retreat, one hopes with minimal effort from you.

Normal household sounds can seem like blasts of noise, which are not just painful but can exacerbate the migraine, so the family needs to minimize sounds from the television, laundry, kitchen, and air-conditioning systems, for example, and to be mindful of noises outside your window, as well. It helps if family members are assigned small duties to ensure that the haven stays a haven. For example, when a migraine comes on, various family members might be onboard to:

- block sources of light, day and night (close the curtains and blinds to block morning sunshine and daylight as well as any outdoor lights that are on at night and, if possible, turn off any timed lights that will come on at dark);
- turn off any "ringers" within earshot, including cell phones, landlines, fax machines, and alarm clocks;
- disable any other automatic timers, for radio and TV, for example;
- keep the room cool, if possible, by adjusting the heat and air-conditioning;

- put a bottle or glass of water at the bedside;
- prevent any odors from invading the environment (for example, remove oils or scented candles from the bedroom, minimize cleansers and air fresheners in the nearby bathroom, and don't cook pungent foods);
- provide medications, cold packs, heating pads, eye masks, and any other remedies that are part of the rescue plan;
- rearrange schedules and cancel appointments for the day;
- make arrangements to take the kids outside or to a friend's house, or, at least, to keep the noise down.

Remember, migraines muddle your thinking. Often, in the throes of a headache, we do not make good decisions. For a variety of reasons, including denial, desperate hope, and the distractions of practical responsibilities, migraineurs often postpone taking their meds. We might think, "I'm just going to finish what I'm doing and then I'll lie down." Or, "I'm going to wait and see if it goes away by itself." Migraineurs—myself included—are famous for making such classically ill-advised decisions. *In such situations, it is most helpful for a primary caregiver to override our bad decisions and take control, to (gently) intervene and encourage us, for example, to take the darn medicine now, not later.*

This is why it is most helpful for support people to know and understand every aspect of the migraineur's treatment plan. This means that they should be familiar with triggers, medications, and fallback plans, and this is why we provide questionnaires and checklists for migraineurs and their caregivers. If caregivers have access to these records, the information can help them handle complex situations for the migraineur. At a minimum, a support person needs to know:

- rescue medication information (which medications the person takes, when they last took any of them, when next to take them, and where to find them);
- other medicines the migraineur takes;
- most common triggers;
- how and when to reach the migraineur's doctors.

Whether to give medication or not is a tricky question. Of course, you must observe the usual cautions:

- Never give anyone someone else's prescription medicine.
- Never take someone else's prescription medicine.
- Never exceed the limits on prescription or over-the-counter medication.

Sometimes, as part of the plan, a caregiver needs to know if and when to take a migraineur to a doctor, urgent care facility, or emergency room. In such a situation, the caregiver might need to speak for the headache sufferer to get information about medications the migraineur has taken, any drug allergies, and details about the current headache, such as when it started, whether the patient has thrown up, and whether it is a typical headache for the patient.

Seven "Don'ts" for the Migraine Caregiver

1. **Don't hover.** Migraineurs know that you love them, that you are concerned and want to help. But they prefer to be left alone when their head is pounding. Confirm this with your migraineur at a time when he or she is not in pain.
2. **Don't interrupt your migraineur's suffering with a "quick question" unless there is an actual emergency.** As difficult as it may be, try to muddle through. Even a simple question increases pain during the asking, and the worry over the answer persists beyond your leaving. Your migraineur desperately needs peace and quiet. Though it seems harsh, the best medicine is to leave your migraineur alone.
3. **Don't play doctor *or* psychiatrist.** Migraines are a real disease, just like diabetes or asthma, and most migraineurs feel bad that their headaches knock them out of commission. Stress is a common trigger, and while a headache may seem like a convenient way to get out of dinner with your mother, it is more

likely the result of the stress of preparing for the ordeal—or any of a hundred other triggers. Remember: *No one endures this kind of pain by choice, nor would they choose physical pain over an uncomfortable night out.*

4. **Don't enlist your migraineur's help in trying to figure out how to carry on the family activities** while he or she is out of commission with a headache. Sure, everybody's plans may have to change, but this is one of those golden opportunities when you can be better than you really are. Whispering a sympathetic, "Don't worry about it. Take care of your head and I'll handle everything else," will elevate you to sainthood while doing a genuinely nice thing for someone you care about. It is hard, I know, but it is much, much better than the alternative.

5. **Don't mess with the plan.** It is the migraineur's responsibility, with their doctor, to develop a headache management plan. Certainly, if appropriate, you should have input. But once the plan is set, do not undermine it. If you think it needs tweaking, suggest changes with the patient and their doctor. A good plan includes lifestyle changes, such as sleep hygiene, regular diet, and routine exercise, as well as one or two preventive medicines and several layers of "rescue" treatment when a headache starts. It is not always easy to stay on plan. It is your job to support the plan, not to be a policeman, armchair critic, or saboteur.

6. **Don't check out.** Some people's reaction to illness is to steer clear of it. In general, this is okay, but when someone close to you has a significant illness, it is your problem as well. This is obvious when the illness is cataclysmic or life-threatening, but sometimes family members ignore a chronic illness until a crisis arises. Migraine affects entire families. It is important to understand as much as possible about the condition, because your awareness can be a critical part of effective management, both in crisis and in the long-term.

7. **Don't blame the victim.** This may seem obvious or even obnoxious. In fact, I wouldn't even mention it if I hadn't seen it happen so many times. Family members do not do this

consciously, but they often give the message that the headache sufferer has some demonic interest in ruining their own life and, by extension, yours. If, in fact, headaches result from overdoing it, then that is a trigger, in the same way that a walk in the park can bring on an asthma attack. Rather than blame loved ones for their genetics, focus on helping them modify their lifestyle based on triggers you observe. The following statements all blame the migraineur:

- "You bring these on yourself by trying to do too much."
- "You get a headache every time we plan to go away."
- "We never do anything because of your headaches."

PART THREE

Put Your Plan into Action: Target Your Specific Triggers

Chapter 8

Headaches
and Eating

Not everyone has a problem with hot dogs or blue cheese or legumes, but some migraineurs certainly do. In fact, not all migraineurs have a problem with *any* foods, but some do. And when they do, regardless of what food triggers the headache, that headache is a migraine, and the treatments are the same as they are for that patient's other migraines. So while I urge all my patients to maintain a headache diary to uncover any specific foods that might be triggering their migraines, there is more to the story.

Without good science to back it up, many migraineurs and their doctors place disproportionate emphasis on the negative effects of certain foods. In recent years, we've also emphasized foods and supplements that might actually *help* with headaches. Unfortunately, we have little scientific justification for these, either.

However, mounting evidence suggests that shifting away from the omega-6 fatty acids to a diet richer in omega-3 fatty acids may decrease headache frequency. Many headache specialists, myself included, also feel that it is beneficial to maintain approximately the same ratios of good and bad fats, carbohydrates, protein, and fiber from day to day. This means maintaining not just a healthy diet, but a *consistently* healthy diet. This does not mean you have to eat the same foods day after day, but it does seem to serve the migraineur well to pay attention to maintaining a relatively steady diet, whether it is high in protein, low in carbohydrates, low in fats, or whichever. Scientists are also currently investigating "anti-inflammatory foods," such as olive oil, walnuts, blueberries, and so forth, but this research is not quite ready for prime time.

Other than *what* we eat, migraineurs need to pay attention to some important dietary issues. Since change itself opens the door to headaches, at the Keeler Center we encourage our patients to try to keep their eating patterns as consistent as possible. So in addition to maintaining those consistent ratios of food groups, meal *timing* is an essential part of most migraine treatment plans. Whether you eat three meals a day or five, keep in mind that most migraineurs seem to do best with a *regular* schedule of mealtimes.

The "Migraine Diet"

Despite books, magazine articles, and infomercials to the contrary, *no scientifically validated diet reduces the duration, frequency, or severity of migraines.* But this is a very attractive idea, so some people have capitalized on migraine sufferers who sometimes search desperately for a cure. So I'll say it again: At this writing, we have no cure for migraines. Only intelligent management.

Still, the question comes up time and again: "What should I be eating?" Aside from the obvious—avoid foods that seem to trigger *your* headaches—we do not have a definitive answer, but we have been looking at this question in our laboratories. Examining migraineurs' cerebrospinal fluid, blood, urine, and saliva during and between headaches, we have found significant differences in the amounts of certain types of fatty acids. This is interesting because fatty acids are an important constituent of the membranes of brain tissue, and they play a critical role in how the nerves in the brain communicate with one another. It appears that omega-3 fatty acids (the "good" ones) are lower in migraineurs than in the general population, and omega-6 fatty acids (the "bad" ones) are higher. We have not determined whether changing a migraineur's diet to one that is higher in omega-3s and lower in omega-6s will have a positive effect on headaches. But it certainly makes sense to increase omega-3s, given the many benefits that have been confirmed in overall good health.

What do we tell our patients? After we tell them that there is no magic solution, we teach them that our basic premise at the Keeler Center is that migraineurs do not handle change well and that consistency seems to be protective in some way. We suggest that they try to keep a fairly consistent diet in terms of both composition and meal timing. We recommend that you start with any diet and routine that already works for you, as long as it meets your nutritional and other health needs. Then superimpose on that a general guideline, a rule, that you will maintain a consistent meal schedule and somewhat predictable proportions of fat, protein, and carbohydrate in your daily diet. Rather than go heavy on the carbs one day and protein the next, just keep it routine. This way, if your diet includes more or less consistent ratios of the various food groups from day to day, you will enjoy more than adequate variety in your diet while maintaining a migraine-preventive regimen that will also help you spot any premigrainous cravings (typically sweets or complex carbohydrates). Whether this will prove to be a valid approach when our clinical studies are complete, only time will tell. In the meantime, it seems like a reasonable and safe course to follow.

Food Triggers

When I started as a headache specialist years ago, I spent some time at a renowned Chicago headache clinic that provided its patients with a special diet and an extensive list of foods known to trigger headaches. It seemed like the right thing to do, so I incorporated a similar list and diet into my headache practice in southern California. After a while, though, one of my patients pointed out that the list removed from her life many of the things that *didn't* give her headaches. So I questioned my patients more closely about their eating habits. Yet again, I learned from them.

Some of my patients get automatic headaches if they drink any alcohol at all. Many of my patients can get a headache from the bits of chocolate in a chocolate chip cookie. Some get a headache from MSG. Some from cured meats. Others, if they eat the famous chocolate-peanut combination of peanut M&M's. But more important, other patients do *not* get a headache from chocolate, MSG, cured meats, or *any* of these things—and rare is the patient who gets a migraine from *all* of them. *There are even some patients who have no food triggers at all.* So why was I telling *every* patient to avoid wine, aged cheese, and legumes, with *no* evidence that those things gave the patient in front of me a headache? When I stopped to think for a moment, I realized that chocolate never gave *me* a headache. So why in the world should I deprive myself of this great pleasure?

I've also learned from my patients that food triggers are usually not subtle. When a trigger is so strong that it will bring on a headache all by itself, it is usually pretty obvious. Most patients whose headaches are reliably triggered by a familiar food will tell me this first thing, practically when they are walking in the door.

For some of us, though, our triggers can be a little harder to detect. Our thinking is more like, "I may be sensitive to some cheeses, because sometimes I get a headache." I think this is probably accurate. Many triggers are not absolute, but in the right setting or the right combination, they can contribute to a headache. These are partial triggers.

At the Keeler Center, we handle food triggers the same way we handle all the other potential headache triggers. *We do not give out lists*, but teach our patients to pay attention to their lives. Again, the best way to do this is by keeping a headache diary for a month or two. Every time you get a headache, you simply write a few notes, recording the foods you ate and any other potential factors that preceded the headache. You will learn a lot from this project and your doctor may well, too. A Zen-like attention to your foods and other daily activities will give you very good information about what triggers your headaches, without making your headaches the focus of all your attention. It is written: Pay attention to your life.

If you find that you get a headache every time you go to your favorite Chinese restaurant, then look closer at that activity. The solution may simply be to ask the waiter which dishes contain MSG. If you find that sometimes you get a headache after eating crab Louis, see if it is made with real or synthetic crab. Sometimes, it really is that simple. Sometimes it is more complicated. When you suspect a food, keep an eye on it, discuss it with your headache specialist, maybe do a little self-experimentation. Try eliminating it and see if you have fewer headaches. You can even reintroduce it and see if it reproducibly elicits a headache. This strategy will give you *objective* evidence to reliably track down nasty triggers, and may keep you from banning innocent foods that you enjoy—which would be a shame.

Deciding whether something is a trigger or not and then figuring out what to do about it can be tricky. Lists of possible food triggers, anecdotes about other people's triggers, and the possibility of coincidence between something and a headache all confound the hunt. Certainly, if you notice that you get a headache every time you are exposed to a particular food, place, activity, or whatever, that "something" should be on your list. And it never hurts to consider the observations of friends, family, health care providers, and other headache sufferers. But keep in mind that everyone's trigger set is unique to that person, and assessing potential "partial triggers" is trickier still. But the same rules apply: How strong is the correlation between that potential trigger and your headaches? There is no easy checklist. But the more aware you are of your environment and physical state, the more likely you are to recognize a trigger when it pops up.

In the end, I find it important to return to the idea of food lists. But the fact is that *all migraine patients should have their own lists*, some of which will have foods on them, others of which will not. Here are my rules:

- Foods definitely can trigger headaches.
- Different foods can be triggers for different people.
- Foods can often be "partial triggers."

Keep in mind that most migraineurs have multiple triggers, and that eliminating one trigger is good, but probably will not be enough to "cure" you.

Meal Timing

While we do not have any universal food triggers, we do have some near-universal agreement that eating meals on a regular schedule reduces the frequency of headaches. But of course, I do have some patients for whom regular mealtimes have absolutely no impact on their headaches. But many migraineurs do much better if they avoid disruptions in the body's chemical balance by eating healthy meals on schedule.

Our bodies secrete chemicals—hormones—on a cyclic basis. In the case of digestion, various chemicals are mobilized in response to food exposure or, on the other hand, fasting beyond an anticipated mealtime. Recent studies have shown that the body produces and stores some of these chemicals in fat cells as well as in the brain. In addition, some of these chemicals play prominent roles in the inflammatory process and in pain modulation.

Maintaining a rhythm to your dietary schedule does not mean you must take your lunch break every day when the clock strikes twelve, whether your work is at a stopping place or not. It just means that you need to pay some attention to the fact that routine is everything for the migraineur. Some patients have found it helpful to carry a small snack in their purses or a few portable foods in the car glove compartment, just in case they work through lunch or are caught in traffic. Since it is also important to get the same sorts of food in a well-balanced diet, you also want to get a variety of food groups every day. This should not become a career. Simply avoid having days when you eat a ton of protein followed by a day of nothing but pasta to make up for it. This is not just a good idea for migraineurs, but for overall health, of course.

An Important Step—Avoid, Modify, or Prevent

When you discover that something definitely gives you a headache, work around it. Easier said than done? Not really. Don't forget, a vital step of trigger management is to "value" each trigger, choosing one of our management strategies: avoid, modify, or prevent. If you won't miss the triggering food, the best way to go is to just avoid it, eliminating the food from your diet altogether. If you don't want to completely avoid it, you can modify the trigger. The most common way to do this is to minimize additional triggers at the same time, but with foods modification strategies might include adjustments to how a food is prepared or the particular brand or quality of the food. Finally, if you prefer to keep the food in your diet—or you have to—and modification is not enough, you can take preventive steps to minimize the headache when you anticipate exposure to the trigger.

For example, if you know that hot dogs are a trigger and so is a hot afternoon, you should avoid eating hot dogs when it's hot out, most of the time. But if you go to the company picnic and your boss made hot dogs from scratch, nitrates and all, he might be offended if you bring your own sushi. In this situation, you might consider pretreating. Whether it's an $800-per-bottle wine-tasting event or that Belgian dark chocolate egg your friends had flown in especially to celebrate your twenty-fifth wedding anniversary, you can't always avoid exposure to your trigger foods. In these circumstances, it is not a bad idea to take a medium- or long-acting triptan (such as naratriptan or frovatriptan) or an anti-inflammatory (such as naproxen or ketorolac) an hour or two before the event.

Increasing evidence suggests that diet and obesity are important in headaches, so most treatment plans will have some component regarding the timing, content, and/or quantity of meals. While some people have specific food triggers, fasting or skipping meals is also a common trigger, and obesity is a risk factor for chronic daily headache.

Use this questionnaire with your headache diary, to look for correlations between diet modification and good or bad headache periods. For example: "My headaches were pretty bad in June while I was on the 'migraine diet,' but hey, I did well when I was on that low-carb diet in August." It is a good idea to repeat this exercise every six months, then compare it to your previous questionnaire. For each question, seek insight into the "regularity" of your eating and diet behaviors to improve your dietary routine.

Do you eat your meals on a regular schedule?

_____

_____

Do you often skip meals?

_____

_____

Are you a grazer?

_____

_____

From day to day, do you have about the same intake of:

Carbs? _____   Fats? _____

Protein? _____   Fiber? _____

Do you notice any effect from too much or too little sugar on your headaches?

_____

_____

Have you identified specific foods that consistently trigger your headaches?

_____

_____

Do you get cravings for carbs, chocolate, or other foods?

_____

_____

Does this seem to be related to headache onset? (Use your diary.)

_____

_____

Do you snack before bed?

_____

_____

Is your caffeine consumption consistent from day to day (including weekends)?

_____

_____

On average, how many glasses of water do you drink per day?

_____

_____

Is this pretty consistent?

_____

_____

Does your weight fluctuate widely?

_____

_____

Chapter 9

Headaches
and Exercise

A patient sat across from me, overweight, and out of breath from the walk into my office from the waiting room across the hall. He looked me dead-on and said, "I can't exercise, because it gives me a headache."

No doubt, this was absolutely true. Exercise can induce headaches. This is well documented. The majority of these are migraines with exercise acting as a trigger. But the problem I have with this statement is that it is a perfect example of the patient letting the headache dictate his life, which is just wrong.

This patient got the first part right: he identified a trigger that made his head worse. But he made a mistake in his approach to dealing with the trigger. Remember, you need to *value* each trigger, and decide whether you should avoid it, modify it, or prevent the headache it can cause. If the trigger is important to you—which it should be—and to your health—which it is—then you want to devise a strategy to keep it in your life and minimize its triggering potential. As migraine sufferers and headache specialists, we aim for that.

Of course, there are about twelve billion reasons to exercise, but what about headaches? Many people with migraine report that exercise will bring on or worsen headaches, and solid, scientific evidence supports the notion that exercise can cause a headache. But this does *not* mean that migraineurs should avoid exercise. To the contrary, there is *more* evidence to suggest that migraineurs who exercise on a daily basis do *better* with their headaches than those who do not exercise.

Recent evidence even suggests that the brain actually "remodels" itself in response to regular exercise, becoming less sensitive to certain disruptions in brain chemistry that can trigger both migraines and other illnesses. This evidence is even more persuasive with regard to tension headaches. In fact, migraineurs should think of exercise as a headache *preventive*.

The Keeler Method employs specific strategies to prevent exercise-induced headaches. That way, we can get the exercise we want and need—without suffering a headache as a result. The bottom line is, if you think exercise brings on your headaches, it is probably not your imagination, but there are ways around it.

For example, Rafi was a high-energy computer programmer who came to us with evening headaches. He was an avid swimmer, one hundred laps three to five days a week. His diary correlated his headaches with his swim days, but not swimming was unthinkable for him. I went and watched him swim. He swam twenty-five laps of butterfly, twenty-five of freestyle, twenty-five of breaststroke, and another twenty-five of freestyle—all strokes that required neck extension. We suggested that he substitute some backstroke (neck flexion) and add some postexercise stretches. Headaches resolved!

Recreation is important for good health and well-being, whether it includes exercise or not. For migraineurs, however, many recreational activities, or certain aspects of them, are often headache triggers. As with exercise, it is important to evaluate recreational triggers to decide if you want to avoid the activity altogether, modify it to avoid headaches, or keep the activity in your life and use an anticipatory strategy, such as taking a preventive measure to avoid headaches. Often, an anti-inflammatory or a long-acting triptan can accomplish this, but it can sometimes be tricky, and merits a conversation with your physician or headache specialist to help you create the appropriate strategy.

Exercise Is Especially Good for Headache Sufferers

mber, once you identify a migraine trigger, you need to evaluate rms of its value to your health and well-being in life. You need to consider whether a trigger is something you can happily avoid or something you want or need to keep in your life, possibly with modifications. It is especially important for migraineurs and, indeed, anyone who has chronic pain to place a high value on exercise—and to develop strategies to keep it in their life.

Exercise raises the body's levels of its own natural painkillers, proteins called endorphins. Among other things, endorphins alter your pain threshold so that a given painful stimulus hurts less. This is a good thing for someone with headaches.

People who subject their bodies to a lot of physical stress, like elite athletes, have very high endorphin levels and, as a result, high pain thresholds. At the other end of the spectrum is your basic couch potato, who gets very little exercise, has low endorphin levels, and feels pain just reaching for the remote. Migraineurs who exercise will have higher endorphin levels and higher pain thresholds, and will be less likely to be disabled by a headache. This gives us an even greater incentive to exercise than the general population.

Of course, all patients must get permission from their doctors before initiating any exercise regimen. If you decide to take on any exercise program, you should make this decision after consulting your physician, and with the doctor's full blessing.

For patients who tend to get tension-type headaches and migraineurs who have tension as a migraine trigger, exercise can be just the ticket. Very persuasive evidence suggests that these headache sufferers do well with stretching and strengthening exercises. Further, people who suffer from tension headaches or headaches resulting from neck problems often improve with proper exercise and stretching. In fact, exercise is an essential component of the treatment for tension-type headaches. Stretching the neck and shoulder muscles not only helps an immediate headache, but also can help prevent occasional tension headaches from transforming into a daily headache pattern. However, the wrong kind of exercise can make tension headaches worse. It is important that patients with this diagnosis work with a trained physical therapist to learn the proper techniques and exercises.

Yes, many migraineurs have trouble with exercise and their headaches, but rather than give up the exercise, a more measured response is called for. It is important to maintain the exercise and devise a way to either eliminate or minimize its detrimental effects on the headaches. For many reasons, migraineurs need to develop strategies to allow them to exercise.

Endorphins

You have no doubt heard someone say, "I have a really high threshold for pain." But what does that actually mean? That headache sufferers have low thresholds for pain? Of course not. Some headache sufferers have really high thresholds, others don't. But different people *do* have different pain thresholds.

How do pain thresholds relate to headaches?

Our bodies manufacture natural painkillers, peptides called endorphins. If we had no endorphins, everything would hurt—the wind on our faces, the shoes we wear, everything. On the other hand, if our endorphin levels were sky-high, *nothing* would hurt. We might not even notice that we had inadvertently severed a finger or were leaning against a red-hot boiler. Since endorphins can be a two-edged sword, our bodies regulate how much endorphins are onboard. While genetics probably play a role in our resting endorphin levels, exercise is the main way the body regulates endorphin levels.

Unfortunately, endorphin levels do not seem to rise in response to *pain*, in which case headache sufferers would have high levels just because of their headaches. It doesn't work that way. Endorphin levels rise in response to physical activity. But low endorphin levels do not explain the whole migraine phenomenon. If they did, Serena Williams, one of the world's greatest athletes, would not experience migraines.

Scientists have measured endorphins in the blood, and studies have shown that high-level athletes, such as marathon runners, have high phin levels, while sedentary individuals have low levels. This is why e runners can complete marathons oblivious to the fact that their e become bruised, battered, and bloody. People like professional athletes, who subject their bodies to lots of physical stress, have very high levels of endorphins and high pain thresholds. Compare this with couch potatoes and other people with very sedentary lifestyles. Such people have significantly lower endorphin levels and lower pain thresholds and, as a result, find the slightest injury to be quite painful.

So in addition to all the other, myriad health benefits of regular exercise, it also increases levels of the body's natural painkillers. The fact is that *incorporating a regular exercise routine into our day will, among other things, gradually raise our endorphin levels, raise our baseline threshold for perceiving pain, and, as a result, reduce the severity of our headaches.*

This is one of many reasons exercise is doubly important for migraineurs. People who exercise actually have a higher threshold for pain, and that means their headaches may not hurt as much, not come as often, and not last as long. With higher endorphin levels and a higher pain threshold, a 7 headache may feel like a 2 and a 10 may register as a 4.

Like all lifestyle changes, these do not come overnight. But the fact is that exercise can be so effective I recommend it as a headache *preventive*. Of course, you have to be careful. For some migraineurs, exercise can be a trigger. In this circumstance, pretreatment with an anti-inflammatory is often successful.

But Exercise Makes My Head Hurt!

Many migraineurs find that physical exertion, even healthy exercise, can bring on or worsen a headache, so they conclude that exercise has a negative impact on their headaches and, therefore, on their lives. However, we all know that exercise is essential to good health. Thus, it is important to turn exercise from a negative into a positive. The Keeler Method shows you how to do this.

One of the ways in which we differentiate migraines from tension-type headaches is that migraines usually worsen with exercise, while tension headaches tend to improve. So if exercise makes an existing headache worse, do not exercise when you have a headache. Also, if exercise makes an existing headache worse and you have a headache every day, talk to your doctor about why you might be having daily headaches, and discuss using a preventive to reduce the frequency of your headaches without limiting your ability to exercise. The popular preventive propranolol, for example, can decrease the frequency of headaches but can also make you tired and prevent your heart rate from increasing when you work out, making you short of breath, so another preventive may be more suitable in this circumstance.

While some people swear that a good workout is the only thing that *helps* their headaches, most migraineurs report that exercise makes an existing headache worse. In fact, exercising when you have a migraine can be an incredibly bad idea. If you are a migraineur and you are feeling "migrainey," right on the edge of getting a headache, or in the middle of one, then exercise is the last thing you feel like doing, and your instinct is probably right. If you have a migraine, exercise will almost certainly make things much worse. Do not exercise until the headache is completely gone and you feel back to normal.

Even when they don't have a headache, many migraineurs find that routine physical exercise can actually precipitate a migraine. If this is you, the bottom line is that it is probably *not* your imagination. The changes that come with exercise—changes in blood flow, hormone levels, and neurotransmitters—are enough to *trigger* headaches in many migraineurs. But for the majority of patients, the connection between headaches and exercise has more to do with *how* and *when* they exercise, not whether they exercise or not. One thing is for sure: avoiding exercise altogether is *not* a healthy solution. But while the benefits of exercising outweigh the downside of getting a migraine, that does not mean that headache sufferers should exercise and just endure the head pain, either.

If you suffer from migraines and find that routine exercise brings on a headache, there are ways around it, and it is useful to explore strategies to prevent the headaches, rather than avoiding exercise. The first step is to determine *why* exercise gives you a migraine. Usually, exercise triggers migraines for one of these two possible reasons:

- Exercise disrupts your body's routines.
- Any amount of exercise is a migraine trigger.

Exercise is a sticky subject for many of us. Clearly, increasing exercise increases levels of endorphins and thus raises our pain threshold, so that a 5 headache may become a 3. Essential to any headache treatment plan, exercise as part of a more active lifestyle also provides many other benefits for our health and happiness. Therefore, we need to know where we are in terms of current exercise, how exercise affects our headaches, and how we can increase our level of exercise without exacerbating our headaches. This questionnaire will highlight obstacles to exercise, and may suggest ways to get around those hurdles. Use this information to build your treatment plan, and return to this form periodically with your headache diary/calendar to see if you have changed your exercise behaviors for the better and to assess any relationship between your exercise changes and your headache frequency and severity.

Do you have a regular exercise plan?

_____

Have you discussed your exercise plan with a health professional?

_____

Does your exercise plan include aerobic activity?

_____

Does your exercise plan include stretching and warm-up?

_____

Do you exercise at approximately the same time each day?

_____

Does exercise tend to relieve a mild headache?

_____

Does exercise tend to worsen a mild headache?

_____

Have you identified specific exercises that either help or trigger headaches?

_____

The first priority is to make sure that your exercise-induced headaches are not a symptom of something more serious, such as cardiac, pulmonary, or vascular disease. If you have avoided exercise for a long time, you should consult your primary care physician to make sure, first, that exercise is safe for you, and second, that your headache is simply the result of exercise acting as a trigger. As with all exercises, if you have other medical issues related to your neck (such as a cervical stenosis or radiculopathy), consult your doctor before undertaking an exercise program that utilizes neck muscles and range of motion.

If there is no medical reason preventing you from doing so, the trick is to block the exercise-induced headaches so you can enjoy the headache-reducing benefits of exercise. You can probably prevent the headaches by taking an anti-inflammatory an hour or so before exercise, but you should talk to a doctor before beginning an exercise program and before starting therapy with an anti-inflammatory.

A Good Exercise Routine

If you do not have any other medical concerns, you can employ useful modification strategies for preventing exercise-induced migraines. With any migraineur's exercise routine, the key word is _routine_. Sporadic exercise is *not* a good idea for migraineurs. We do much better exercising on a regular basis, rather than episodically. Twenty minutes every day or three days a week is much better than four hours only on Saturdays. Migraineurs do best with regular schedules, so, ideally, we should exercise at about the same time and for the same amount of time *every* day, and that time should *not* be just before bed. This kind of regularity is fundamental to the antimigraine lifestyle. To avoid an exercise-induced headache:

- maintain routine in your exercise regimen, ideally every day at the same time and for the same amount of time;
- hydrate aggressively, because dehydration combined with exercise can be a "double whammy" for migraineurs;
- minimize all other potential triggers when and where you exercise: work out in a cool environment with good circulation, no loud music, and no fluorescent lights;
- start with a measured stretching regimen before beginning any aerobic exercise.

For all exercise, regardless of type, it is crucial that you stretch before and after a workout. Warm up slowly and work your way into the session gradually. Not only will it protect you from painful muscle pulls and joint injuries, but it will also make your workout less likely to trigger a headache. This is because going slowly allows you to monitor your body more carefully, watching for any telltale signs that you are heading for headache trouble.

Many headache sufferers feel that certain exercises exacerbate their headaches, but if you do not have a complicating injury, this should not be the case. More often, the problem is that the offending exercise is working a muscle that you have not stretched and warmed up adequately. Just because you are twenty minutes into a workout, you cannot assume that every muscle is loose and ready. Before a workout or in your initial warm-up session, be sure to systematically and thoroughly stretch your entire body.

In general, headache sufferers tolerate aerobic exercise better than anaerobic exercise, but proper breathing is a most important factor. This may have something to do with energy metabolism or oxygen exchange. No one knows for sure. For many headache sufferers, holding your breath is not just poor exercise form, but also bad for your headaches. If you are unsure about when and how to breathe during exercise, talk to a trainer, physical therapist, or other expert in the field.

With aerobic exercises, migraineurs should avoid any jarring or pounding. The less jarring the motion, the better for your head. Swimming is an excellent aerobic exercise for migraine sufferers, and other good options include bicycling, elliptical machines, and StairMasters or similar equipment, which are often better tolerated, for example, than jogging, treadmills, and traditional aerobics classes. Finally, programmed exercise, such as yoga or tai chi, is excellent.

For weight training, free weights are probably better for overall conditioning, but machines may offer a more balanced alternative, particularly for novices. If you are working with machines only, go with less weight and more reps, taking care to exhale as you lift and inhale as you relax. Move quickly through the different machines, making multiple circuits rather than more sets on one machine. The idea is to be a little out of breath at the end of your session. Pay close attention to how your body responds to each specific exercise. *If it hurts, don't do it*. You can try to come back to it later with less weight or a less extreme range of motion. If you notice a particular movement or exercise brings on a headache, report this the next time you see your doctor.

Pretreating

If you modify your workout routine and still find that exercise gives you a migraine, or makes your headaches worse in general, you can employ several other strategies to help prevent exercise-induced headaches. Often, the easiest thing to do is to treat or medicate before you begin exercising.

Most headache experts think that when exercise brings on a migraine it is due to an inflammatory response. Thus, it follows that one way to block the headache is to block inflammation. If you do not have any medical reason why you should not take nonsteroidal anti-inflammatory drugs (NSAIDs), these are the medications of choice for preventing exercise-induced migraines. Available in both over-the-counter and prescription strengths and formulations, they include:

- acetylsalicylic acid (aspirin, Ecotrin)
- aspirin with other antiplatelet medications (Plavix, Aggrenox)
- choline magnesium salicylate (Trilisate)
- Cox-2 inhibitors (Celebrex)
- diclofenac (Voltaren, Cataflam, Voltaren-XR)
- diflunisal (Dolobid)
- etodolac (Lodine)
- fenoprofen (Nalfon)
- flurbiprofen (Ansaid)
- ibuprofen (Advil, Motrin, Medipren, Nuprin, PediaCare Fever)
- indomethacin (Indocin, Indocin-SR)
- ketoprofen (Orudis, Oruvail)
- meclofenamate (Meclomen)
- nabumetone (Relafen)
- naproxen (Naprosyn, Naprelan, Anaprox, Aleve)
- oxaprozin (Daypro)
- phenylbutazone (Butazolidin)
- piroxicam (Feldene)
- salsalate (Disalcid, Salflex)
- tolmetin (Tolectin)

Some of these medications are available over the counter, while others are by prescription only, and still others are available in one strength over the counter and in stronger doses by prescription. Prescription medications in this class that can also help:

- Indomethacin is probably the most effective but also the hardest on your stomach.

- Naproxen is an excellent alternative in the prescription strength of 500 mg or 550 mg.
- Toradol is another prescription NSAID that is quite potent.
- Celecoxib (Celebrex), the only COX-2 NSAID on the market, is very effective as well.

Most of the NSAIDs are known as COX-1 inhibitors. COX-2 inhibitors work on another branch of the same biochemical pathway. Celebrex is the only one of these now available in the United States.

NSAIDs can block the inflammatory response and prevent it from triggering a headache, but they are also very useful late in a headache, when there is central inflammation and triptans may be less effective.

To protect the lining of your stomach, it is best to take NSAIDs with some food or a stomach-protecting medicine. This is something to discuss with your doctor, particularly if you will be taking NSAIDs on a frequent basis. Of course, if you are going to treat before exercise, you don't want to eat or take medicine just before working out, so it is wise to eat something light and take your NSAID about an hour before exercising. This gives your stomach time to settle and allows the medication to get into your system.

Some patients describe a more classically "migrainous" onset to headaches with working out, such as a typical aura followed by a typical migraine or, in patients who do not have auras, their typical throbbing, one-sided pain, nausea, and light sensitivity. These migraineurs may benefit from taking one of the triptans before exercising. If you use a triptan for migraine rescue, some headache specialists advocate pretreatment with a long-acting triptan, such as naratriptan (Amerge) or frovatriptan (Frova).

However, this can be problematic. It's best for migraineurs to exercise on a daily or near-daily basis, but you should not take triptans more than two days a week. So patients who consistently get migraines with workouts should discuss with their doctor the possibility of starting a preventive medication to help minimize or eliminate exercise-induced headaches. With continued, regular exercise, you can expect to reduce the frequency and severity of your headaches, and as your body adjusts, exercise might stop acting as a trigger. After about three months, you will probably be able to stop taking the preventive medication.

Similarly, if you get headaches every day and exercise makes them worse, you should talk to your doctor about why you might be having daily headaches. And again, discuss the use of a preventive to reduce their frequency. Make sure your doctor understands that you don't want a preventive that will limit your ability to exercise, as some preventive options are not suitable in this circumstance.

Most preventives do not have any effect on exercise. The most notable exception to this is a class of drugs known as beta-blockers. Medicines like the popular preventive propranolol (and others ending in "ol") are in this class. While it can decrease the frequency of headaches, propranolol can also make you tired. Beta-blockers tend to slow the heart rate and prevent it from increasing in response to the body's demand for more blood and more oxygen. When you exercise, your muscles call for more and more oxygen, and the blood supply shifts in that direction, so less goes to the brain. This can result in light-headedness, nausea, and an overwhelming need to lie down on the floor of the gym. This, in turn, will cause others to stand over you and ask loudly if you are all right, which can be embarrassing.

Other medications used for headache prevention, for example, calcium channel blockers and ACE inhibitors, also lower blood pressure by different mechanisms. These do not have a dramatic effect on pulse, and may be a better choice if you also require blood-pressure control, but are not suitable for people with low blood pressure. For people with normal blood pressure, a better alternative for a daily migraine preventive might be topiramate, valproate, or nortriptyline. Of course, every medication has side effects, and the choice depends on other coexisting medical conditions, lifestyle, and other factors. You should have this discussion with a doctor who can help you manage your headaches.

Many migraineurs use nonprescription preventives such as butterbur, feverfew, or coenzyme Q10, with good results. So far, no one has looked at the effectiveness of these agents in preventing exercise-induced headaches, but there does not seem to be any danger in using them while pursuing an exercise program.

Therapeutic Exercises and Warm-up Stretches

Stretching is a good idea for everyone but is critical for people who get headaches—whether before a workout or just for the sake of stretching. But all patients must obtain permission from their doctor before doing any exercises, even these. If you decide to take on this or any exercise program, this decision should *follow* your medical evaluation, *not* replace it.

A physical therapist experienced in treating headaches, neck and shoulder myositis, scapular stabilization, and craniosacral work can be invaluable to a migraine treatment plan. Just as some medicines can worsen headaches, so can some yoga postures, stretches, and exercises. Always ask if your therapist is experienced in treating headache patients. You can easily learn these and other physical therapy maneuvers in just a few sessions. If your physician prescribes physical therapy, most insurance companies will cover these consultations.

As a general rule, when you stretch one muscle, be sure to stretch the muscle that opposes it. For example, if you stretch your biceps, also stretch your triceps; if you stretch your anterior (front) shoulder muscles, stretch the posterior (back) shoulder muscles; if you do crunches, do back extensions.

Often, headache sufferers carry a lot of tension in the neck and shoulders, so you should give special attention to these areas before exercising them (and, in fact, any time). Begin every exercise session with stretches to prepare your neck and shoulder muscles and, when stretching your neck, never roll it. Instead, systematically stretch each individual set of muscles in the neck.

WARM-UP NECK STRETCHES This is a good stretching regimen for your neck. As long as you have your doctor's clearance, always perform this stretching regimen before a workout and repeat it several times per day. Sit upright in a chair or on an exercise ball and:

- Tilt your right ear to your right shoulder, taking care not to turn your chin toward the shoulder or down toward the chest, hold for ten seconds, then slowly return to an erect position.

- Repeat on the left side for ten seconds.
- Rotate your head on an axis, looking over your right shoulder with your chin over your shoulder, hold for ten seconds, then return to the face-forward position.
- Repeat on the left.
- Drop your head, chin to your chest for ten seconds.
- Tilt your head up and look at the ceiling for ten seconds.*

Remember: Six movements, ten seconds each. That's just one minute of your life. Once you have a good range of motion with these stretches, you can modify them for a more advanced stretch to increase your range of motion. When you move your head to each position, stretching comfortably, place a hand on your head on the same side to which you are turned, and press your hand gently *against* your head for five seconds, then remove your hand and let your head move farther into the stretch. Replace your hand, push it against your head for another five seconds, remove it, and let your head drift farther still. Repeat this gentle pressure in each of the six positions described above.

CHEST PRESS   Stand in a doorway with both arms out to your sides, elbows and forearms up each side of the doorjamb and hands toward the ceiling. Your upper arms should be parallel to the floor and your elbows should be bent at 90 degrees. Lean your upper body forward, pushing your shoulders and chest a few inches through the doorway, for a ten-count. Relax. Repeat five times. Then stand away from the doorway with your arms in the same position, forearms parallel to the floor, elbows bent at 90 degrees, and hands toward the ceiling. Keep your arms in this 90-degree angle as you slowly press your elbows, forearms, and hands together in front of your chest. Repeat ten times.

*If your headaches are due to cervical instability or dissection, looking up could be disastrous. That is just one reason why you need a diagnosis and medical evaluation before you do physical therapy.

DIAGONAL ARM LIFTS   This physical therapy maneuver is a great warm-up before any exercise program. You can do these arm lifts with or without light weights (two to five pounds maximum). Stand with erect posture. Start with your right arm straight down, diagonally across your body, with your right hand in front of your left thigh. Without bending your arm, slowly lift it up and diagonally across your body, until it is straight up with your hand pointing at the ceiling above your right shoulder. Slowly lower the arm diagonally to the starting position. Repeat ten times, then do the other arm.

ARM PULLS   Standing a few feet from a tall dresser, put your left hand against the edge of the dresser and lean your upper body slightly forward, resting on your arm. Stretch your right arm down, reaching toward your left foot, then pull the arm up in a "sawing" motion, tucking your hand up toward your right armpit and pushing your elbow toward the ceiling. Repeat ten times with each arm. As you get stronger, lean on a lower surface, such as a counter or sturdy desk, or you can even lie down over an exercise ball. You can also do this using a stretch band attached to a low drawer, cabinet leg, or closed door.

ARMCHAIR STRETCHES   Sit straight up in a sturdy armchair. Hold your chin down and in, and press your upper back and shoulders back, into the chair. Place your forearms on the chair's armrests, palms down, and press your forearms down onto the armrests. Hold this position with your chin in, shoulders back, and forearms down, feeling the stretch through the shoulders. Then, continuing to hold the position, slowly nod your head in slight, one-inch movements up and down. Continue the nodding movement, and gradually tilt your right ear toward your right shoulder. Continue the gentle nodding as you gradually return to center and slowly nod and tilt toward the other shoulder. Slowly repeat, alternating right and left sides, five times.

Easy on the Neck

There are no specific exercises that all headache sufferers should avoid, but anyone who has headache and neck problems should avoid any exercises that stress the neck. For example, running, jumping, and contact karate can all worsen headaches when the neck is not properly stretched and warmed up. When a patient's neck is tight, even light exercise can worsen a headache. When exercise is done without the supervision of a personal trainer or physical therapist, proper warm-up, stretching, nontraumatic exercise, cool-down, and postexercise stretching are essential.

Caution!

Consult your doctor before you begin any exercise program.

Chapter 10

Headaches and Sleep

Many headache sufferers have a big issue with sleep, and clinical experience tells us that sleep and migraines are closely related. Migraineurs who do not keep to a fairly predictable sleep pattern tend to do worse than those who do. We also note that a disproportionately high number of headache sufferers have trouble falling asleep and/or staying asleep. And, when a headache strikes, the first thing a migraineur wants is to go to sleep.

The Keeler Method uses a wide variety of strategies to improve sleep hygiene and maximize the potential benefits of sleep for migraine management. For some migraineurs, it is as simple as not lying awake in bed watching television for hours, but trying to go to sleep and wake up at the same times each day. Others need to be evaluated for sleep apnea, teeth grinding, or parasomnias (sleep disorders that disrupt normal sleep cycles). Often, addressing and rectifying a migraineur's sleep issues can dramatically improve their headaches.

In our research laboratories, we examine cerebrospinal fluid (CSF), comparing the spinal fluid of migraineurs with that of people who do not get migraines, and those who have other pain syndromes and other neurological conditions. We also look at the changes in migraineurs' CSF during headaches compared with their nonheadache state. We have seen that even when a migraineur is headache-free, her spinal fluid is different from that of a nonmigraineur, with striking changes in the levels of a certain prostaglandin that is associated with sleep. (So much for those who say migraine is a psychiatric problem.)

Learning about the effect of prostaglandins and sleep proteins on headache, researchers are intensely interested in the relationship between sleep and headache. For example, we know very well the story of estrogen and headache, but what about other hormones, such as cortisol? Since we know that changes in estrogen levels can trigger a migraine, what about changes in cortisol levels? One of the body's natural steroids, cortisol is the "stress hormone," and it fluctuates in a pattern throughout the day. Our sleep cycle apparently regulates cortisol to a significant degree, with levels dropping to their lowest just before we wake up. Researchers postulate that when we don't sleep well cortisol levels are thrown off enough to trigger a headache. Undoubtedly, the picture is much more complicated than this, but the clinical evidence is firm: Poor sleep is a frequent and common trigger for headaches.

While these data are new and exciting, in our labs and elsewhere we are just beginning to explore the full implications for treating headaches. But it certainly appears that there is a good, biochemical explanation for the benefits of sleep in migraine. The potential for modulating prostaglandins to treat migraine is very promising, and drugs that can do this already exist. It is now a matter of determining how and whether these drugs cross the blood–brain barrier, and measuring their effect.

Research in our labs and elsewhere has shown that sleep and headaches are biochemically linked. Indeed, sleep is an issue for many headache sufferers. The relationship between your headaches and sleep may suggest important treatment options. This questionnaire will help you sort out whether a sleep problem is causing or contributing to your headaches, or if it is a consequence of your headaches. Either way, improving sleep hygiene is always a good idea, and this questionnaire will help highlight any areas where there is room for improvement.

While most of these questions call for simple Yes/No responses, any observations might help you and your doctor with effective migraine management.

Do you consider yourself a good sleeper?

_____

A subjective question, this is a very reliable indicator of overall sleep quality.

Do you feel rested when you wake up in the morning?

_____

This information may provide insight into your "internal clock" and help guide changes in your sleep hygiene.

Do you often have a headache on awakening?

_____

Specific headache types are associated with headaches on awakening, so this can help with diagnosis.

Does your jaw ache in the morning?

_____

Jaw clenching and grinding can be subtle, but a painful jaw in the morning is a clue not to be ignored.

Are you an "active" sleeper?

_____

Restless leg syndrome can interfere with sleep quality and worsen most headaches. Treat the restless legs, and that becomes one less trigger.

Do you snore?

_____

Snoring can be a symptom of sleep apnea, which is often associated with morning headaches.

Does your bedmate snore?

_____

This is just plain annoying, and can disrupt your sleep, worsening your headaches (and your relationship).

Does your dog/cat/bird/other pet or a child sleep in your bed?

_____

Like it or not, sharing your bed with anything other than a like-minded adult can be disruptive to your sleep and bad for your headaches.

Do you have a pretty consistent bedtime?

_____

We all have a biological clock that resets during sleep. When that clock is constantly being reset, the changes it causes in the body can trigger migraines for many people.

Do you watch TV in bed?

_____

Do you eat in bed?

_____

Do you read in bed?

_____

Do you do anything else—other than sleep and make love—in bed?

_____

These questions are the heart of "sleep hygiene." The brain learns to associate actions and behaviors. If the "getting into bed" action is associated with "Let's go over my day," or "Let's see how my favorite late-night soap opera is going," or "Now let's think about all the things I have to do tomorrow," then your bedtime behavior is activating, not sleep-inducing.

Do you have a high-quality pillow?

_____

Sometimes, it is just that simple—a good pillow.

Is your mattress really old?

_____

A mattress that does not support you will cause muscle tension, which often triggers headaches.

Is your bedroom dark and quiet?

_____

Migraineurs are sensitive to environmental stimuli. We are often "light sleepers."

Do you awaken with an alarm or radio?

_____

A "natural" awakening is often a good indicator of a well-set sleep cycle.

Do you awaken at the same time every morning?

_____

This is the flip side of going to bed at the same time. Migraineurs do best with predictable, reproducible cycling.

On the weekends or on your days off, do you sleep in?

_____

This is the most common cause of weekend headaches.

Do you nap regularly?

_____

There is nothing wrong with napping, so long as you do it on a regular schedule.

Sleep Routines

When I was a medical student, Fridays were usually our light days, and on Saturdays we were in the cadaver lab, doing what medical students do. Throughout the time I was learning my dissections of the human body, I did so with varying degrees of headaches. When I talked to my professors about this, they waved me off with an explanation about formalin. I would get used to it, they said. I managed to get through Gross Anatomy (well named, I might add) and moved on to the following year's coursework. But to my dismay, my Saturday headaches persisted, long after the formalin was gone.

Years later, many of my patients complained of weekend headaches and, they often added, "when the week's stress was largely gone." Well-described "letdown" headaches could explain weekend headaches, but in my case, Gross Anatomy was anything *but* stress-free. "Caffeine withdrawal" is another explanation that has been bandied about as the reason for weekend headaches, since many people have a perpetually refilled coffee cup at work but then they relax on the weekend and end up with a withdrawal headache. Still, this didn't answer my question about my medical school headaches. Given how late I would stay up the night before Anatomy lab, there was little danger of my showing up without a healthy jolt of caffeine coursing through my veins.

So what accounted for my Gross Anatomy headaches? How could they help explain weekend headaches in my patients? The answer became clear when I began collecting information about sleep patterns from my patients. Most people, especially parents, tend to keep pretty regular hours during the week. But they enjoy socializing or going out on Friday or Saturday night and, often, this runs well past their usual bedtime, so they sleep late the next morning to get their seven or eight hours of sleep. The problem is, they're not the *same* seven or eight hours.

We know that the body releases certain hormones on a diurnal (daily) basis and that cortisol fluctuates with our twenty-four-hour cycle, with the highest levels present in the early morning and the lowest levels present three to five hours after the onset of sleep, typically around midnight. When we mess with our biological clock by pulling an all-nighter or sleeping in, we change this internal cycle and disrupt our cortisol levels. In some people, this disruption is more than enough to trigger migraines. It turns out that, for many migraineurs, it is not enough to get the same *amount* of sleep, but we also need to get our sleep at approximately the same part of the twenty-four-hour day.

Sleep patterns, or chronobiology, are a problem for many headache sufferers. Too much or too little sleep can predispose to migraines, as can frame shift or changes in the timing of the sleep cycle. When you track your sleep pattern in your diary and look for correlations with headaches, you can identify sleep-related triggers.

In today's world, sleep problems create many problems for migraineurs, particularly for shift workers and frequent travelers. For the average person (without headaches), it takes about one full day to make up for each hour of time-zone change or sleep-cycle shift. This means if you are traveling from, say, New York to Amsterdam (six time zones), you can expect almost a week of jet lag before you are adjusted to your new schedule. We think this slow adjustment is the body's way of protecting our delicate hormonal cycles from sudden change (which, if too sudden, can result in inflammation). In migraineurs this protective mechanism does not appear to work as effectively as we might prefer. Thus, changes in sleep pattern (or time zone) are more disruptive and can trigger headaches.

Other sleep disruptions are also common headache triggers, and headache sufferers are vulnerable to several potential pitfalls around sleep. These include sleep deprivation for any reason, including child rearing, staying up late, pulling an all-nighter, getting a bad night's sleep, and sleeping in. This last is one of the most common mistakes headache sufferers make.

Often, the migraineur's reasoning goes something like this: Sleep helps migraines, so more sleep is better, so sleeping in should generally help my migraines. Sounds good, but wrong, wrong, wrong. For headache sufferers, regularity is an important feature of a migraine-free lifestyle, and regularity means you need a structured, healthy rhythm to your day, including regular sleep patterns as much as regular mealtimes and regular exercise.

This raises the issue of what we doctors call "sleep hygiene." Good scientific data as well as clinical evidence support the assertion that *good sleep hygiene is probably the most important element of lifestyle for most headache sufferers.* The whole idea behind sleep hygiene is to use nonpharmacologic methods to promote sleep, and we have many. Most migraineurs are very sensitive to medications, whether prescription or natural, so I prefer to treat sleep issues with lifestyle modification whenever possible.

Many migraineurs find that too much or too little sleep worsens headaches. Other patients find that difficulty falling or staying asleep is a nightmare (pardon the pun) that contributes to their headaches. We know that for many migraineurs it is not enough to get the same amount of sleep every night. We need to get it in approximately the same part of the twenty-four-hour day. By creating good "sleep hygiene," sleep can become a positive element in managing your headaches and improving your life. Clinically we have worked out much of the strategy for using sleep to manage headaches.

Migraine sufferers generally do best when things are nice and orderly and routine. That is not because we are all type A, obsessive-compulsive neurotics. In the same way that migraineurs do better in a well-controlled environment in terms of light, sound, and so forth, so, too, we do better when we maintain our "internal environment" in a steady state, as steady as possible.

Your body is used to beginning the day at a certain time, so your sleep cycle and cortisol levels are entrained for that pattern. When you sleep in, you disrupt the pattern and, often, that is enough to trigger a headache. Even when you have stayed up late the preceding night, sleeping more than a half-hour late the next morning is not a good strategy. A better plan might be to premedicate with your headache medicine before you engage in a potentially headache-triggering behavior such as staying up late. Your headache doctor can direct you toward medications with long half-lives that will offer protection through the next day.

If you get a lousy night's sleep and, at three a.m., decide to kill the alarm because you still haven't fallen asleep, you are adding one problem on top of another. Even in this situation, sleeping in can trigger a headache just as easily as staying up late. It is not just a matter of getting your six or eight or ten hours of sleep. They need to be the *same* six or eight or ten hours, every night. So, if you have trouble falling asleep, you need to have a strategy for doing so, perhaps a medication, natural remedy, or behavioral approach. Your health professional can help you select the alternative that is best for you. Regardless of which method you choose, or what hour you finally fall asleep, you should always get out of bed at approximately the same time every day.

"Sleep Hygiene" Involves Behavioral Modifications

One of those medical buzzwords you hear on *Oprah* and the *Today* show, "sleep hygiene" has a lot of good, hard science behind it. In fact, as stated before, for most headache sufferers, *sleep hygiene is probably the most important element of their lifestyle.* Both scientific and clinical data support this. Sleep hygiene includes strategies for keeping a routine of good habits around your sleep patterns, primarily with regular hours to optimize your sleep.

Again, the idea behind sleep hygiene is to use nonpharmacological approaches to promote sleep, and we have many wonderful nonmedication strategies to help. In my clinic, I always try to go this route. Most migraineurs are very sensitive to medications, whether prescription or natural, so I prefer to treat with lifestyle modification whenever possible.

What is a healthy sleep pattern for a migraineur? For the most part, it is the same as a healthy pattern for anyone else. The goal is to get a good night's sleep, awaken refreshed, go through your day without dragging, napping, or self-medicating to stay awake, and go to bed relaxed, clear-headed, and ready to sleep.

A good sleep environment—a quality pillow and mattress, and light and sound control—can be very important, but the most important element in a good night's sleep is how we prepare in the hours before going to bed. It's best not to eat, ingest caffeine, smoke, exercise, or take on projects just before bedtime. Use the hour or two before retiring to wind down and calm down, rather than fill up your evening until you get into bed. If you spend your evening being productive, you tend to take the next few hours to do a postmortem on your day, obsessing on what you didn't get done and what you need to do tomorrow. Then bed becomes the place where you think about things, rather than where you sleep.

With a reliable sleep pattern, your hormone levels will be consistent, and your body can coordinate the rejuvenating effects of sleep. Since sleep is a major component of an antimigraine lifestyle, here are some basic guidelines that will help most migraineurs establish and maintain a healthy rhythm in their sleep cycles:

- Go to bed at the same time each night, more or less. If you have kids, go to bed an hour or two *after* they do.
- Get up at the same time each morning, even on weekends, regardless of how well you slept (or didn't sleep) the night before.
- If you are a napper, take your nap at the same time every day and for the same length of time.

Sleep Problems

If headache disrupts your sleep, either with difficulty falling asleep, mid-cycle awakening, or early awakening, you should discuss this with your doctor, as it is likely a significant contributor to your daytime headaches and requires attention. In this circumstance, your doctor may consider jaw clenching, sleep apnea, parasomnias, and medication effects.

If you have other sleep problems, such as a hard time going to bed and waking up at the same time every day, and your headaches are out of control in both frequency and severity, it is well worth the effort to work on your sleep hygiene *before* you try using any sleep aids. If your sleep routine is not at all routine, you may have a hard time making it so. But by focusing on your sleep hygiene, you *can* regulate your sleep cycles. If you adhere to the following regimen for a few days, you should have no difficulty falling asleep.

Insomniac's Guide to a Good Night's Sleep

1. Create a comfortable, dark, quiet sleeping environment.
2. Pick a specific bedtime and stick to it.
3. Pick a specific wake-up time in the morning and stick to it.
4. Do not nap during the day. Or, if you must nap, try to do it at the same time each day and for the same amount of time each day.

5. Do not eat, read, or watch TV in bed. Ever. Use your bed *only* for sleep and sex.
6. Do not eat or exercise just before bed.
7. If you are still awake twenty minutes after going to bed, get out of bed, sit in an upright chair, and read something boring. Do not do anything that is the least bit stimulating. When you get tired, go back to bed. Again, if you are still awake after twenty minutes, get up and read again. Repeat as necessary throughout the night, but still get up at your regular time in the morning.
8. Get up at your regular time and drag yourself through your day, regardless of how you slept—or didn't sleep—the night before.
9. Repeat all the preceding steps every night until you find that you fall asleep within twenty minutes of your chosen bedtime. This may take a couple of days.

After adhering to this schedule religiously for about two or three days, most people sleep well enough to be over the problem. It works amazingly well. If these strategies don't resolve your sleep problem, you might need to get medical help for your specific issues, distinguishing between physical problems, such as sleep apnea or restless leg syndrome, and psychological problems, such as anxiety or depression. When sleep disturbances rise to the point of being a significant health care issue, it is time to seek advice from an expert, starting with your primary care doctor. However, keep in mind that if a solution includes the possibility of taking sleeping pills, migraineurs should consider some important headache issues.

Sleep Meds and Migraine

When you experience an occasional night—or run of nights—of poor sleep, you might consider a sleep aid. Lots of medicines out there can make you sleepy. Unfortunately, they don't all promote *quality* sleep, and many can actually *cause* headaches in some people. While some of the offending medicines are available only by prescription, others are available over the counter or at health food stores. But before you consider taking a pill for sleep, you must exercise special care regarding your headaches. For migraineurs, the two primary problems with sleep medications are headaches as a side effect, and medication overuse headaches.

NATURAL REMEDIES While most of us in Western culture are used to quick fixes for our problems, there are many "slower" natural remedies for sleep. These are a good alternative because they are less disruptive to the natural sleep cycle, and they tend to be gentle and not particularly potent sleep aids. In my experience, these natural products are most effective when used in conjunction with a concerted effort to improve sleep hygiene.

The most popular of the natural remedies are valerian and chamomile teas. Valerian is a plant that can be purchased as a 300 mg capsule or taken as tea. It tends to calm and relax without dramatic side effects in most people, though too much valerian can upset the stomach. We often use valerian as a transition from prescription sleep aids or benzodiazepines to natural sleep. Chamomile tea has been used as a calming beverage to settle the stomach and ease anxiety for hundreds (probably thousands) of years, again without side effects.

Melatonin is a natural product very similar to the body's own sleep-inducing protein. As we age, and probably under stress as well, the body's levels of melatonin drop, and some patients find it effective to take melatonin supplements, available in health food stores, usually in 3 mg doses. An analog of melatonin, trade named Rozerem, is also available by prescription.

Kava kava and hops are other natural supplements used to help sleep, but we know very little about their effect on headache. Licorice, an ingredient in many "natural" sleep aids, can be a potent trigger for headaches and, if you are sensitive to this food, you should avoid these products.

OVER-THE-COUNTER SLEEP AIDS Since most natural products generally do not provide enough help for patients with significant sleep issues, many patients turn to over-the-counter products for help. Unfortunately, headache sufferers don't usually find them very beneficial.

Antihistamines have a strong side effect: sleepiness. Available over the counter, antihistamines, such as Benadryl and Tylenol PM, are common sleep aids. But in addition to making you sleepy, antihistamines can disrupt your sleep cycle and leave you feeling tired and unrested in the morning. Worse, particularly with habitual use, antihistamines can promote an unwelcome morning headache and worsen headache in general. Indeed, with regular use, many of the over-the-counter sleep medications can have this effect, as can the nonprescription stimulants used to counteract the effects of the sleep aids.

PRESCRIPTION SLEEP AIDS   Most patients who exhaust all the options will need to discuss the advantages and disadvantages of prescription sleep aids with a doctor. But it is important that headaches are part of this conversation.

Newer prescription sleep aids have several advantages, the most striking of which is greatly reduced "hangover." Two relatively short-acting medications, Ambien and Sonata, effectively treat simple insomnia. In other words, they help you fall asleep and can sustain sleep for about four hours. Then you are on your own. This is an excellent solution for someone with difficulty falling asleep but no problem sustaining sleep, once achieved. While no formal studies have looked at this class of medication in migraineurs specifically, it is widely used by the population as a whole and I have not seen problems with it in our patients.

In addition, three even newer medications boast up to eight hours of sleep with a single dose. One of these is a reformulated Ambien called Ambien CR, in which half the tablet dissolves quickly and the other half dissolves about four hours later. There have been reported cases of sleepwalking and other parasomnias with Ambien CR. Lunesta is another agent that can rapidly bring on sleep, then maintain it for up to eight hours, without a hangover in most people. Rozerem, which is very similar to the body's own melatonin, offers up to eight hours of sleep. Again, these medications have yet to be studied in a population of migraineurs, but empirically and in my clinical experience their judicious use does not seem to cause worsening headaches and, in fact, can substantially improve sleep hygiene, which in turn improves the patient's headache pattern.

Tricyclics—like amitriptyline (Elavil), nortriptyline (Pamelor), and desipramine—were originally developed as antidepressants. But these medications are not often used for that purpose anymore, because they have a reliable side effect: sleepiness. Popular and inexpensive sleep aids, these prescription medications also modify pain perception, so we use them as headache preventives. Some are not recommended for use in the elderly, but as a class, they are largely safe and effective. With a wide therapeutic range (meaning that many different dosages can be used safely), their main side effect at higher dose, besides sleepiness, is dry mouth. The only significant downside is that these medicines can make you feel a bit "hungover" in the morning, but patients can usually compensate for this by taking the pill earlier in the evening.

Amitriptyline or nortriptyline may be other good choices for patients who have frequent headaches and trouble sleeping. These medications have a significant propensity for causing drowsiness that can last for six or eight hours or more. With a very wide therapeutic window (meaning that the dose can vary from 10 mg to more than 100 mg), these medications are relatively safe to use on a regular basis.

Sometimes, when daytime drowsiness is a prominent side effect with the other choices, protriptyline can be a good substitute. Many other headache-preventive medications list drowsiness as a potential side effect. For many of these, the effect is temporary or never manifests in the first place. Sleepiness as a side effect is definitely more common with some preventives than others. If sleeping too little is a problem for you, discuss this with your doctor when you are selecting the most appropriate preventive.

On the other hand, patients who have the opposite problem, sleeping too much, should also look carefully at their medications and, obviously, avoid those that are sedating. Unfortunately, none of the medications presently approved for headache prevention fight sleepiness. Protriptyline, which is similar to amitriptyline, is relatively nonsedating, but I have not found it particularly effective as a headache preventive.

Caffeine

Caffeine is a very interesting substance. From a pharmacologic point of view, it is an adjuvant, meaning that it promotes or enhances the actions of various other medications. It is also a stimulant, an appetite suppressant, and a diuretic.

Caffeine is also very interesting in terms of headache. An ingredient of certain combination headache remedies such as Fioricet and Fiorinal, caffeine enhances the effect of its muscle-relaxant and analgesic elements. Caffeine also contributes to medication overuse headache. Caffeine in beverages can abort a headache, if used early in the headache's development. But when habitual caffeine use is interrupted or increased, the change can trigger a headache. And, in certain rare headache types such as hypnic headaches, caffeine before bed can actually prevent headaches and allow a normal night's sleep.

Usually, though, the relationship of caffeine to sleep is less complicated. For the vast majority of people, caffeine either postpones sleep or significantly disrupts sleep "architecture" (the structure of sleep through the night). For this reason, most sleep specialists discourage caffeine intake in the evening. Of course, some people swear they can drink coffee at night and still sleep, but strong evidence suggests that their sleep quality would be better if they didn't.

Some headache specialists feel strongly that no migraineur should ever, *ever* have caffeine. However, excessive use of caffeine (like almost anything else) or erratic use of caffeine (like anything else) has the potential to get a migraineur in trouble.

For most headache sufferers, the best way to deal with caffeine is to have a consistent, day-to-day intake. If you are a two-cup-in-the-morning-and-one-soda-in-the-afternoon person, stick to that schedule, day in and day out, week in and week out, *including weekends*. Be aware of the caffeine content in your medications, some sodas, and other caffeine sources, so you know that you need to get that amount of caffeine every day. No-Doz or other over-the-counter caffeine pills can be an acceptable substitute in situations where you cannot maintain your usual intake of caffeinated beverages. Examples of such circumstances include when you must fast for a blood test or another medical procedure, when you are traveling and have no access to your usual morning beverage, or when you just don't feel like a coffee or a soda. If you only take caffeine when you feel a headache coming on, do not have an entire pitcher of caffeinated tea while you sit out in the sun. Disruptions to routine will often trigger a caffeine headache, which is really a migraine triggered by caffeine or caffeine withdrawal. The exception to this is the patient with chronic daily headache. Someone in this position should eliminate all caffeine until her headaches are under control.

If you go to bed anytime before midnight, it is best to have your last caffeinated beverage around six or seven, or at least three hours before you will go to bed. If for some reason you need to stay up late, caffeine is not a bad alternative, but if you know it is a trigger for you, it might be a good idea to take a triptan or other migraine rescue medication along with your double nonfat half-caffè Frappuccino latte.

Chapter 11

Headaches and Hormones

Sometimes, headaches do go away. Sometimes, forever. The most common circumstance is when a woman reaches menopause. Anywhere from 30 to 70 percent of women reportedly stop getting migraines after menopause, or their headaches improve dramatically. We find that menopausal patterns tend to run in families, so if your mom's headaches went away in her fifties, there is a good chance that yours will, too. Unfortunately, many women also find that their headaches spin out of control during the windup to menopause, perimenopause.

Another golden period for some women is early pregnancy. About half of all women with migraines report that their headaches dramatically improved during pregnancy and even disappeared during the headache-free zone, the second and third trimesters. But the headaches typically returned (sometimes with a vengeance) after delivery.

About three times more common in women than in men, migraines are most active during what we myopically call the reproductive years. As far back as the mid-1970s it was demonstrated that fluctuations in estrogen levels led to headaches in many women.

So are hormones a factor in migraine? It's a safe bet they are.

But just how hormones (especially estrogen) trigger migraines is complicated. We know that sudden changes in estrogen levels are bad for headaches, and that changes in estrogen are not even close to the whole story when it comes to migraine, since guys get migraines, too. But between these two facts is a world of experience dealing with hormones and headaches, and we've learned many lessons that can help women better manage their headaches.

The relationship between reproductive hormones and migraines is, perhaps, the best *and least* understood aspect of headache management. Best, because it has been studied extensively. We know the contributions of estrogen (huge), progesterone (minor), the timing of menarche, and the relative effects of chemical, surgical, and natural menopause on headaches. Least, because we have yet to consistently apply this knowledge to clinical care.

As far back as the 1970s, researchers were looking carefully at the relationship between sex hormones and headaches. Of particular interest were the hormones estrogen, progesterone, and, later, follicle-stimulating hormone and luteinizing hormone. These early studies showed that when estrogen levels dropped, migraine headaches were triggered in most women; given estrogen, these women could prevent or at least postpone the headaches that typically accompanied their periods. On the other hand, if progesterone was given, it postponed the period, but not the headaches. The fact that for many women headaches get much better during late pregnancy, when estrogen levels remain consistently high, supported these observations. And further studies showed that dramatic fluctuations (usually drops) in estrogen were associated with worsening migraines; when estrogen remained fairly constant (as in pregnancy or with replacement therapy) headaches improved. So we know that migraine is not a response to high *or* low estrogen levels, but to dramatic *changes* in estrogen—up *or* down. Of course, estrogen is *not* the only player in the migraine game, but for many women it is a major player. Certainly, compelling arguments support the use of low-dose birth control or hormone replacement, but *with respect to migraine, it is more about maintaining consistent levels of circulating estrogen.* When there is a significant menstrual component to a patient's headaches, the Keeler Method focuses on this objective. Sometimes when a low dose of estrogen is used in a woman who still has her ovaries, fluctuating levels persist, as do headaches. When higher doses are used, the ovarian production of estrogen is completely suppressed and the levels are steady.

Like all diseases, migraine has what is known as a natural history, a progression across the spectrum of our lives. In women, migraine is often tied to the hormonal changes of reproductive life. Migraines often begin with menarche (the first menstruation), change with pregnancy and childbirth, change again as menopause approaches, and again with completion of menopause. Examining each of these stages in recent years at the Keeler Center, we have developed strategies for anticipating these changes and coping with them as they begin to occur. The medications we might offer a woman anticipating pregnancy, for example, are very different from what we use to prevent headaches in a woman beyond her reproductive years.

As you live through these stages of life, discuss these health care strategies with your doctors. Your primary care physician, gynecologist, and headache specialist can help you design the best headache management plan for your specific needs throughout your reproductive years and, of course, beyond.

Are your headaches affected by your menstrual cycle?

_____

If so, at what age did you begin menstruation?

_____

Did the onset of menstruation affect your headaches?

_____

For many women, estrogen change is a huge trigger, and the relationship between the two must be explored.

Are you pregnant?

_____

Are you planning to become pregnant?

_____

When?

_____

This is important for both medication decisions and planning for lifestyle changes.

Have you ever been pregnant?

_____

If so, did this affect your headaches?

_____

How you responded to pregnancy (headache-wise) in the past can be helpful in predicting future responses to changes in estrogen levels with future pregnancy or menopause.

Are you perimenopausal?

_____

Postmenopausal?

_____

If so, when did your periods become irregular?

_____

Perimenopause can begin as many as fifteen years before actual menopause. For many women, this is when headaches start to get out of control.

Was your menopause natural, chemical, or surgical (hysterectomy)?

_____

How you get to menopause often tells a lot about how your headaches tie in to the change in life.

Did this affect your headaches?

_____

If you had a hysterectomy, did you also have your ovaries removed?

_____

This can have a huge impact on hormonal status and the cycling of your headaches. It can help guide hormone replacement therapy.

Menstrual Migraine

Fortunately, not every child of migraineurs gets headaches, but unfortunately, if you get hormonally related migraines, there is a good chance that your daughter will get migraines when her periods start. Your son, too, may well become a migraineur when he hits puberty.

Many women can trace the beginnings of their migraines to puberty. In girls, migraine often starts with menarche, the onset of menstruation, the first menstrual period. In the majority of women who get migraines, menses trigger their attacks, though most women also have attacks with other triggers.

These are just probabilities and patterns we see. At present, we don't know for sure because we don't have blood tests or imaging modalities that can predict who will or will not suffer from migraine.

Many patients describe themselves as having several types of headaches: menstrual headaches, sinus headaches, and tension headaches. While these kinds of headaches certainly do exist, it is more likely that these patients have one kind of headache (migraine) with several different kinds of triggers. While this is a hot area for research just now, current thinking is that dramatic fluctuations in estrogen levels can trigger migraines. For this reason, when we see that hormones—whether estrogen, cortisol, or epinephrine (to name a few)—play a role, we try to develop strategies to level out or minimize the fluctuations.

True menstrual migraine is a headache that occurs in women *only* around their periods. Headache specialists usually distinguish these from menstrually related migraines that occur in women whose headaches are worse with their periods but who also get migraines at other times and from other triggers. In fact, no scientific evidence suggests that menstrual migraines differ in terms of pathophysiology from migraines triggered by other things. However, many women describe their menstrual headaches as being the most severe of all their headaches. Menstrual migraines can also last longer and can be more resistant to treatment. This may be because the trigger (estrogen change) is a potent trigger in these women and is difficult to manipulate once the change has begun.

It is possible that the severity of menstrual migraines is related to the fact that these headaches occur during periods, when there are a lot of other changes and stressors, a kind of perfect storm of triggers. But it appears that these headaches are pathophysiologically similar to migraines that occur at other times. However, this may turn out to be an artificial distinction. Fluctuations in estrogen levels remain one of the most consistent triggers for migraines, and for both menstrual migraines and menstrually related migraines, the treatment goals are the same: to decrease the severity and duration of these headaches.

A little background may be helpful. Different parts of the body communicate and regulate one another in a very complex way, sending urgent or long-lasting information signals with a feedback regulation. Urgent messages, needing to transmit over milliseconds to seconds, travel through nerve impulses and through chemicals called neurotransmitters. Slower but longer-lasting messages are transmitted via hormones. The longest-lasting messages come through very slow molecular (genetic) changes. The hormones are in between, transmitting reasonably quickly, but lasting a while. Hormones cycle and fluctuate in a rhythm. Cortisol, which cycles along with sleep cycles, fluctuates on a roughly twenty-four-hour basis. Gastrin cycles on a six- to eight- to twelve-hour basis. Estrogen fluctuates on a twenty-eight-day cycle.

Remember, migraine is a response to a change in the environment that the brain perceives as hostile. What's that you say? Hormones have nothing to do with the environment? Hah! The body must keep track of changes in the *external* environment, to be sure, but it is also very sensitive to changes in the *internal* environment. Just as external changes— fluorescent lights, noxious smells, or movement—can trigger a migraine, so can changes in the internal environment. Thus, just as swings in gastrin during fasting, or cortisol after the proverbial all-nighter, can trigger headaches, fluctuations in estrogen before, during, and after menses can also cause cyclical migraines.

Once we understand that dramatic changes in the environment— including our internal environment—are likely candidates as triggers, we need to identify *which* changes lead to your headaches and then set out to control them as much as possible. In the case of estrogen, this often means regulating the hormone to smooth out the monthly fluctuations. We can do this in a number of ways.

For migraine, the overall best strategy is to treat a headache before it becomes a headache, and we focus most of our management plan on this objective. But when a headache is upon you, you should begin rescue treatment as early in the headache as possible with your usual migraine rescues. For acute relief, rapidly acting triptans (such as rizatriptan or sumatriptan) remain the mainstay of treatment. You might start with a triptan in combination with an NSAID, or follow it, if necessary, with a longer-acting triptan (such as frovatriptan) a couple of hours later. Your doctor can help you with appropriate rescue treatments, which will generally be the same as for your other migraines, regardless of the trigger. Again, the best headache management helps you *avoid the hormonal swings that set you up for cyclical migraines, so our strategy focuses on preventing or minimizing these headaches in the first place.*

Hormonal Intervention

Several different approaches can help decrease the monthly fluctuation of estrogen. Migraineurs often improve when they are on constant hormone replacement and, for many women, an estrogen supplement smooths out the variation during the month. In the case of menstrual migraine, this may involve one of many estrogen formulations (or estrogen plus progesterone, if the patient still has her uterus), some of which are bioequivalent. Some are taken as a pill, but we prefer those that maintain levels of the hormone for long periods of time, like estrogen patches, rings, or depot injections. As a rule, the lowest effective dose with the steadiest release over time is the way to go.

Birth control pills are a very common option for treating menstrual irregularities, preventing pregnancy, and yes, helping control migraine headaches. When considering this option, keep a couple of things in mind. First, 20 percent of migraineurs have "classic" migraines (migraines preceded by an aura—visual, sensory, or otherwise), and *these migraineurs should not take birth control pills.* If they do, it increases their risk for stroke, and this appears to be particularly important for women in their childbearing years. If you get an aura with your migraines, be sure to discuss this important point with your doctor.

If you do not get an aura with your migraines, birth control pills may be an option. Most birth control pill regimens are designed around a "21/7" model, meaning that you take twenty-one days of estrogen followed by seven days of placebo pills, which contain no estrogen. While this is a highly effective means of birth control, it will likely mean that many women will get a headache every three weeks. Therefore, neurologists and gynecologists often recommend using birth control pills to suppress menstruation in a "63/7" configuration. Using this strategy, you would take the estrogen-containing pills for sixty-three straight days and *then* take seven days of placebo pills. In this case, the woman has her menstruation every two months instead of every twenty-eight days, which decreases the frequency of the estrogen-letdown headaches. Compared with the 21/7 regimen, this regimen does not appear to have any additional adverse side effects. Unless a woman is trying to become pregnant, it appears that women do not need to have periods, nor does it appear that suppressing periods for prolonged lengths of time does any harm. Of course, if this interests you, discuss it with your doctors.

Considering birth control pills, migraineurs should also keep dosing in mind. From a headache perspective, patients should use the lowest effective dose to achieve smaller day-to-day estrogen fluctuations. Whether the pill is a combination of estrogen and progesterone or simple estrogen does not appear to affect the headache pattern, but for other health reasons, you should discuss this important question with the prescribing doctor.

The more your headaches are tied to your periods, the more likely it is that you will see improvement with some form of estrogen regulation. However, some women do not see improvement with birth control pills or other estrogen replacement programs. We don't have a very good explanation for why this is, but we see it. If you are in this group or if for any reason you do not want to take estrogen, we do have other options. One alternative is to take a headache medication for a short period before and/or during the start of menses, while other women will benefit from taking a daily preventive throughout the month.

Pulse Prevention

Many women's menstrual cycles are as reliable as night following day. Their periods may come every twenty-three days or every thirty-one days, but these women could set a calendar by their cycle. For some of these women, the migraine that comes with it may be equally predictable. In terms of headache management, these women are actually lucky. By knowing when their headaches are likely to come, they can act to minimize or even prevent them.

When we can anticipate that a trigger is likely to generate a headache, we can use a headache abortive or preventive medication for a short period of time to avoid getting the headache. This approach is called pulse prevention. In the case of menstrual migraine, women take the medication during their PMS days or when their period starts. To be sure, the headache may surface anyway, but it is likely to be less severe and more responsive to the usual rescue treatments.

We have a couple of alternative strategies. Some women can simply take a nonsteroidal anti-inflammatory drug (NSAID) like ibuprofen or naproxen on a regular basis for a couple of days before they would typically experience the menstrual migraine, and continue it for the first few days into that period. Women often need to experiment but this is often enough to effectively prevent or minimize the menstrual migraine.

If pulse prevention with an NSAID doesn't work, we can try using a long-acting triptan (like frovatriptan or naratriptan), beginning two days before the patient expects the headache and continuing for the duration of the menses. For some women, it may be very effective to simply take a long-acting triptan the night before their period, or before they expect the headache. It may still be necessary to take the usual rescue medication, or even a second triptan, if the headache does come, but generally, the headache will be less severe and more easily treatable.

Frequently, my conversations with my patients include comments along the lines of "I get a headache the first four days of my period, but I am only supposed to take my triptan two days a week. What about that, Dr. Fancy Neurologist?" (My patients are very comfortable with me.) True, taking triptans *preventively*, at night before bed, even for only a few days, is controversial. Some doctors feel that this will lead to medication overuse headache (MOH). This has not been my experience with this particular strategy. Many headache specialists, myself among them, find that *this is the one circumstance in which daily use of triptans for more than the prescribed two days per week is appropriate.* One possible explanation for this is that the menstrual migraine is one really long headache episode, and the central windup that is felt to be responsible for MOH is not induced with this single episode and its treatment. At this writing, we do not have a generally accepted explanation for this observation. Also, mixing triptans, such as taking a long-acting triptan as a preventive at night and then a more rapid-acting triptan for rescue the next day, is outside the FDA-approved uses. Again, I have not seen problems with this approach, but you should discuss this with your doctor.

Having said that, if a woman's headaches are predictable with every (or almost every) menstrual period, and they are reliably four-day headaches, daily use of triptans during this time appears safe and effective. We have used frovatriptan in such situations for up to ten days without apparent MOH. However, on a number of occasions, we have seen emergence of the headache for a day following cessation of the medication, although this does not seem to correlate with the number of days the triptan is taken. We have not been able to predict which patients do well with this kind of pulse prevention and which patients find that it only delays the headache. Again, this approach to managing menstrual migraines is outside the FDA-approved recommendations for triptan use, and you should not undertake this or any treatment without the complete support of your treating physicians.

Some studies have also looked at pulse prevention with migraine preventives, such as divalproate (Depakote) or topiramate (Topamax). Unfortunately, since both of these medications require titration over time to attain the proper blood levels in the body, the studies had issues getting to the therapeutic dose quickly enough to help. Depacon, an IV form of divalproate, has been used to rapidly titrate to therapeutic blood levels, which is then followed by oral divalproate for the duration of the menses.

In menstrually related migraines, the trigger is pretty straightforward and so is the solution. To be sure, it is not a perfect solution, but for most women, it works well. Unfortunately, some women do not have cooperative, predictable cycles or predictable headaches within the cycles. These migraineurs may benefit from other preventive strategies.

Other Approaches

For women who do not get their periods on a sufficiently regular basis to know when to use a pulse preventive, estrogen treatment to help regulate their cycles and to prevent their headaches might be a good idea, but this may not be an option, either. Other women are severely affected by menstrual migraine and also have headaches at other times throughout the month. For all of these women, another alternative is to take a daily preventive medicine such as topiramate, propranolol, or another choice throughout the month, which can be most beneficial (see the thorough discussion of preventive options on page 153). Remember, the Keeler Method is a three-part strategy of lifestyle modification, prevention, and rescue. And all three of these apply as much to menstrual migraines as to any other primary headache.

Those who strongly prefer to start with more "natural" treatments might try butterbur, magnesium, or feverfew. While these are valid and effective treatments, as a rule herbal preventives and supplements take a long time, up to three months or more, to show a therapeutic effect. Everyone is different. My best advice is to be open to alternatives—both traditional and otherwise.

For any given individual, lifestyle changes, whether they have ten thousand years of precedent or just came up on the Internet, may be worth evaluating. Specifically, with menstrual migraine, my patients have had good success with regular exercise, and yoga in particular, as an adjunctive therapy. I have also found that regular sleep and good hydration during menses are beneficial. Biofeedback and psychological counseling, both effective tools for migraine in general, have been less effective for menstrual migraine specifically, and I have not found acupuncture or herbal remedies to be particularly effective. However, they are safe alternatives and I am not aware of any danger in experimenting with them.

Finally, pregnancy often will solve the problem of menstrual-related migraines, at least temporarily. But then, it can also create many complications and might be a bit extreme as a treatment strategy.

Pregnancy

For many women, migraine frequency and severity often improve dramatically during pregnancy, particularly during the last two trimesters. As many as two-thirds of women experience an improvement in their migraines during pregnancy. Think of this as a nice bonus, just partial compensation for the months of nausea, weight gain, and mood swings. Some headache specialists feel that the more closely your headaches correspond to your periods, the more likely you are to experience improvement during pregnancy. For some women, their headaches do not change at all during pregnancy and, unfortunately, other women actually *begin* to get migraines during pregnancy.

Every woman with migraines should consider several issues *before, during, and after* pregnancy. Whenever possible, it is very important to talk with a doctor about your migraines when you are hoping or planning to conceive. In general, women should taper off preventive medications *before* becoming pregnant, except for patients with complicated migraine. Some preventive medications are relatively safe during pregnancy, and some are much more dangerous. By the same token, some rescue medicines can be used during pregnancy, but these are usually quite different from the medicines we use in nonpregnant headache sufferers.

During the first two trimesters of pregnancy, estrogen levels are high, and they remain high. But as delivery dates approach, estrogen levels begin to decline, then they can fall precipitously postpartum. Headaches can return with a vengeance, so women who plan to nurse their babies have still more medication questions to consider. Not all medicines cross over into breast milk, but some do, and some of these are more dangerous to babies than others. For example, it appears that sumatriptan (Imitrex) is safe to take while breast-feeding. It is important to discuss every medication—prescribed, over-the-counter, herbal, or supplemental—with your ob-gyn. This is definitely not an area where a migraineur should wing it.

Menopause

Different people use the word "menopause" differently, and even use different words to refer to it. Commonly, we think a woman is going through menopause, or the "change of life," when the physical changes of midlife become evident. Technically, menopause itself is that point in a woman's life when she no longer menstruates. When a woman has not had one menstrual period in twelve months, we say she has "gone through menopause." Then, she is postmenopausal.

The premenopausal phase that leads up to menopause is called perimenopause. This is the problematic phase, when the prominent and famous symptoms arise: weight gain, hot flashes, mood changes, depression, longer and more irregular periods, and, often, symptoms of migraines. For most women, perimenopause occurs around age fifty and lasts about two years, but it can begin as early as a woman's thirties or as late as her sixties, and can last ten years. In any case, the hormonal changes actually begin many years before we notice the symptoms, and long before menopause itself.

For as many as two-thirds of women with migraines, headaches *decrease* dramatically or even stop completely with menopause. But remember, menopause is that point when you no longer have periods. Perimenopause, the approach to menopause, can be tough—and many women experience a worsening of their headaches or a change in headache character, sometimes with increased auras but decreased head pain.

In most perimenopausal migraineurs, the *quality* of the headaches does not change, but the *frequency* and *severity* do. Among some migraineurs, however, the migraines do change in specific ways as they move from perimenopause into menopause and beyond:

- For some women, the pain component of the migraines goes away with menopause but the auras or visual changes continue from time to time.
- Women who have classic migraines (migraines with aura) may experience less dramatic changes than those with common migraines (migraines that begin without a warning), but this is not always the case.
- According to some recent reports, women whose migraines were worse during their periods might have a harder time with headaches during perimenopause.
- In a subgroup of women, the migraines they have known most of their life disappear but are replaced by "late-life migrainous accompaniments." These curious episodes begin with a series of visual changes (distortions or auras) or sensory changes in the arms and legs, sometimes associated with a headache, and they come in flurries over days, lasting from fifteen minutes to a half-hour. Sometimes, these are confused with the symptoms of a stroke or transient ischemic attack (TIA), so if this happens you should seek immediate medical attention. Once a doctor rules out a stroke, I suggest you see a neurologist to discuss late-life migrainous accompaniments, which you—and your doctors—might consider a benign curiosity, rather than a life-threatening crisis.

But the first clarification we must make is to determine whether a woman's headaches are due to perimenopause or something else. Headaches can be due to a number of causes, and just because you are "of an age" does not automatically mean that your headaches are due to hormonal changes. For example, it is very common that approaching menopause increases the frequency or severity of a woman's headaches and, often, a woman will start overusing headache medications. Before we know it, she is having medication overuse headaches—and all the estrogen in the world won't fix MOH.

In perimenopause, it turns out, estrogen levels fluctuate pretty widely. That is why periods become erratic and many of the other annoying sensations we associate with that time of life emerge. It is also one of the reasons that many women use hormone replacement, either estrogen alone (if they have had a hysterectomy) or with progestin if they still have their uterus. Once menopause occurs, estrogen levels stabilize again, at a much lower level, and headaches often settle down.

All of the phenomena of perimenopause are almost certainly related to changes in estrogen, and possibly progesterone, during this stage of life. When we suspect that perimenopause is causing changes in the headache pattern, we can measure estrogen and other hormones and, to minimize these headaches, we can manipulate estrogen levels. But how you come to menopause will be relevant to how your headaches respond. Today, with various medical interventions, perimenopause can vary from natural to chemical to surgical. These distinctions are important, particularly from a headache perspective.

Natural menopause is when a woman allows the process to progress naturally, with a gradual decline in estrogen levels. Eventually, her periods will end without medical interventions such as surgery or hormone replacement. Natural menopause can take two to ten years. To be sure, this gradual decline in estrogen can be a very rocky course and, often, headaches worsen during this time. However, good scientific data show that, for headache sufferers, the body much prefers a gradual decline over surgical menopause, when estrogen production is cut off abruptly.

"Chemical menopause" refers to the use of hormone replacement therapy to help the body adjust more gradually to hormonal changes and minimize the symptoms of menopause. Also, sometimes, physicians will advocate using certain drugs to stop the body's production of estrogen, essentially hormonally simulating a hysterectomy. The thinking is that this medical hysterectomy will indicate the woman's possible response to a hysterectomy, and aid in the decision whether to undergo the surgery, but the literature is not clear as to whether this is a valid indication of how an individual will respond to removal of her uterus.

At the extreme, when a woman's uterus is surgically removed in hysterectomy with or without oophorectomy (removal of the ovaries), we call it surgical menopause. In this case, the body abruptly undergoes major hormonal changes, adjusting suddenly to the postmenopausal state. If your menopause is surgical with a hysterectomy, it is likely that your headaches will worsen, often for many years, more than if you undergo a natural menopause. Eventually, receptors die off and estrogen production trails to near zero. At this point, the estrogen becomes moot in terms of being a trigger. If the only reason for considering hysterectomy is to improve headaches, I strongly recommend you consider other options. There is very strong evidence that this is not appropriate. However, if there are other compelling reasons for hysterectomy, then someone experienced in headache should be part of your medical team.

If you are unsure of your menopausal status, your physician can order blood tests to clarify your levels of the various hormones that change during menopause. Often, however, these tests can be somewhat vague, and your symptoms might be most informative.

As a migraineur, keep in mind that as you get older, headaches *can* be due to some other cause, and *anytime you get a headache that seems different from usual, you need to bring it to your doctor's attention.*

During perimenopause, a lot goes on in your body. While hormones drive many of the changes you experience, your body also has an intricate interaction with your environment. Your mood, energy level, sleep pattern, diet, weight, and physical condition are all in a rather fragile balance. And—surprise! All of these factors have a striking effect on the frequency, duration, and severity of migraines. So when headaches are an issue, we need to define the various elements that might be contributing to worsening headaches, probably with the help of a physician. Once you understand the contributing elements, it becomes pretty clear where to focus treatment.

Natural Menopause

We do not treat menopause. Menopause is a naturally occurring life event. Now, we may want to treat some of the *symptoms* that come with perimenopause, and a worsening of migraines can certainly be one of those symptoms.

In natural menopause, the decline in estrogen levels is *gradual*. The changes that lead to menopause begin *years* before a woman begins to notice the signs and symptoms, but once changes begin—irregular periods, hot flashes, and change in headache pattern—it takes an average of about two years for most women before menstruation ends. Then the woman is through menopause. Though it can be a very long, rocky course, good scientific data show that for headache sufferers the body much prefers this gradual, natural decline in estrogen production. Of course, this is consistent with our philosophy that migraineurs do better with less disruption to their body's rhythms, internally and externally.

But during menopause, even natural menopause, a woman's estrogen levels fluctuate pretty widely, which is why women experience erratic periods with many other annoying symptoms and, possibly, changes in their headaches. To make matters that much worse, many menopause symptoms can disrupt life enough to increase a woman's headaches even more. Very often, such symptoms might not be menopausal, but a symptom of something else, and treating the underlying cause will often take care of it, so it is important to check with the appropriate physician. To treat these symptoms as well as the headaches, I like to start with lifestyle changes.

For example, when night sweats and hot flashes disrupt a woman's sleep, I suggest that she first go through the basics of sleep hygiene, rather than turn reflexively to the latest sleeping pill. Working on sleep hygiene can almost certainly help. If hot flashes are the problem, see a good gynecologist. Medications such as clonidine can help both hot flashes and headaches, but a woman should make such decisions with input from her gynecologist or endocrinologist.

Another big issue at this time of life is exercise. Menopause comes just when many women are in the busiest and most productive years of their lives, with less time, less energy—and so much more to do. Often, we sacrifice our exercise and leisure time. Needless to say, this is exactly the wrong thing to do. Exercise is critical for a number of reasons. Particularly with respect to headache, exercise causes the body to produce endorphins, our natural painkillers, so I urge all my patients to make exercise a regular part of their day, every day, just like eating and sleeping.

As soon as you realize that your headaches are more frequent and you're moody, you're having hot flashes, or your periods are getting more irregular, check with your doctor, who will be able to run blood tests to determine whether, in fact, you are perimenopausal. If you are, you can take steps to minimize the symptoms—especially the headaches.

The good news is that, with few exceptions, migraine rescue and preventive medications get along pretty well with perimenopause. Well tolerated, the treatments are more effective in natural menopause than in chemical or surgical menopause. Migraine medications and other strategies that worked for you in the past usually continue to work during perimenopause. In fact, if your treatment plan stops working or changes, that is reason enough to sit down with your doctor and reevaluate what might be happening in your body and in your treatment strategy. Properly managed, perimenopause symptoms can become relatively innocuous. The important thing is to realize that these symptoms, including headaches, are not something you just have to live with or ride out until you're through menopause.

Hormone Replacement Therapy in Menopause

If you are perimenopausal, you might want to consider estrogen replacement (with progestin if you still have your uterus), but this is a complicated issue. Certainly, strong evidence supports a beneficial effect on headache frequency, severity, and duration in some women. However, hormone replacement therapy (HRT) is not without risk, and the decision to go on it is complicated. You must have a discussion with your gynecologist and your headache doctor before you decide to start HRT.

It is usually not necessary to be on HRT just for migraine prevention through perimenopause, but with few exceptions, migraineurs tolerate hormones for perimenopause very well, particularly the low-dose, steady-release formulations. And estrogen preparations do not have adverse interactions with most migraine medications.

As with any therapy, you need to weigh the risks versus the benefits of hormone replacement, and these will be different for different people. On the plus side, HRT has several advantages, including possibly reducing bone loss and protecting against certain neurodegenerative diseases. So, for example, if osteoporosis is important in your medical chart or family history, this should factor into your decision. Some women—

among them smokers, women who have had a partial hysterectomy, and women with a strong family history of certain kinds of cancer or cardiovascular disease—will have different risks associated with HRT. And a woman in her thirties has a very different risk profile from that of a woman in her seventies.

Specifically regarding HRT and migraines, you should know that not all women are hormone sensitive, and not all migraine subtypes respond to the stabilization of estrogen levels that HRT can provide. In general, if you had a strong association between your headaches and your menstrual cycle from your early teens through your early forties, your headaches are likely to be hormone sensitive and more likely to respond favorably to estrogen replacement.

Similarly, if you typically get an aura before your headaches begin, you may be more likely to benefit from HRT than is a woman whose headaches begin without such a warning. However, you and your doctor *must* weigh this against admonitions based on the increased risk of stroke among women who have migraine with aura and who use hormone replacement. Except in extreme cases, most headache specialists will avoid HRT in women who get migraine with aura. In young women, stroke risk is increased, but still relatively low, if they have migraine with aura. However, if high-dose estrogen (greater than 50 micrograms) is added, the risk goes up, some estimating as much as twelvefold. In young women without other risk factors for stroke (like smoking), low-dose estrogen (35 micrograms) appears to be safe. This is a complex and important area, so this is a conversation is best left to each migraineur and her treating physician.

Estrogen comes in a variety of preparations and several delivery forms. There are natural estrogen preparations, pharmaceutical preparations, creams, pills, patches, rings, and depot (under the skin) formulations. While no one choice is right for every woman, the option you select can directly impact your headaches.

In migraineurs, estrogen replacement raises several other considerations. Perhaps the most important is to select the formulation and delivery system that will keep estrogen levels steadiest. As with birth control pills, it is best for migraineurs to use the lowest dose of estrogen that provides symptomatic relief. The rule of thumb is: Start low and go slow.

A low-dose, continuous-release formulation of HRT is a good choice with respect to headaches. One option for some women is continuous use of cyclic preparations. For example, the most commonly prescribed HRT formulation is twenty-one days of estrogen followed by seven days of placebo, essentially blank pills that have no estrogen.

The patch is another antimigraine approach. The patch releases a steady supply of estrogen over an extended period. When replaced on a regular basis, the patch keeps estrogen levels pretty even. Some people can be allergic to the adhesive, but if that is a problem it is worth experimenting with the several different brands on the market.

Keep in mind that despite a regular estrogen supplement your body's natural production of estrogen is decreasing, so estrogen levels will still change unless the estrogen dose is high enough to completely suppress your body's estrogen production. Therefore, it is important to reevaluate now and then, both with blood tests and with your diary, to see how you are doing on a given dose.

Once the tumult of hot flashes and headaches with perimenopause has passed and menopause is complete, you should revisit the issue of estrogen replacement with your doctors, who may again suggest blood tests to assess hormone levels as a guide for dosing. They may also recommend supplements such as niacin, which may affect your headaches as well.

Surgical Menopause: Hysterectomy

We often call hysterectomy "surgical menopause" because the result is similar: no more periods and less fluctuation in estrogen levels. However, surgical menopause is very different from natural menopause, especially if you are a migraine sufferer.

Of course, many women have to undergo hysterectomy for other reasons. If you are contemplating hysterectomy, discuss with your health care team the very real possibility that your headaches may worsen. You might consider starting a preventive medication a month or more *before* the surgery. Hormone replacement strategies might also help manage migraines that may occur following hysterectomy, and the triptans and other migraine rescue medications remain effective strategies.

There are certainly valid medical reasons to consider a hysterectomy, but headache control is not one of them. Studies of women migraineurs who undergo surgical menopause show that they are much more likely to experience worsening headaches that can persist for months or years, compared with women who go through natural menopause. The most important point is that *a migraineur should never consider hysterectomy as a treatment for migraines.*

Some physicians advocate a trial medical hysterectomy, prescribing certain drugs that will simulate menopause, giving both doctor and patient a preview of how the patient might respond to menopause. However, the literature is not clear as to whether this is a valid indication of how an individual will respond to hysterectomy. Again, if the only reason for considering hysterectomy is to improve headaches, I recommend caution. At the very least, a woman should get several opinions from experienced gynecologists, headache specialists, and endocrinologists.

Unfortunately, hysterectomy is not simply a matter of cutting off estrogen, because, whether women use hormone replacement immediately after surgery or not, headaches do not improve. The estrogen picture is complicated. Estrogen receptors (distributed to many parts of the body, including the brain) are in a delicate balance, depending on many factors in addition to the body's estrogen supplies. At present, we do not have the capability to reproduce the perfect hormonal environment to simulate natural menopause. Maybe someday, but for right now hysterectomy should not be an option for headache control.

In Due Course

In medicine, we talk about the natural history of a disease, the course it will take if we don't alter it or don't know how to intervene. Some changes arise along the way—pregnancy, perimenopause, and menopause itself—but the natural history of migraine usually starts with puberty and, unfortunately, continues into old age. As a woman goes through these phases, the frequency, severity, and duration of headaches often change. While everyone is different, headaches frequently worsen with midlife changes. But often, after the very rough period during the windup to menopause, migraine improves for about two-thirds of women. As migraineurs, each of us is charged with the task of learning about our own headaches as we go along.

Chapter 12

Headaches and Work

What can you do if your job gives you migraines?

You could buy a lottery ticket.

If that doesn't work and you have to continue working like the rest of us, you need to break down your work environment into components and assess each part as a possible trigger. Very often, just the act of parsing out your workday will highlight your problem areas. Then you'll be able to decide whether you can avoid the trigger or modify it, or if you'll have to take other measures to prevent a headache. For example, I have a patient who teaches third grade. On the surface, one would think that this entire experience would be one giant trigger, but my patient genuinely loves teaching third-graders—noise, chaos, and all. However, the flickering fluorescent lights in her classroom drove her crazy. She was able to persuade her administrator (without the threat of a suit under the Americans with Disabilities Act) to install full-spectrum bulbs and even some lighting appropriately anchored to the walls. Her headaches became much more manageable.

Common migraine triggers in an office might include a coworker's perfume, poor posture when sitting at your desk, or the flash-rate associated with a computer screen. These are very different triggers from the pressure of a deadline or a psychotic boss. Sometimes, multiple triggers or a constellation of triggers—like a "bad day"—might result in a headache. Teasing out the various elements can be tricky, but with a little thought it is usually doable. Then, you can take steps to minimize their triggering effect. Such solutions might be as simple as installing filters on computer screens, using less noxious bathroom disinfectants, or quieting loud noises. So tracking triggers in your work environment, and then figuring out what to do about them, is well worth the investigation.

Remember, migraine is *not* a psychological problem but a true medical disease. As such, you *must* be accorded the same consideration as employees who have asthma, diabetes, or any other chronic condition, and you are *legally* entitled to expect appropriate modifications in the workplace to allow you to work effectively around your condition. If this means you need to take a ten-minute break from your computer every hour, then that is what you should do. If it means you need to shift your hours or your employer needs to change the lighting around your work area or adjust the placement of your desk, you are protected in asking for these things. Your physician can be a great help in documenting as well as facilitating necessary changes, and *you should not hesitate to ask for such help.*

Migraine costs our country $14 billion each year. But less than 15 percent of that is in the direct costs of health care—doctor appointments, medications, and ER visits. The rest, $12 billion, comes in missed workdays and "presenteeism," decreased productivity when we show up for work despite a headache, or when we get a headache during the day and just try to power through. Almost every migraineur has experienced such days.

Given that most of us must work and, for many of us, elements of work either trigger or worsen headaches, we need to figure out ways to minimize the effect of work on our headaches. And, yes, it is easier said than done.

Workplace Triggers

The Keeler Method approaches workplace triggers on two levels. The first level addresses changes the headache sufferer can make in work activities to minimize triggers. The second focuses on changes to the workplace that employers can make, often at the employee's request and, with hope, without their having to invoke the Americans with Disabilities Act. Examples of the first type include identifying work-related triggers, keeping rescue medicines at work and taking them early, varying activities to avoid prolonged computer use, and maintaining daily exercise. On the employer side, equally simple modifications include eliminating triggers (perhaps changing fluorescent bulbs to full-spectrum bulbs that fit in the same fixture) and providing workers with access to a quiet, cool, odor-free environment when necessary. We have developed a variety of strategies that can improve almost any work environment.

When the work itself is the problem—the stress of the job or an incompetent coworker—you might have a more difficult challenge. Whatever the issue, identifying it is half the battle. Once you identify the stressor, you can develop a conscious strategy, whether it is an organizational, interpersonal, or even a competency issue. Counseling might help, or you might need to consult your employer, union representative, doctor, or colleagues to find a workable solution.

Many people think that a headache triggered by work is automatically a tension-type headache. This is not necessarily so. The issue of whether a headache problem is primarily migrainous or tension-type is best decided during a long discussion with your doctor, but the essential fact is that stress is a common trigger for both types of headaches, and work is right up there among the most common sources of stress. If work-related stress is a significant migraine trigger for you, and a new job is not an option, the task becomes one of stress management.

So, for migraineurs, the first step is to define those elements in the work environment that contribute to headaches. Sometimes this can be tough. There may be a manager who hates you or a fellow employee who lives for sabotage. Sure, a psychotic boss or jerk in the next cubicle can be triggers, but what if it is the work itself—the stress of the job or the pressure of deadlines? These problems are common in the workplace. The difference for you is that they contribute to worsening health, and that becomes a different issue that your employer must address.

It is not uncommon for migraine sufferers to notice in their headache diary that most of their headaches tend to occur toward the end of the workday or workweek. Often, this means they are not dealing with work pressures as they increase over time. One very effective method for overcoming this trigger is to frequently reassess the level of stress by taking a short break every hour, using this time to stretch, take a walk, or briefly change activities. For office workers, it is easy enough to set an hourly alarm in Microsoft Outlook or a similar program to remind you to take a break.

If you have stress management issues at work, your response to these challenges may include a headache, so it is important to address such problems. Often, these are human resource issues and you can—and should—deal with them in that arena. It is important to document any offenses and then bring them to the attention of your ombudsman.

The next chapter addresses stress as a migraine trigger, so this chapter focuses on workplace triggers that have less to do with work relationships and more with the work environment, for the elements of the environment can, when you properly address them, improve your headaches. For office workers, lighting issues are common, and your employer can address these fairly easily. Similarly, filters or screens can be installed to block a computer monitor's flicker rate, though these are generally built in to the newer CRTs. Other office modifications might be trickier, but with a little creativity, you can deal with nearly every office trigger.

One of my patients, David, is a talented software designer who works for an enormous company that makes computer games. Apparently, he is so valuable to them that they actually listened when he told them that his doctor wanted to change his department around, provide him with a quiet place to go, and modify his computer screens, lighting, and work schedule. To the company's delight, David went from an average of six missed days of work per month to less than one. Of course, he is doing a lot of other things with medications, exercise, and his family dynamics, but he (and we) credit the lion's share of his success to the changes to his workplace, where he spends about twelve to sixteen hours a day.

Tracking the triggers to your work environment and subsequently figuring out what to do about them is well worth the investigation. To identify triggers at work, the best place to start is with the *location* of the work and then to narrow that down to identify the precise trigger. To do this, it helps if you break "work" down into its components. Once you narrow down *where* your triggers are, then you can begin to look at the specific triggers.

Elements of Work Environments

Most people work in one of three environmental situations: an indoor workplace with continuity, outdoors, or mobile jobs without continuity. Those who work indoors, in a set workplace each day, have the best chance of controlling their environmental triggers. They can easily assess the environment, such as their offices, common areas, and restrooms, to look for potential triggers. Maybe it's the lobby (too cold or hot), the conference room (stuffy, smelly, or overly bright), the office (dusty, poorly lit, or noisy), or the desk (bad ergonomics). In these situations, the headache diary can help point out areas where the migraineur needs changes.

Outdoor workers, such as construction workers, laborers, delivery people, and forest rangers, have much less control but can probably characterize their work sites to a degree, and take measures to mitigate exposure to triggers, such as using masks, sunglasses, and earplugs as appropriate. A common example is the construction worker who, during the demolition phase of a remodel job, gets a headache toward the end of the day. Even if he is not directly involved in the demolition, the dust may be the trigger. If he wears a mask, the problem can be corrected and the trigger reduced or eliminated. Similarly, wearing low-grade earplugs can reduce noise enough to protect against a headache but still allow you to hear someone speaking directly to you.

The third group is the toughest. People who travel, make office calls, spend time in airports and hotels, or change time zones and altitude on a frequent basis can have trouble identifying their specific triggers because they change their lifestyle patterns so much and experience so many variables.

Anyone who finds that work contributes to migraines will do well to:

- examine the components of "work";
- consider all sensory inputs;
- consider any disruptions to the body's routines, especially sleep, diet, and exercise.

Once you identify a specific trigger, you need to *value* it and decide whether you can avoid or modify the trigger or whether you need to anticipate and prepare for headaches, so you can minimize the pain and disruption they will cause.

COMPUTERS   Computers can be a great aid to the migraineur, saving time, helping you maintain your schedule, and even serving to remind you to take breaks and medication. Computers can also be a trigger for headaches if the screen flickers, pops, or is too bright. Computers can also affect migraines when we are compelled to look too long and focus too hard on what we are doing, without taking appropriate breaks. Treat your computer as a potentially dangerous ally, and be sure to get away from it now and then.

PHYSICAL STRAIN   Physical strain should not be confused with physical *exercise*. Strain comes from exerting without proper warm-up or from overtaxing muscles. This not only refers to hefting ninety-pound bags of cement, but also to holding a particular posture for an unnaturally long time. The musculoskeletal and nervous systems are intimately involved with each other, and it is a very short distance between neck stiffness and head pain.

SHIFT WORK   Shift work can be a particularly sticky work situation for migraineurs. We are generally very sensitive to variations in our sleep patterns, so disruptions to our daily schedules are likely to increase the frequency and severity of headaches. If a migraineur works swing or night shift on a permanent or semipermanent arrangement, most can adjust. The problem arises when the shift shifts, when a person works night shift for a period of time and then works days for a while, then changes to swing. This is one of the few situations where intervention from your physician may be necessary. Given the choice between paying out for disability and adjusting someone's schedule to provide regularity in terms of hours, breaks, and mealtimes, most employers will do everything they can to accommodate your need for a regular pattern (as they do with diabetics).

EYESTRAIN   This is one of those vague headache attributions that has persisted along with other pseudo-diagnoses. Certainly, if you over-use your eyes, either by virtue of poor lighting or prolonged focus, the muscles that you use to focus your eyes will fatigue and ache. Whether this represents a true migraine trigger or muscle tension is difficult to say, but if your individual experience is that prolonged use of your eyes in some circumstances consistently leads to a migraine, that is hard to argue with. However, generally eyestrain resolves with "resting the eyes," as my father used to say. And there is nothing wrong with taking a break when your eyes hurt.

LIGHTING   Almost everyone who has experienced a migraine knows how painful bright lights can be when you have a headache. In headache circles, we call this photophobia. It is actually one of the International Headache Society's criteria for defining migraines. In my clinical experience, I find that many people who do not meet other criteria for migraines also experience light sensitivity when their headaches are severe.

But it turns out that not all light is noxious (painful) to headache sufferers. Some light is worse than others. For example, fluorescent lighting with standard bulbs seems to be universally hated, while full-spectrum, incandescent, indirect lighting is often better tolerated. Studies have shown that certain wavelengths of light are better tolerated than others in headache sufferers. For individuals with extreme photophobia, special contacts can even be fabricated, allowing them to get out of a dark room and function reasonably well outside.

While most migraineurs experience photophobia when in the throes of a headache, light sensitivity *between* headaches has been less well studied. Again, in my clinical experience, bright or fluorescent lights can be a potent trigger for headaches in some people. In others, the combination of these light sources with any other potential trigger—a really hot day, a crowded, tense room, or after a bad night's sleep or some wine—is often enough to set the headache wheels in motion.

Some recent research in Japan suggests that specific preventives are better for people with severe light sensitivity. Lamotrigine, an antiseizure medication often used for headache prevention, has been reported to decrease photosensitivity.

For sensitive migraineurs, it is well worth the effort to exercise some control over the lighting in your home, workplace, and other places where you spend much time. When indirect incandescent lighting is an option, go for it. When overhead fluorescent lighting is all there is, ask about full-spectrum, nonflickering, or Ott bulbs to replace the standard fluorescent type. When all else fails, I encourage light-sensitive patients to keep sunglasses with them at all times. The best are dark red, if you can get them, and online sources are available for these specialty glasses and contacts. Remember, it is better to endure a few stares for wearing your sunglasses indoors than to suffer through a monster headache. Besides, people will think you're cool if you wear sunglasses indoors.

Resolving Workplace Triggers

Every work environment has potential triggers. Usually, once you identify a trigger, you can also identify a solution—not a cure, but a way to eliminate the trigger or reduce its impact. The idea is to modify triggers to minimize their triggering potential.

You can likely effect many of these changes quietly, on your own, but others may require that your coworkers or employer actively participate. Sometimes, it helps if you provide literature to your employer and colleagues, just as you would if you had epilepsy, diabetes, or severe allergies to bee stings. You can find such materials on the Web or get them from your physician.

To minimize the impact of headaches on work, early intervention and anticipatory measures are important. Modifying triggers is the first step and, for mobile workers, this can require intense planning, with special care to arrange schedules, take preventive steps, and devise backup plans. Especially important for people who work on the go, these are good rules to live by for all migraineurs.

Those who work in an outdoor environment are just as entitled to accommodations for their headaches. This includes, for example, access to and opportunity for adequate hydration and, very important, eye, ear, and respiratory protection in dusty, noisy, or very bright environments.

At your request, your employer can (and should) take steps to help you. It is in the employer's best interest to accommodate employees' needs. If this means modifying the workplace, most employers *will* be willing to make the necessary changes. It is important that you present your request through proper channels, with documentation and a logical plan. Demands and threats tend not to work nearly as well as rational presentations.

Many of us spend a third or more of our lives in our work environment. Our performance there has a direct impact on our economic survival, our social standing, and our general health. It is only common sense for the worker and the employer to band together to make this time as productive and pleasant as possible.

THE AMERICANS WITH DISABILITIES ACT When rational discourse does not work, legal channels exist, and you can use these to force your employer to make appropriate changes. In my experience, this rarely works out well for either party, so you should use this leverage only as a last resort.

Rescue in the Workplace

If the day is shaping up to be a bad one, whether you are at work or anywhere else, it is a good idea to take your anti-inflammatory, triptan, or other designated rescue medicine before the headache gets going. Rather than power through the beginnings of a headache, notice and address it as early in the process as possible. This might mean that along with your rescue medicine you need to take a short break in a quiet, cool, dark place. This can often make the difference between getting through the day and going home sick.

The most important part of your rescue plan is the availability of your rescue strategies, whether they are minute meditations or the latest pharmaceutical agents. *It is critically important that you have your rescues readily available to you at all times.* Do not just keep your rescue meds in your bathroom at home. You may need to keep several locations stocked. If you commute or drive a lot in your job, keep a rescue medication (not one that will impair your ability to drive) in your car's glove compartment. If you carry a purse, keep your rescue medicine in it. Keep medicine in your desk and in your valise or suitcase. Also, make sure you always have access to your other rescue aids, such as sunglasses, mask, earplugs, or cold pack, for example.

With migraine, it's important that you always have an escape plan. Everywhere that you spend significant time, have a place where you can go that is cool, quiet, private, and dark. Understandably, this is not always possible, but if you spend significant time in one location, odds are that sooner or later you will need such a refuge. Worst case, this can be your vehicle. If so, always keep a windshield screen in your car.

Chapter 13

Headaches and Stress

Perhaps the most striking change in headache management in the last five years has been the realization that most headaches are migraine. Pure tension headache is a relatively uncommon condition, although some people have a mixed headache pattern with elements of both tension and migraine. But for the majority of headache sufferers, the headache is migraine.

This is important because when the headache is present we want to treat the *pain*. If we focus on the trigger, we are a day late and a dollar short. The time to work on the trigger is *before* the headache starts.

So what about all that tension in your neck? Certainly, *tension is the most common trigger for both migraine and tension-type headaches*. Most of us carry stress in the muscles of the neck and shoulders. The nerves that cause these muscles to contract originate in the cervical spinal cord, separated by only a millimeter or so from the nucleus of the trigeminal nerve, which mediates sensation in the head and just happens to be the pathway for migraine pain. Stress causes tension. Tension triggers migraine.

Identifying the sources of stress is not a task to undertake in the throes of a headache, but with a cool, calm head that is in proper working order. Note that both good stress and bad stress can be associated with migraine—again, not in everyone, but in some people. Whether you are one of these people requires a little observation and introspection. Once you know if you are such a person, modification is not too difficult.

Remember, migraineurs do best when they maintain a predictable environment. We often react badly to change, whether it's a fluctuation in sleep patterns, hormone levels, or stress. For example, many migraineurs experience letdown headaches. These patients are fine during the highly stressful workweek, but when the weekend rolls around, *boom!* The headache crashes into their otherwise peaceful Saturday. Friday-night beers, late parties, or Saturday-morning caffeine withdrawal might explain many letdown headaches, but good evidence suggests that the sudden *decrease* in stress, perhaps associated with a crash in epinephrine and cortisol, triggers this headache in some people.

So, like most triggers, stress in and of itself may not actually be the trigger. Rather, *changes* in stress—like changes in estrogen, barometric pressure, or sleep pattern—correlate with the onset of headaches in susceptible individuals. And like many other triggers, stress is pretty much impossible to eliminate from your world. Remember, when you can't eliminate a trigger or modify it, your only option is to manage it.

Probably the most common trigger for migraines, not to mention for tension-type headaches, stress can be psychological, situational, physical (such as exercise), or endogenous (meaning that some people are wired to respond to seemingly innocuous stimuli as stressful). Chronic illness itself can be a tremendous stressor, and migraine is not exempt from this association. By classifying your stressors into those you can eliminate, those you can modify, and those you can avoid, you can begin to get a handle on this most troublesome trigger. As you go through this questionnaire and identify your stress triggers, consider whether you can avoid the stressor to eliminate the source of the stress, or if you need to figure out a way to modify the stress, such as taking little breaks during a stressful time, meditating when the stress starts to build, or medicating before embarking on a highly stressful activity.

Go over this questionnaire every three to six months, comparing it with previous questionnaires. It's a good way to monitor long-term progress in getting your stressors under control.

List your five most significant stressors at home, at work, and in general.

1. _____
2. _____
3. _____
4. _____
5. _____

Do you feel that stress is a trigger for your headaches?
_____

Do you monitor your stress level on a regular basis?

_____

Do you have a reliable means of reducing stress?

_____

Do you have more or fewer headaches on vacation?

_____

Do you feel stressed at night before going to sleep?

_____

Do you make lists of daily tasks and monitor your accomplishment of them?

_____

Does this add to or reduce your stress levels?

_____

Are there individuals in your world who create stress for you?

_____

Managing Stress

Stress is the result of being trapped in a situation over which you have no control, say, when you're attending your sister's wedding and your husband's beautiful ex-girlfriend shows up with her millionaire boyfriend. You can't always avoid exposure to your triggers.

We all carry our stress with us until we find a way to dissipate it. Many of us carry our stress in our shoulders and neck, physically hunkering down against the onslaught. Others of us carry our stress in our stomachs and get ulcers, or we externalize it with sweating, crying, or being nasty to other people. One way or another, stress works its way to the surface and finds a way to dissipate. For headache sufferers, this will sometimes mean that the pain becomes so bad that we have to remove ourselves not just from the stress, but from the environment as well.

Often, employing better ways of managing stress will lead to fewer headaches and dramatic improvement. But migraineurs usually have other triggers in addition to stress. So, while stress management does help manage headaches—and there are about a million other reasons to practice stress management—it does not "cure" migraines. But managing stress does not come naturally to most migraineurs—or to most *people*, for that matter.

What, exactly, is stress management? I have a patient who says her idea of stress management is to get a headache, excuse herself from the cause of the stress, and retreat to her room to lie in the dark for a few hours. To me, that is like driving your car off a cliff to avoid a traffic jam. Yes, it gets you out of the situation, but at what price? In this sense, migraine is the ultimate stress management program because it gets you away from the stress, at least for a while. But the cost is too high. Besides, in most cases, the stress will still be there when you return to your life.

Stress management should be both effective and proactive. It should prevent the stress from building to the point where your body shuts down with a headache. A good stress management strategy requires that you recognize, anticipate, and, ideally, avoid the stressor (whatever is causing the stress). When you can't avoid the stressor, it is good to have a plan to modify it, to dissipate or lessen its effect. It can be useful to break these plans into several parts: I use internal, external, and situational strategies.

Meditation, yoga, visualization, and prayer are examples of internal strategies. Not everyone is comfortable or suited to these approaches, but if they work for you, they can be very helpful. To get started with these, a teacher or guide is often more successful than a book, audiotape, or video program.

External strategies have more to do with modifying your environment with, for example, appropriate music, furniture, lighting, and privacy. When you have control of your immediate environment, you have more control over what comes at you, so to speak.

Situational strategies attempt to relieve stressful situations before they add up. It is good to have a generous supply of these strategies on hand because stress tends to multiply on itself, and these tools can help defuse the stress before it explodes into a headache. For example, it is effective to:

- schedule breaks for downtime;
- plan to take a five-minute walk every two hours;
- offer to return to an issue after you have had time to process it;
- make lists and check things off;
- pace yourself.

Some stress management techniques can be positive, practical, and healthy: meditation, sex, or exercise, for example. But a wide variety of the techniques that we use to defuse stress can be negative, like displaced anger or compulsive eating. It helps to step back, look at your priorities, and take a breath. Such simple skills are critical for migraineurs and essential parts of your migraine management plan.

I saw a patient a few months ago who was the CEO of a medium-sized tech company. His headaches were escalating and his old treatments no longer worked, and he felt there was no rhyme or reason to his headaches. His business was doing well and his home life was happy, so he came to us for a "fresh approach." We asked him to keep a headache diary, and when he brought it in a month later, there was a pattern. His headaches clearly escalated as the week progressed so that by Friday he was in real pain. When we explored his work pattern, it became obvious that "business doing well," meant growth, more work, and longer hours. While he was very conscientious about limiting his employees' work hours, his own workload was going up and up and up. We asked him to start treating himself like one of his employees, enforcing the five-minute breaks every hour that he imposed on his workers, no mandatory overtime, incentives for using the gym, and so forth. Within two weeks, his headaches were back under control. This worked well for him, and it was a home run for us. The answers are not always so apparent, but whenever you identify your stress and develop a plan for defusing it, you can usually keep it from spinning out of control.

If stress is a significant trigger for your headaches—whether you get migraines or tension-type headaches—these techniques should help you modify your lifestyle, reduce some of your stress, and minimize the effects of stress on your headaches. The Keeler Method emphasizes stress management techniques, including methods for defusing stress, from meditation and neck stretches to support groups and individual counseling. Since some of these work better in certain contexts and for certain patients, and since every migraineur is a little different, the Keeler Method does not have a fixed stress-reduction program, but all of our stress management plans incorporate several helpful principles.

NAME YOUR STRESS   When we replace what is known as free-floating anxiety with a specific concern (or concerns), we can better manage it, so it helps to define precisely what is causing you stress. This is not always easy to do. Very often, we don't know what we are stressed out about. Other times, we know very clearly the source of the stress, but feel there is no remedy (at least no legal remedy) available to us. Still, making a list of the stressors, "naming the enemy," is an important first step that can actually alleviate some of the stress. Sometimes, this requires the help of a counselor, sometimes, not. Your list may change from day to day, or it may seem set in stone. That is fine, but it is also a good idea to prioritize your stressors from greatest to smallest.

BREAK IT UP   It helps if we divide our major stressors into smaller, more manageable parts. For example, if you are stressed out over a deadline by which you must complete a particular project, break up the project into smaller components, and create a timeline for each milestone so that you will finish the overall project on time. If you are worried about finances, make a list of all your debts and make a plan for dealing with each one. If it is a relationship issue, map out the specific problems in the relationship and begin addressing each one in an order that seems to make sense to you.

ESCAPE PLANS Try to balance your stress with other, more pleasurable aspects of life. For example, as stress quietly accumulates, give yourself small breaks from the stress, typically just five or ten minutes every hour or so during the workday. You can do "minute meditations" or yoga stretches, or take short walks, fiction breaks, and music breaks, for example. In addition, make sure that your stress management plan has a grander escape, something you look forward to in the evening, before work, or on the weekend. This can be a hike, a sporting activity, a bike ride, a massage, a class, or just an undisturbed period with the newspaper, a crossword puzzle, a movie, or a book. The only essential ingredient is that it must be an activity you genuinely enjoy and something you will look forward to.

ROUTINE All our stress management plans incorporate regular exercise, sleep, and mealtimes. Scientific studies show that these elements significantly reduce stress and improve our ability to manage it. Coincidentally (or not), these very same things reduce the frequency and severity of headaches. Go figure.

Stress Management Techniques

Whole books describe stress management techniques, so that is beyond the scope of this one. Certainly, patients can avail themselves of the many wonderful methods of stress management that are out there. I have not found one approach that works for everyone. With a little bit of meditation practice, some people do well with guided imagery and melt away into a wonderful Zen state, while others stare straight ahead, tapping a nervous foot, unable to comprehend the point. Some people find that various kinds of biofeedback allow them to bring a steamrolling headache to a stop, while others can't seem to make the connection. Some people find that craniosacral therapy lasts for weeks, others just until the end of the session.

Matching the right stress management technique to the person is an art. At the Keeler Center, we have a therapist whose full-time job is to help our patients find just the right approach. Fortunately, the Internet can be a rich source of options for stress management. Often, what feels right *is* right. What does it comes down to? Everyone needs to have a conscious, articulated plan for managing stress. Whether they run ten miles a day, meditate for twenty minutes, or talk with a psychiatrist every week, people need to dissipate their stress. Stress demands attention. If you ignore it, it only gets worse.

Keep in mind: Not all stress is out "there" in the ether. Pure muscular tension can be a potent trigger for migraines, not to mention its obvious role in tension-type headaches, so migraineurs do well to pay attention to physical stresses that set them up for a headache. In medical school, when we dissected the neck, we learned that the trigeminal nucleus, which is the nerve center for pain in the head, extends from the middle of the brain stem all the way down into the middle of the cervical spine. And guess what sits right next to the lower part of the trigeminal nucleus? Cervical nerves, which are the nerves that go to the muscles of the neck and shoulders. We also learned in medical school that nerves firing right next to other nerves can cause those nerves to fire too. So this means that if your neck muscles are all knotted up they can irritate the nerves that make your head hurt. And if your head hurts, that can irritate the nerves that tense your neck and shoulder muscles.

The point of this little anatomy lesson is that we can use good posture, breathing, and mobility work to help prevent headaches and we can use physical relaxation techniques to help stop a headache. Again, it is beyond the scope of this book to set down the techniques of biofeedback, physical therapy, massage, craniosacral work, and other methods that can help dissipate physical stress or prevent it from building in the first place. Perhaps it is enough to make you aware of this and to encourage you to seek out these treatment modalities as part of your treatment plan.

Chapter 14

Headaches and Social Events

I t is nice to have a glass of wine with dinner. It is fun to stay out late and close a nightclub. It is relaxing to spend a day at the beach. While many migraineurs think these activities are off-limits to them, for the majority of us, this is not so. We can still do these things. We just need to take measures to minimize the likelihood that a headache will result, and to minimize the headache, if it does materialize. The trick is anticipation and preparation.

Some social triggers are very common, but others, of course, can be tricky to uncover. Many social activities will have a ripple effect, causing disruptions in your lifestyle rhythms. As usual, sleep, diet, and exercise routines are at the top of the list. Changes in these areas can be triggers, or can combine with other partial triggers to push you over the edge. Be careful to examine objectively the activity itself as well as its components. The most important thing is to validate that something really is a trigger before you eliminate it from your life based on a possibly false assumption. Remember, the best way to do this is by keeping a good headache diary.

Whether changing your social life can help your headaches depends on your triggers. When you know ahead of time that a certain behavior may lead to a headache, you can go into it with your eyes open and act accordingly. For example, if your social life involves staying out late on Friday nights and you get headaches on most Saturdays, then modifying your social life can certainly help. The key is to identify the specific trigger and evaluate it. When you decide how important something is to you, you can also decide whether to avoid the trigger, modify your plans

❖ 339

to minimize your headache risk, or pretreat to avoid or minimize the headache. In any case, with a few simple strategies, you can do the things you want to do and enjoy a good life—without paying for it with a wicked headache.

Avoid or Modify the Trigger . . . or Pretreat the Headache

Sometimes, modifying your plans results in unexpected but welcome changes. Whether it's a break in the Saturday night routine or a change of venue, it's a real bonus when you don't get your usual headache the morning after. So you might go to the party, abstain from drinking alcohol, and graciously offer to be the designated driver. Or go to the dinner and leave early enough to maintain a reasonable sleep schedule. These are certainly better alternatives than skipping the outing completely for fear of triggering a headache.

In some cases, we can't avoid a known trigger. In other instances, no amount of modification will be enough. And, other times, we just don't want to avoid or modify it. That's fair. But going into these situations we know that the activity is going to give us a headache. In such a case, we can pretreat by taking a medication to avoid or minimize the headache. For me, the combination of a plane flight east followed by exercise (skiing or cycling) is deadly. When I go on such a vacation, I take a long-acting triptan and an NSAID before I leave, and try to give myself a day before I start aggressive exercise. Some of my patients anticipate headaches and pretreat before visiting relatives, running marathons, or going to the beach. Whatever your triggers, once you recognize them, you can address them, one way or another.

Many triggers work through an inflammatory pathway to generate a migraine. Often, a simple nonsteroidal anti-inflammatory like naproxen or ibuprofen can provide an added buffer between a trigger and a headache. One of my patients uses an anti-inflammatory like naproxen before a night of light drinking. Some of the triptans, too, can be very helpful for patients who are going into a situation that is likely to trigger a headache. While many physicians (not headache specialists) think that all the triptans are alike, one of the triptans, frovatriptan, surprisingly lasts four to five times longer than all the others. This is a great choice for pretreating when a migraineur anticipates a trigger and the headache that follows.

For migraineurs who find that their headaches consistently interfere with their social lives, perhaps the most important "modification" is initiating preventive therapy. Whether this is a prescription medication or a natural agent, its effect is to make your head less sensitive to your triggers. While no preventive can eliminate 100 percent of your headaches, if you properly select and utilize a medication, it will often allow you to pursue activities that you could not enjoy otherwise. Even if a headache follows, it will probably be less severe, of shorter duration, and more responsive to your usual rescue medications.

Food and Drink

Many of us enjoy a nice glass or two of wine, but we know that the drink increases the likelihood of a headache the next day. Reluctantly, many of us automatically give up the wine for fear of the headache. But in the Keeler approach, we first ask: Is this activity important to you? If the answer is yes, we develop a strategy that will allow you to have the wine and avoid or minimize the headache.

If you seem to get many headaches related to your social life, you will need to look closely at the individual elements of your activities. Usually, one of those elements is food. Everyone's triggers are different, and this is certainly true of food triggers. The only way you can know that a specific food is a trigger is to be a careful observer of your life, which leads us back to the headache diary, an invaluable tool to help you accomplish this. For this reason, I urge all my patients to keep a diary for a month or two, especially if they are crossing all their favorite foods off their list of pleasurable things in life.

Again, in terms of our social lives, food *timing* might also be an important trigger. To minimize food-related triggers, try to eat meals at roughly your normal times, even when you're going on a day trip, to a party, or anytime you stray from your routine. Do not eat a late dinner or let yourself go hungry. Some patients find it helpful to keep a few snacks in the car for emergency situations, when food might not be available.

An obvious culprit, alcohol is a trigger for many migraineurs. Though that is downright unfair, it makes sense. If we view migraine as the body's way of alerting us to potential dangers in the environment, we might see the headache as an indication that too much alcohol is not good for our internal environment. While some people, obviously unhealthily, can drink all day and not get a headache, others of us cannot even get away with a single after-dinner drink. But again, if you enjoy drinking now and then, or like to have a glass of wine with dinner, you might want to narrow down your investigation to determine your precise trigger.

There's a popular belief that the nitrites and/or tannins in red wine are an absolute migraine trigger, but no hard science supports this. While a lot of people can handle white wine but not red, a significant number cannot drink wine at all. Similarly, many people claim that "clear" alcohol, like vodka and gin, is less likely to trigger headaches than rum, say, or tequila. In fact, this has not been well studied and no one knows. Recently, a group at the University of California, Berkeley, developed a method for testing an alcoholic beverage—such as red wine—to determine the content of chemicals thought to be associated with hangover headaches. We don't know whether this will prove to be useful for migraineurs, but the identification of the migraine-causing component of wine and other alcoholic beverages remains to be discovered.

One thing, though, is for sure. As a migraineur, whenever you add alcohol to the mix, you *may be* flirting with headache danger. Whatever else you do to modify or pretreat, at least you can hydrate aggressively when you drink alcohol. This doesn't cost you anything.

Finally, remember, with alcohol consumption and medications, it is recommended that moderate daily drinkers of alcohol do not take acetaminophen (Tylenol). Many over-the-counter migraine rescue medications contain acetaminophen, as do some prescription rescues. To avoid liver damage, heed the warnings about alcohol consumption and the use of acetaminophen products.

Nightlife

If the occasional late night is essential to a patient's pleasure in life, we can develop a strategy to accommodate that and employ other strategies to prevent (or at least minimize) the headache that might result.

It is important to identify the specific trigger, rather than to blame the entire activity, so you can modify your social life to minimize the risk. For example, some migraineurs are very sensitive to perfume, strobe lights, loud music, or other aspects of parties and social situations, such as crowded, overheated, or smoke-filled rooms. One hint to identifying the specific trigger is to consider which of the elements bothers you in another environment. If you got a headache after you were exposed to fumes or smoke from a fire, or you know you get a migraine when you walk by the perfume counter in a department store, it may well be that odors and bad air in a stuffy nightclub are headache triggers for you. If you got a headache after attending a loud concert, it might be the noise of the nightclub that bothers you, more than the late night. Or if you often get a headache when you spend any time under bright sunshine without your sunglasses, it might be the strobe light, not the night of dancing, that triggers your headaches. Some objective investigative work can pay off in important awareness, and then you can decide whether to modify your plans by changing to a different venue, to eliminate another partial trigger, or to pretreat, if you really have to go to that certain club.

Since nightlife is by definition at night, the obvious lifestyle issue that might be a contributor is your sleep schedule. Especially in combination with other elements of partying, sleep disruptions can cause a problem. Among sleep triggers, staying up unusually late and sleeping late in the morning after are common. But this is not to say that people with this trigger should never vary their sleep patterns. I have a patient who can occasionally stay up late without a problem, or have an occasional drink without incident, but when he does both he will definitely have a headache the next morning. Now when he goes out, he modifies the trigger: he tries to do one or the other, but not both, which works well for him. Another patient finds that taking a long-acting triptan before staying up late works well for him, so he doesn't have to give up the social life he prefers.

If you sleep late the morning after a night out, this change in your sleep schedule may also be a trigger for you. If you are a coffee drinker, you could wake up to a splitting headache. If you drink coffee every weekday morning, you need to drink about the same dose at about the same time on Saturdays and Sundays, too, to avoid the potential trigger of caffeine withdrawal. If you happen to wake up before the headache sets in, get your coffee as soon as possible. If you just can't drag yourself out of bed to put on the pot (or can't stomach a cup), things could get worse fast. Caffeine pills, such as No-Doz, can be a good solution for this "emergency." If the headache is already blazing, you will likely need migraine rescue as well as caffeine to keep the headache from steamrolling.

"Not tonight, honey, I have a headache"

This old saw was thought to be a thinly veiled excuse to avoid sex, but the fact is that any kind of physical exertion, including sexual activity, will usually worsen an existing migraine. For a smaller percentage of migraineurs, sexual activity consistently *brings on* a headache. Fortunately, today, we have effective strategies to allow migraineurs to pursue activities that in the past would have been off-limits, because of their reliable association with headaches.

Weekends

Many migraineurs are puzzled by the timing of their headaches. One of the great riddles is often the "weekend migraine." The story usually runs like this: "I don't get it. I work like a dog all week, under incredible pressure, and get through the week just fine. Then the weekend rolls around and I'm set for a well-earned break and *bam!* I get smacked with a head-ache. What's the deal with that?" Remember, my clinic is in California. That's how people talk in California.

I usually respond with the following questions:

- Do you go out for a celebratory drink or other recreation on Friday night?
- Do you stay up late on Friday night?
- Do you sleep in on Saturday morning?
- Do you have as much caffeine Saturday as you do during the week?
- Are you more physically active on Saturday than you are during the week?
- Are you less stressed on Saturday than during the week?
- Is your diet radically different on the weekends?

By the time I run down a handful of these questions, my patient gives me the vertical push-up gesture, saying, "Okay, okay. I get it."

The Outdoors

When we venture out into the world, we expose ourselves to many potential triggers. But keep in mind that locking ourselves in a cool, dark, quiet room would not guarantee a headache-free existence, and it *would* promise a pretty boring life. And so we go forth, armed with a plan to protect ourselves the best we can from the onslaught of migraine triggers. Still, common sense tells us that the more control we have over our environment, the less subject we are to the whims of nature. Thus, going to football games or picnics, or visiting mountaintops or beaches, can be risky. But these outings are part of our lives, and most migraineurs would like to find a way to experience them without fear of headaches.

Remember, preparation and anticipation are the keys to successful outings. Think about where you are going. Think about what you will be doing and what kinds of resources are available to you. For example, if you are going to the beach, will you have access to a shaded retreat from time to time? Will you have access to sun protection, adequate hydration, and medication? If you are going to a picnic, will meals be served on a schedule to which you will be able to adapt, or should you bring something along? Will your food triggers likely be served? Will you be exposed to allergens or hot sun or altitude changes?

The external environment is filled with potential triggers for headaches: foods, weather changes, pollutants, anything. Our brains respond to a hostile environment with a headache, and remember, nonmigraineurs can get headaches too, but it takes a stronger stimulus than it does for migraineurs. We are just very sensitive to those environmental changes that our brains perceive as hostile.

The migraine-triggering effect of extreme heat, sunshine, and altitude changes is widely known, and some recent studies have confirmed that headaches can also be influenced by weather changes, particularly changes in barometric pressure with approaching storm fronts. Many headache sufferers, of course, have known this all along. The problem remains, though, that weather changes are difficult to predict, much less control, so we need to employ strategies to avoid a headache when the weather is likely to be a trigger.

For example, in regions where a predictable rainy or monsoon season occurs, pulse prevention, using a preventive medication on a short-term basis, is a good strategy. With the newer, long-acting triptans and anti-inflammatories, many migraineurs now pulse for a few days or a week when a known trigger is on the horizon, or might use the preventive for even a few months, depending on their period of increased headache risk. In this circumstance, we walk a fine line, because we must balance the risk of medication overuse against the benefit of avoiding a known trigger and, likely, a whopper of a headache.

In the same way, when taking a business trip across time zones or traveling to a significantly higher or lower altitude, shorter pulses of preventives for a few days or a week can be very useful. It is always a good idea to start the pulse therapy a few days before you travel. Your headache doctor can help plan pulse prevention.

Many patients feel daunted contemplating these kinds of questions, and throw their hands up and decide that it is just too much. But we migraineurs are a hearty lot. With a little anticipation and preparation, we can fully enjoy outdoor events, and we should not allow the potential for a bad outcome to discourage us. Most of all, headaches should not be the focus of our lives, but a footnote.

SUNGLASSES For light sensitivity, certain shades of sunglasses work better than others. Dark oxblood-red sunglasses provide the best protection against light sensitivity. Keep in mind that with red-tinted glasses you won't see green—as in traffic lights. Contact lenses are best because there is no leakage of light around the edges, but wraparounds are a good, practical alternative. Lamotrigine, an antiseizure medication often used for headache prevention, has been reported to decrease photosensitivity.

Travel and Vacations

Vacations, particularly when they involve air travel or altitude change, cause a lot of anxiety in some headache sufferers. While some migraineurs simply don't travel, most grin and bear it. And unfortunately, "bear it" often means enduring an excruciating headache. This significantly cuts into vacation time, not to mention pleasure. But travel and vacations can become quite manageable, even enjoyable, if you understand the relationship between travel and headaches, break the adventure down into its components, and develop specific strategies for the suspect elements.

Travel includes many potential triggers because it involves changes, *lots* of changes. For any given trip, these may include fluctuations in stress levels, time zones, sleep cycles, altitude, barometric pressure, mealtimes, diet, and physical activity.

We can modify some of these—like sleep cycle, mealtimes, and physical activity. We cannot modify others, like changes in barometric pressure and altitude. But we *can* anticipate them. In the Keeler Method, we break the travel down into similar components, and look at each one for its triggering potential.

Disruptions to Your Routines

Stress around travel can be significant in preparing for a trip, while on the road, and upon returning. Some attention to the timing can help a lot. A couple of buffer days before and after a major trip can make it much less stressful, so it helps if you can take a few extra days off work, so you do not work right up until you leave town, and also plan to delay returning to work until a day or two after coming back from vacation. It also helps if you begin your trip planning well in advance of your travel dates, so you can gradually accomplish all the tasks necessary to get out of town. If anxiety or muscle tension are part of your travel behavior, discuss possible medication remedies with your doctor before traveling.

Some things should not change with vacation. For example, if at all possible, maintain your regular mealtimes, sleep patterns, and exercise patterns. Keep your caffeine intake and medications as consistent as possible. Tempting as it is, we should not sleep in or party late into the night on vacation. But if we must, we might anticipate a headache—and take preventive measures (such as an anti-inflammatory or long-acting triptan) to circumvent the headache.

While we can anticipate and try to prevent these problems, unexpected things do happen that make vacations so much fun. Adventures with new foods, new flora and fauna, really old buildings, and so forth can be part of vacation travel. It is not possible to plan for everything, nor should we. But if we keep to our routines around eating, sleeping, and exercise, if we stay prepared with our rescue plans in mind and available, and if we plan for an accessible refuge if a bad headache occurs, vacations can be successful, interesting, and fun.

Time Zones and Altitude Changes

Plane flights can be problematic for a few reasons. First, traveling across time zones disrupts your sleep cycle. To minimize this disruption, try to strategize when to sleep and for how long—in the days leading up to, the day of, and the day after your flight. When you are preparing to travel across time zones, move your bedtime up or down, depending on the direction in which you are flying, to adjust your internal clock to the new time zone. Ideally, you want to be on schedule for the time you arrive at your destination. So, if you will arrive in Rome or Tahiti in the morning, you want to adjust your clock during the days before so that you will sleep on the plane (perhaps with a short-acting sleep aid) and awaken upon arrival. Similarly, if you are planning an evening arrival, arrange to be at the "end of your day" as you arrive. As a rule of thumb, figure that your body and brain need *one day of adjustment for each time zone you cross*. So if you are crossing four time zones, traveling east, advance your bedtime by one hour each day for four days before traveling.

Some migraineurs are very sensitive to altitude changes. Even for nonmigraineurs, a throbbing, pounding headache is a common symptom of "altitude sickness," and dramatic fluctuations can be a potent—and very common—trigger for migraineurs traveling by air, pressurized cabins notwithstanding. For migraineurs, the trigger and the headache can ruin a vacation.

If you know that altitude changes cause you problems, often you can use preemptive strategies to block this trigger before going on a plane flight or even a long uphill drive. Acclimatization, in which you accomplish changes in altitude very gradually rather than precipitously, is an example of such a strategy. Sensitive migraineurs may benefit from premedication with a mild antihistamine, an anti-inflammatory (like aspirin or a nonsteroidal anti-inflammatory such as naproxen sodium or ibuprofen), a long-acting triptan (such as frovatriptan or naratriptan), or a carbonic anhydrase inhibitor. I have had more than one patient assure me that chewing gum is highly effective. Another reliable strategy is to hydrate well, preferably with water. And it is very important to maintain all your usual patterns of food intake, sleep schedules, and exercise during travel, and to avoid combining the altitude change with other known triggers, such as alcohol.

For some people, almost any change in altitude—even just a couple thousand feet—can trigger a headache. For others, it takes a more dramatic change. Like all triggers, this is an individual question. One hint will be to notice your reaction when you drive up to the local mountains. If this triggers even a small headache, it is not your imagination. This is a clue that you need to use prevention strategies when you plan to travel to a higher altitude.

Migraineurs traveling to mountain destinations for skiing or back-packing vacations can get very nasty headaches. To acclimatize gradually, be careful to adjust to altitude change before you exert yourself. This means you may need to arrive a couple of days before skiing or hiking, to help prevent headaches. I suggest about one day for every twenty-five hundred feet in elevation change, but everyone is different, and some people are more sensitive to this. Moreover, the higher you go, the more time it takes to adjust. A change from sea level to twenty-five hundred feet may not be a problem, but from ten thousand to twelve thousand five hundred may take several days. Mount Everest climbers adapt at base camps along the way for weeks at a time. If you can't add the extra time, or don't want to change to a lower elevation, premedicating can often block the trigger.

Scuba diving headaches are more complicated. While we do see headaches as a result of pressure changes, these are uncommon, particularly in shallow, recreational diving. More commonly, stuffed sinuses can worsen pressure equalization across the eustachian tube, the anxiety of a dive can cause muscle tension, or shallow breathing while diving can cause a carbon dioxide–retention headache. Scuba-diving migraineurs should also keep in mind that migraine medicines can increase the risk of nitrogen narcosis, and should *always* discuss their medicines with a physician experienced in diving medicine.

Chapter 15

Other Illnesses, and Headaches and Aging

Migraine does not exist in a vacuum. For many patients, it is just one of several or even many chronic illnesses. Because migraine is so common, we often see it in concert with other common conditions. But when two conditions frequently "come together," they are considered "comorbid." No, comorbid does not mean you are going to die. The term refers to medical conditions that we often see together in the same person. Several conditions are more common in migraine sufferers than in the general population. Among these are asthma, depression, irritable bowel syndrome, obesity, and a variety of others.

Whether all these conditions are related in some way, or whether it is simply the sheer numbers of people suffering with them, is a matter of some controversy. We do not understand the exact reasons for these associations, but interestingly, each of these conditions does reflect an "abnormal" relationship with the environment. It is also interesting that when we treat one of these conditions, we sometimes see improvement in the others. Unfortunately, not always.

In any case, patients and their doctors need to keep comorbid conditions in mind when developing treatment plans, in terms of looking for some of these other conditions and developing treatments that do not make other conditions worse but, ideally, address more than one problem at a time. For example, you don't want to go on a preventive that will help the headache but make the asthma worse. If there is a medication that will control both seizures and headaches, then you can reduce the number of medications that a patient needs to take.

Some Complications Need Special Handling

Many patients who get migraines also live with other medical conditions and take other medications. If this is you, it is critical that you work with your doctors, *and* that they work with each other, so your treatments do not interfere with one another to your detriment. Headaches as one component of multiple medical conditions can present very complex issues. And migraines themselves can progress into situations that need special care. All of these situations require appropriate and ongoing management by a team of physicians and other health care professionals.

SIDE EFFECTS   Headaches are frequently listed as a side effect for a wide variety of medications, including those used to treat common conditions like hypertension and depression. Headaches may also be a symptom of other common conditions, and migraine medicines might cause side effects of other conditions that the migraineur suffers.

One common example is the medication propranolol. In the class of blood pressure medications called beta-blockers, propranolol is often used to help prevent migraine. But asthma is more common in migraineurs than in the general population, and propranolol can make asthma worse, so propranolol should never be used in people with that condition. Not only that, propranolol can also worsen existing depression and make exercise difficult. Still, in the right patient, it is a great drug.

The common triptan, the mainstay of headache rescue, is another example. Patients on certain kinds of antidepressants, called monoamine oxidase inhibitors, should not use triptans. Anti-inflammatories can cause problems in patients with irritable bowel syndrome. The list goes on and on, and obviously, it can be very complicated. This is one of the principal reasons why it is important to enlist the help of someone who knows a bit about medicine—like a physician or a pharmacist—when developing your treatment plan. In a candid moment, many of my colleagues will say that this is why doctors get the big bucks. It is complicated business, and the stakes can be very high.

Asthma

Asthma and other respiratory disorders are common in the general population, as is migraine. Therefore, it is likely that a significant proportion of people will have both conditions. Through the miracle of statistics, we can actually predict how many migraineurs are likely to have respiratory difficulty and how many people with respiratory problems are likely to have headaches. It turns out that the association between the two conditions is greater than we would expect on a purely statistical basis. The incidence of asthma in the general population is approximately one hundred asthma patients for every thousand people. Among headache patients that number is more like 150. So comorbidity is about 50 percent more common. Trust me, in the world of statistics, that is a big number. It means that it is more than coincidence that headaches and breathing problems seem to go hand in hand. Obviously, not for everyone, but for many of us.

Of course, the obvious question is: *Why?* What is it about the two conditions, or the people who have these conditions, that sets them up for this comorbidity? As you might expect, we don't have a definite answer. But we have some good theories, which can help us control the conditions. Several biological explanations for the comorbidity of asthma and headache have been suggested. The first and most obvious is that there is a genetic predisposition. This means that the same genes that set us up for one condition also set us up for the other. To date, we have not found the gene or genes responsible, but this remains the most likely explanation.

Another, perhaps more intriguing, explanation is mast cell activation. Mast cells are part of the immune system, and are very reactive to "assaults" from the outside. In one sense, asthma and headache are both exaggerated responses to external stimuli or triggers. One of the body's first responders to these triggers is the mast cell, and in both migraine and respiratory illness, mast cell response may be abnormal. Another possible common ground would be a functional abnormality in smooth muscle. Blood vessels and airways are covered with similar receptors. That is why some headache medications are a problem for people with asthma (like some anti-inflammatory agents and the beta-blocker propranolol), and certain other medications have been noted to help treat both headache and asthma (like corticosteroids). Clearly, there is a relationship here, but these conditions are not the same entity. On a more specific level, many researchers are studying vasoactive mediators such as calcitonin gene-related peptide (CGRP), neurokin A, substance P, and others to determine their role in the reactive brain and lungs. Others are looking closely at arachidonic acid metabolism and fatty acids for their role in triggering these "attack disorders."

It is also intriguing to note that stress is often a trigger for both asthma and headache. This raises the possibility that a common disorder underlies both conditions. But other than the observation to support this, we have no evidence of it. It does underscore the importance of recognizing the potential role of stress in these conditions and, if it is a trigger, managing stress to reduce the frequency and severity of attacks. Similarly, a growing body of literature suggests that sulfites are a trigger for both migraine and breathing disorders. When a patient makes a dietary change, we can track improvement in both conditions and then judge whether the offending agent was significant or not.

Many commonly used asthma treatments list headaches as a side effect. It is important to bring your headaches to the attention of the physician who is treating your asthma (or any other medical condition) so that, together, you can weigh the risks against the benefits of taking each medication—and explore other options. By the same token, your headache doctor should be aware of any other medical conditions, and you should discuss the potential impact, positive or negative, of any medicines or other treatments the doctor recommends.

Depression

Depression and headache, especially chronic daily headache, seem to go hand in hand. In fact, depression is *four times* more common among headache sufferers than it is among the general population. But is this simply because it gets depressing when your head hurts all the time? Or is there something more to the connection?

Psychiatrists like to talk about two kinds of depression. The first, often called reactive depression, washes over you when your cat dies or you lose your great-grandfather's heirloom watch (to give a couple of personal examples). Reactive depression is in response to a specific event or series of events, and generally, it is time-limited, meaning that it will eventually get better. The second kind of depression is called endogenous depression. In this type, the depression has no obvious reason, and yet the feeling is undeniably there. People with endogenous depression usually have a long history of feeling blue, or worse. Intriguingly, in both circumstances, the brain chemistry appears to be very similar: not enough serotonin is getting to where it needs to be. In the simplest terms, people with reactive depression chew up their serotonin more rapidly than normal, so they don't have enough to go around. People with endogenous depression, probably for genetic reasons, don't *make* enough serotonin to go around. In either case, they don't have enough serotonin, which is probably why the class of antidepressants called selective serotonin reuptake inhibitors (SSRIs) works well for both groups.

In headache, the question is whether the associated depression is endogenous or reactive. As with so much of this headache business, the answer is neither simple nor clear. Studies have looked at this relationship, and it does appear that endogenous depression is more common among migraineurs than reactive depression except among certain subsets, such as those who develop their headaches suddenly after a car accident or other head trauma. This is not to say that it isn't depressing to have frequent headaches, only that there appears to be more to the picture for many headache sufferers. Again, regardless of what kind of depression the patient has, the treatment is often the same, though reactive depression may resolve as headaches are brought under control, eliminating the need for treatment, while endogenous depression is more likely to persist, requiring long-term treatment.

The good news is that many migraine treatments also help treat depression, and vice versa. This might tend to suggest that one condition is "caused" by the other and that treating one condition is the reason the other condition improves. This has been studied in several different ways. For example, one study found that in a group of depressed patients suffering from headache, their condition improved significantly only when the medication (in this case amitriptyline) improved the depression as measured by psychometric testing. However, other studies have shown that treating the depression with SSRIs often improved the depression, but either did not affect or actually worsened the headache condition.

The relationship between headache and depression is important because you and your doctor must be mindful of both conditions in developing a medication strategy. For example, long-term use of propranolol has been associated with worsening depression. On the other hand, propranolol is often used to treat the symptoms of anxiety often seen in migraineurs. Many antidepressants list headaches as a common side effect, and other antidepressants alter sleep patterns, weight, or other parameters that are critical to the migraineur's well-being. With all medications, it is important to review the most common side effects with an eye toward their impact on your other medical issues. While I can't discuss specifics in this text about the many medications out there, you can search the Internet for any medication you are considering and identify any concerns in two minutes. Once you identify them, you can discuss them with your doctor.

Addressing depression, both during the diagnostic process and when developing the treatment plan, is essential to good headache care. Monitoring for depression during treatment is also critically important. Depression, anxiety, and bipolar disease all can complicate headache treatment, so the migraineur, together with the doctor, needs to consider these when planning their treatment. In almost every case, an optimal combination of medications and other therapies will address all the comorbidities without improving one at the expense of the other. The first step is to identify the players, *then* the strategy will follow.

Medications are not often the source of depression, but some headache medications *have* been associated with worsening depression. Any patient who experiences a worsening depression should consult a doctor who is qualified to address it. Worsening headache or the effects of worsening headaches on a person's life may certainly be the source of depression. In this case, careful selection of a headache medication is critical.

Irritable Bowel Syndrome

Despite the fact that the head and the gut are some distance away from each other, irritable bowel syndrome (IBS) shares many features with migraines. Studies have reported that IBS is more common among migraineurs than among the general population, and migraine is more common among people with IBS. Like asthma and migraine, IBS appears to be an exaggerated response on the body's part to something in the environment. IBS has triggers, just as migraine does. And not everyone has the same triggers. This makes IBS difficult to treat—just like migraine.

As with other comorbidities, it is important to be mindful when treating one condition so as not to make the other worse. For example, medications that contain belladonna, often used for IBS treatment, can worsen headache. Similarly, many medications used in headache, such as the NSAIDs and steroids, can worsen stomach problems.

A "gut–brain" connection is a hot topic among researchers. It is interesting to note that there are more serotonin receptors in the lining of the gut than there are in the brain. While we do not understand the exact relationship, serotonin is clearly a major player at both sites. And while the specific subtype of receptor differs, the serotonergic system is active in both disorders. For our purposes, the "designer drugs," like the triptans and the SSRI antidepressants, are very specific for *brain* serotonin receptors and do not appear to be active at gut receptors. Most patients with IBS do not have problems with these medicines.

I have had more than one patient report that improving her IBS has had a positive effect on her headaches. Interestingly, I have seen fewer examples go the other way. To my knowledge, this has not been studied formally. Whether the stress of active IBS is a trigger for migraines or whether there is a more direct connection, we simply don't know at this time. But the connection is clear: Addressing one condition without the other rarely results in a satisfactory outcome.

Obesity

Perhaps one of the most widely misunderstood concepts in migraine is the role of foods, dietary patterns, and weight. Very recent research suggests that the overall makeup of diet may be important. During the recent low-carbohydrate craze, many patients reported that their headaches were better and, indeed, we saw this in their diaries. But we do not clearly understand the role of carbohydrates (or fats or proteins, for that matter) in headache pathophysiology. Recent work, however, has shown that migraineurs may have too little of the good omega-3 fatty acids, and a relative excess of the less desirable omega-6 fatty acids in their spinal fluid. We do not know the clinical significance of this, but it is likely another good reason to shift our diets toward the omega-3s.

Other recent research has shown that obesity correlates with chronification of migraine, but not with migraine in general. The reason for this appears to involve some of the chemicals that are stored in and released from fat cells. These chemicals, called cytokines, promote inflammation—and inflammation promotes headache in susceptible central nervous systems. Fat cells also produce other chemicals called leptins and interleukins that modulate the immune response and alter inflammatory reactions.

Unfortunately, many of the medicines we use in headache treatment plans can increase appetite (as with valproate or amitriptyline) or decrease it (as with topiramate). So we need to be mindful of the patient's weight issues when we select headache treatment medications. The obverse is also true: Some weight-loss medicines, particularly phentermine and any of the amphetamine class, can worsen headaches for many migraine sufferers. Again, we must always weigh the risks and the benefits of a treatment before making a decision.

Migraine and Other Chronic Pain Syndromes

This is one of the most difficult areas of headache management. What happens when someone has *both* migraine and chronic pain due to a failed back, fibromyalgia, cancer, or arthritis, for example? If daily use of pain medication, especially narcotics, is associated with worsening headaches, how can we take care of these patients' chronic pain? Most headache specialists give one of two answers:

- For some reason, it is okay to take daily pain meds when there is coexisting nonmigrainous pain.
- Patients with both chronic pain and migraine must learn to live with one or the other.

These are not satisfactory answers. At the Keeler Center, we try to find preventives that will help *both* the chronic pain and the migraines. We have had good success with pregabalin (Lyrica) in this regard, as well as other antiepileptic agents. We also try to use local agents, such as lidoderm patches, nerve blocks, and similar interventions, to control the local pain. Also, at least clinically, we do not see medication overuse headache in migraine patients who use NSAIDs daily for arthritis. This is a very gray area, and much more work needs to be done before we can generalize about this situation.

Until then, we need to manage whole patients, not a collection of syndromes. This means that doctors need to communicate with each other, doing their best to make sure that medications are compatible and that, whenever possible, they use nonmedicinal solutions.

Headaches and Aging

In 2007, the American Academy of Neurology asked me to give a lecture on migraine changes with menopause *and* andropause. I had spoken on migraine and menopause many times, but never on andropause. When I began to research for the talk, I found out why. There have been few rigorous studies on andropause in general, and the literature on andropause and headache is even more scarce.

As the average life expectancy increases in this country, and older individuals' physical activity increases, the natural histories of their diseases and medical conditions will change. At the same time, medication regimens evolve and complicate their lives, and all of this further complicates their migraine picture.

Men in their fifties or sixties often lose their migraines, although we haven't studied this as well as we have the changes in women. In fact, we do not entirely understand the reasons why headaches improve with aging, but it most likely has to do with the fact that as we age our hormonal fluctuations even out and, at least for some of us, our lifestyle becomes routine and more constrained, with less exposure to triggers.

Unfortunately, for a percentage of migraineurs, headaches persist well into their seventies and eighties. For some, there is no substantive change in the character of their headaches, so management remains much the same, perhaps with minor adjustments dictated by any limitations in mobility, renal function, or other illnesses and conditions. For many elderly migraineurs, the very nature of the headache changes. Whenever there is a change in the character or frequency of headaches, it is a good idea to discuss these changes with your health care providers.

Headaches in Midlife

Happily, some of us do actually outgrow our migraines. For about two-thirds of women (and probably a similar portion of men), migraines disappear or improve dramatically after the menopause (or andropause). For others, headaches continue as before or they simply change in character.

Sleep issues can become common in middle age. As we get older, we produce less and less melatonin, a sleep-inducing protein, and taking 1 mg to 6 mg of this over-the-counter supplement to augment your body's production is a natural approach. It's important to discuss the best dose and duration of treatment with your doctor, especially if melatonin doesn't work. Other possible disorders might be causing sleep problems, so you should talk to your doctor and perhaps explore thyroid disorders, breathing disorders, and depression.

Depression commonly flares in middle age, and headaches may

flare along with it. Many of us tend to sit, eat, and sleep when we are depressed, and this is bad for headache. If depression seems to be a factor in your life at this time, talk with a health care professional and be sure to remind them that you have headaches. Counseling or a short course of antidepressants may make a world of difference. But use caution because some antidepressants are more likely to worsen headaches than others.

NEW HEADACHES IN MIDLIFE   Less than 3 percent of migraines begin after age fifty. On the other hand, many medical problems can present with a new headache during middle age. And as we get older, secondary headaches are more common. Secondary headaches are due to some other cause, so any headache that seems different from usual is worth discussing with your doctor. If a middle-aged or perimenopausal woman starts to get headaches, she should also consult a doctor.

That does not mean all new headaches are something serious, either. Such problems can be disorders of the immune system, problems with blood vessels in the brain or in the head or neck, heart problems, sleep disorders, breathing disorders, thyroid problems, depression, and even infections. Though very rarely, even brain tumors can first present with head pain. *Many* diseases and medical conditions can first present with headaches. Most of these are benign, meaning that they are not dangerous—only annoying—but others require medical attention. *The most important thing is that someone with headache expertise should make the diagnosis.*

Migraine in Older Patients

One example of a headache change in elderly migraineurs is "late-life migrainous accompaniment," which replace a patient's common migraines with a characteristic pattern of numbness and tingling that begins in one hand or leg and marches up the body, followed by visual changes and perhaps a headache. The phenomenon occurs in this very stereotyped way, lasting sometimes for hours, and then it resolves. The first few times it happens, the patient will—appropriately—go to the emergency room and be evaluated for stroke. Frequently, older individuals who have a history of migraine come to their physician concerned that they are having a mini-stroke, also known as a transient ischemic attack (TIA). To be sure, people in this age group are more prone to stroke. But when these patients are imaged with diffusion MRI, MRA, or true angiography, the tests are negative for stroke. So it is unlikely that these are vascular events. When the ER doctor finds nothing amiss, the patient goes home, only to experience an identical event a day or a week or a month later because, in fact, for some migraineurs, their typical migraines can change with age to this pattern. With luck, these patients will eventually see a neurologist who is familiar with the phenomenon, and the patient will be relieved with the diagnosis of late-life migrainous accompaniments, which present with:

- typical classic migraine auras (without subsequent headache in 50 percent of cases);
- gradual buildup of symptoms
- typical duration: twenty to thirty minutes
- age at onset typically between fifty and sixty years
- complete resolution between episodes.

This transformation produces a neurologic deficit that doesn't change significantly from episode to episode. Described in individuals (male and female) between the ages of forty and ninety, LLMA consists variously of visual changes, numbness, and tingling on one side of the body, speech difficulty, and other neurologic deficits. LLMA follows the time course of migraine, rather than that of TIA, as it can last from minutes to hours, while TIAs are typically seconds to minutes. Characteristically, the migrainous accompaniments build over time (unlike cerebrovascular events) and may progress from one symptom to another. The episodes often recur. A benign syndrome, this diagnosis can spare the patient from repeated hospitalizations, emergency room visits, workups, and unnecessary medication changes. However, this is a diagnosis of exclusion and requires a thorough investigation at first presentation.

Ophthalmic (Ocular or Retinal) Migraine

In this condition, patients can experience a transient (passing) episode of disturbed vision, often lasting up to twenty or more minutes. While this is a variant of migraine, it is not typically associated with pain. In fact, patients with this usually go to their ophthalmologist first. But in reality, the problem is not in the eyes but in the visual processing centers at the back of the brain. It is a good idea to have your eyes checked, however, to rule out other eye problems that might mimic the migraine. Typically the episode begins with an enlarging blind spot on one side or the other. If you close either eye, the spot remains (that is how you know the problem is in the brain rather than in the eyes). In almost all cases, ophthalmic migraines are not dangerous, and they usually require no treatment. However, if they are greatly interfering with a person's life, a preventive agent may be used to decrease their frequency and duration.

Other Headaches in Older Patients

Of course, older patients can also have *non*migraine headaches, and some of these can be symptoms of something much more serious than migraine. Temporal arteritis or tumor headaches, for example, can have grave consequences if left undiagnosed and untreated. Sadly, even migraineurs can suffer such headaches, though no more frequently than the general population.

GLAUCOMA Glaucoma can present with severe eye pain and a pupil that does not respond to light. The headache from glaucoma is typically in one eye only, and even feels as if it is in the eyeball. The eye is red, and the cornea (the transparent part covering the iris and pupil) may appear clouded. The use of tricyclics, sometimes as a headache preventive, can precipitate an attack of one kind of glaucoma, acute angle glaucoma. Any patients who have glaucoma in their family history should see an ophthalmologist if they experience unexplained decline in visual acuity or pain in one eye.

GIANT CELL ARTERITIS (TEMPORAL ARTERITIS) A disease of older people, temporal arteritis should not be diagnosed in someone under sixty years old. It can affect any of the large, extracranial arteries, and head pain is one of the more nonspecific presentations, often involving pain in the neck, face, head, jaw, or tongue, along with joint pain, anorexia, weight loss, and malaise. Patients often describe it as a constant pain with frequent lancinating exacerbations. Occasionally the artery can be felt as a hardened, throbbing vessel at the temple. A laboratory test, called an erythrocyte sedimentation rate (ESR), can strongly suggest the diagnosis, which can be confirmed by biopsy. Still, if the biopsy is normal, it does not rule out the diagnosis, which is important to consider because, untreated, the condition can lead to blindness. The treatment for temporal arteritis includes oral steroids and monitoring of the ESR.

HYPERTENSION, CHRONIC PULMONARY DISEASE, AND CARDIAC DISEASE A variety of other diseases in older people can present with headache, including hypertension, chronic pulmonary disease, and cardiac disease. Generally, though, headache is not prominent in hypertension until the blood pressure surpasses 220/120. This headache tends to be at the back of the head. Present upon awakening, this headache improves once the patient is up and about.

Also, nitrates such as nitroglycerin, which are commonly used for cardiac purposes, can often result in headaches.

STROKE Headache with the onset of a stroke is not common. Headache occurs with stroke in 25 to 50 percent of patients, depending on where in the brain the stroke occurs and whether the stroke is the result of a blockage or a ruptured vessel. It is unusual to see headache with small strokes; headache with stroke is almost always a large stroke. Of course, headache is very common with other, more dramatic neurologic events, but in this circumstance neither the headache nor the neurologic deficit is typical for the patient nor is it seen in isolation (without other signs or symptoms).

TUMOR   Headache resulting from a mass lesion (such as a brain tumor) is a concern when the headache is just in one place and seems to be getting progressively worse. It is particularly worrisome when the headache is also associated with a neurologic deficit. Note that the classic triad of headache, nausea, and waking with pain is relatively uncommon, and any patient sixty years old or older with a new or different headache should see a neurologist.

Other Causes

Often, older patients take multiple medications, so it is very important to watch for interactions. A great many of the medications commonly used in the elderly (vasodilating antihypertensives, isosorbide dinitrate, and bronchodilators, to name just a few) can exacerbate headache, so patients and their doctors need to pay attention to medication issues.

Other headaches in the elderly can be due to degenerative changes in the cervical spine, which can result in pain at the back of the head and top of the neck. Often, this pain is worse on awakening or is made worse by movement.

Chapter 16

Adjusting Your Treatment Plan over Time

Nothing stays the same. Not in the outside world, not inside your body. What worked for you last year may not work for you now, and what didn't work five years ago may be the perfect solution now—or at some point in the future. I know this makes it hard, but you can never confidently say, "Been there, done that," nor can you take a giant sigh and say, "Finally, I have the answer."

As the patterns of our lives change, for better or worse, our headache patterns change, too. Hormone levels shift over time, sleep patterns adjust to family needs and work schedules, environments change with the season, and exercise varies with general health and time limitations. By staying alert and flexible, your headache management can evolve along with your life. As you incorporate changes and modify your plan, you can maintain control and continue to live the life *you* choose. So you periodically need to review your treatment strategy, triggers, and lifestyle questionnaires to keep on top of your headaches.

Really, the ultimate goal is to keep headaches at bay without thinking about them all the time. We need to keep it real, to accept and incorporate headache management into the background of our lives, by being aware, being vigilant, and staying in tune. Or, as Ram Dass (and later, the rock band Oasis) said, "Be here now." For migraineurs, this means checking in regularly with your inner headache specialist.

Just as your life with headaches is living and organic, your treatment plan must be, too. If you learn to perceive reassessment not as a setback or failure, but as part of the process, then you can continue to make healthy modifications. When you see your migraine management in this way, life becomes much easier.

There is good evidence that migraine is a *progressive* condition, meaning that it both changes over time and, for a significant portion of migraineurs, gets worse if left untreated. But there is also evidence suggesting that with proper management, migraine that has progressed to daily or near-daily headaches can *regress* to a less frequent or episodic pattern. So it is important that your treatment plan keeps pace with your headaches. Certainly, as you implement a good management plan, your headaches will change. They may also change simply because of the natural history of the condition. It is important to monitor your changes so you can modify your plan over time. That means we need to reevaluate, looking at all three components of our comprehensive migraine management plan: lifestyle, prevention, and rescue.

Improve Your Strategy

Life is dynamic, and your headache plan will naturally change over time. But there are several common changes that we need to guard against. One is the patient who says, "On this new plan, I have so few headaches, I think it is time to change the plan." This usually means, "I think I'll stop taking my medicine." Most of us do not like to take medicines. We take medicines when we are sick, because we have to. But when we are feeling well, they seem to be a nuisance, and if they have side effects, they *are* a nuisance.

But imagine that you have diabetes instead of migraine. Your doctor puts you on insulin, and in a few weeks your blood sugar is perfect and you feel great. Would you stop the insulin because you feel so well? No! The same thing often applies in migraine. The daily preventive medicine is the thing that is cooling off your brain and making it less reactive to your usual headaches triggers. True, sometimes, after a long period of being headache-free, particularly if you have made lifestyle changes to avoid and minimize your triggers, then, maybe, you can slowly wean off your preventive.

Another common mistake is to think that your new strategy makes you immune to headaches so now you can do all the things you have avoided for fear of a headache. I wish we had a medication or a lifestyle change that could protect us 100 percent from further headache suffering, but we don't. No matter how good the plan, for the vast majority of us, an occasional headache will break through.

It is important to give each strategy a chance to work. This means you need to periodically review your management plan, on the basis of new things you learn about yourself, your headaches, and the plan itself. You can modify everything, to some extent, for the better, from what time you wake up in the morning to the timing of your medicines. But you don't want to constantly tinker. Only by settling into a strategy can you know if it is working. Still, every so often it is good to step back and look at where you were, where you are, and where you want to be.

The Evolving Treatment Plan

Patients frequently ask, "Will I need to take this medication or maintain this regimen forever?" Well, no. But some people do remain on preventives for many years. Others find that after six months or so their headaches have "cooled off" to the point where they can revisit management with rescues and lifestyle modification only. Still others find that over time one plan morphs into another, either because of decreasing effectiveness, changes in lifestyle, or the emergence of new options. The fact is that not many migraine treatment plans work forever because bodies change, lifestyles change, and triggers change.

As a function of aging, the natural progression of the disease, and the changes we make in caring for our headaches, our headache patterns will change over time, so our prevention plans need to be organic and flexible, adapting to our ever-changing headache profile. In other words, finding the right prevention plan is only the beginning. By maintaining a headache diary, meeting regularly with your headache doctor, and staying vigilant toward triggers, the prevention plan will continue to evolve and serve you well.

I generally encourage my patients to reevaluate the treatment plan at least every four months when things are going well, and more often when they are not. Every reevaluation should look at all three components: lifestyle, prevention, and rescue. How you then change the plan depends on how the headache pattern has changed since the last time you monitored it. For example, if in reviewing the last four months, you see no change in severity or frequency but notice that the headaches are now clustering around the latter part of the workweek, you might want to alter the lifestyle part of your plan, emphasizing relaxation techniques to diffuse the tension that builds as the workweek winds up before the weekend. Or, if your headache diary shows that headache frequency is increasing but severity is not, this suggests either a lifestyle change or a change in preventive response. Without periodically reviewing your diary, you might respond to either of these scenarios by simply increasing your rescue medication, which could easily result in medication overuse headaches.

Periodically, patients should review their migraine management progress with a headache specialist or experienced health care provider. Interpreting headache diaries and questionnaires can be a little like reading a spreadsheet or the ticker tape that squiggles across the bottom of one of the financial networks. It doesn't mean a whole lot unless you know what you're looking at, even if you know what the numbers and letters stand for. Between visits with a headache specialist, you can follow a few general guidelines.

If the number of headache days per month is increasing, consider:

- medication overuse
- new or increased trigger exposure
- loss of lifestyle rhythms (sleep, eating pattern, exercise)

If rescue medications don't seem to be as effective as they were, consider:

- the timing of your medication;
- the frequency of your taking your rescues (never more often than two days/week/medication unless your doctor tells you otherwise)

If your headaches seem to be going away but returning when your rescue wears off, consider:

- changing or modifying your rescue regimen
- including a long-acting triptan

Of course, there are many other possible things to be gleaned from studying your headache diary, but these are broad trends that you can observe. Just as diabetic patients must monitor their blood sugar levels and asthmatics must be mindful of pollen and pollution levels, so must migraine sufferers monitor the things that worsen their headaches. You can accomplish this with your headache diary, other questionnaires, and (since migraineurs are superior) your own excellent powers of observation.

Education

Migraineurs walk a fine line. We should not make a career out of our affliction, but denial will get us into trouble in very short order. Unprecedented resources are available to headache sufferers today. Across America, many communities have brick-and-mortar headache specialists, support groups, and, as a last resort, even the good old library.

It is extremely valuable to stay current and involved with the headache community. A great way to do this is by joining the American Council for Headache Education (ACHE), which will direct you to a headache specialist in your area, and which has a newsletter for headache sufferers. You might also join a local support group, visit online chat rooms, or, possibly, sign up for an online news service. For example, some sites are devoted entirely to advances in neurology, including headache updates. PubMed is a site that provides searchable abstracts from published scientific papers. Among the best migraine sites in the medical community are those provided by Magnum, a nonprofit website with good headache information, as well as ACHE. When you find websites with which you are confident and comfortable, bookmark them to stay current on the newest headache research.

The Internet doesn't check credentials when someone puts up a website, so, yes, there is a lot of bunk out there. When you look for information on the Internet, you'll hear from everyone—from the crazies to the experts—but this is better than burying your head in the sand. Besides, the Internet also provides a world of experience and insight, and whatever information you learn on the Internet, you can sift through it with your doctor and *absolutely* run anything by your health care professional before you try it.

From virtual support groups and headache blogs to sites sponsored by pharmaceutical companies, as well as authoritative sources from within the medical community, the Internet provides tremendous resources for education and up-to-date information. Several sites provide question-and-answer services, although no reputable site will give specific medical advice. Since the Internet changes so rapidly, reviews of specific sites will soon be outdated. Instead, here are some general guidelines for researching migraine on the Internet:

- Be wary of sites that appear in highlighted boxes either above or to one side of general listings. Generally, these are paid listings from companies trying to sell you something. It may be a good product, but you are not likely to get a balanced view from the vendor or their site.
- Listings are usually ranked by how many people have accessed them, and following the crowd is not always the best way to go. A site may be high on the list because they "know how to play the game." Again, it may be a perfectly good site, but being the most popular is not the same as being the best. Take time to read the summaries enough to identify the origin and agenda behind the site.
- University sites, well-known medical groups, not-for-profits, and consumer advocacy groups will generally serve you well. Often, the pharmaceutical companies will have good information, but remember, they have a product to sell, too. Increasingly, many communities have brick-and-mortar headache clinics, online support groups, and live chat rooms.

Every patient's treating physician should be an ally in patient education. Ideally, this should be a two-way street, in which patients educate their caregivers about their headaches, and caregivers, in turn, offer information and options that patients can employ to improve their situations.

The Future of Migraine

Less than twenty years ago, migraine was treated with narcotics and other painkillers. We had no migraine-specific drugs. Migraine was thought to be a relatively rare occurrence, and there was no epidemiologic data about the prevalence of the disease. Many physicians believed that headache was a "psychological" condition, and many patients believed that headaches represented some flaw in their character or personality.

Today, we have a clear understanding of the prevalence of headaches and their cost to individuals and society. Employers and workers alike are beginning to recognize the wisdom of creating an antimigraine work environment, and headache sufferers are learning to understand how to take control of their headaches. We also have an entire class of migraine-specific drugs and are about to have a second. It is likely that sometime in 2009 the first calcitonin gene-related peptide receptor antagonist will be approved by the FDA. If the triptan evolution is any indication, it is likely that more will follow in rapid succession.

Our understanding of what goes on in the brain during a migraine is expanding at an amazing rate, and headache science is moving pretty fast. New classes of molecules are being described in relation to migraine, and molecules known in other contexts are now being evaluated for their role in migraine. Understanding these relationships will, inevitably, lead to new and better treatments. Treatments are becoming increasingly effective, and alternative/traditional lines are blurring as doctors devise holistic treatment plans—in the best sense of the word. Basic research scientists and clinical caregivers are even collaborating more closely than ever. As a result, new advances occur almost daily, and any one of them may provide a key to improving your headache situation. So stay with it. While we have a long, long way to go, things can only get better.

Your Headache History

Headache History

This questionnaire provides a foundation upon which you and your doctors will build your entire program. It is intended to aid your communication with your doctors, not to replace your physicians' medical history interview and physical examination. Take your time.

How old were you when you *first* got headaches of *any* kind?

_____

_____

This is important. Long-standing headaches are more likely to be primary (not due to anything else, like a brain tumor or infection). First-time headaches in an adult raise some red flags.

At what age did your headaches begin to interfere with your life?

_____

_____

This gives an idea of progression, and helps focus on life stages and their connection to your headaches.

Typically, where on your head do you feel your headaches?

_____

_____

Different kinds of headaches have different distributions of pain. Migraines are more often on one side than the other, while tension-type headaches tend to be in the neck and temples. These are not absolutes, but they help flesh out a picture.

On average, how many headache days do you experience:

Per week?_____ Per month? _____

Headache frequency helps determine whether someone needs a daily preventive, and can suggest the possibility of medication overuse, toxic exposure, or chronification. Discuss with your doctor if you experience headaches more than two days per week or fifteen days per month.

Describe the quality of your pain and what it feels like:

_____

_____

Many headaches have "typical" pain qualities. For example, migraines often throb, while tension headaches are often pressure-like. Cluster headaches are often stabbing in quality. None of these observations by themselves can make the diagnosis, but each is a piece of evidence and helps solve the puzzle.

If you feel that you have more than one kind of headache, describe what makes them different from one another:

_____

_____

While some people have more than one headache type, more often patients have a single headache type with different presentations. These descriptions can help clarify this.

Using the pain scale (0 is no pain and 10 is the worst pain imaginable), how do you rate the pain of your *typical* headache?

_____

Using the pain scale, how do you rate the pain of your *worst* headache?

_____

This important information provides a reference point down the road when evaluating whether your headaches are getting better or worse. Don't worry whether your 7 means the same thing to anyone else, including your doctor. By definition, pain is subjective. This means that only you can decide what number your pain deserves, and you can never be wrong, argued with, or dismissed. It is your pain. You get to decide (if you need a little guidance on this, see Pain Scale, page 95).

How long does your typical headache last?

_____

_____

Does your typical headache start quickly or gradually?

_____

_____

This very useful information can help your physician select an appropriate rescue medication, because some rescues come on quickly but don't sustain, while others come on slowly but last for a long time.

During your headaches, are you highly sensitive to:

Light? _____   Sound? _____

Smell? _____   Something else? _____

These features help classify the kind of headache you are having and suggest lifestyle changes to avoid triggers.

At any time before, during, or after a headache, do you notice exquisite sensitivity to touch in your:

Skin? _____   Hair? _____

Scalp? _____   Teeth? _____

The presence of these sensitivities is important in the selection and timing of rescue medications.

Before or during a headache, do you experience:

Excessive yawning? _____

Nausea? _____

Vomiting? _____

Yawning, an often-ignored warning of impending headaches, should signal that it is time to take a rescue. Nausea and vomiting are important because they can dehydrate you and worsen your headache. Their presence changes the management recommendations to include antinausea medication and other strategies.

List any other nonpainful symptoms:

_____

_____

These can tip you or your doctor off to unsuspected triggers or other illnesses that may need attention.

What seems to soften a headache or make it go away?

_____

_____

It is important to integrate the things you find useful into the treatment plan. It is also important to make sure that a seemingly effective short-term solution does not have long-term untoward consequences.

Do any of the following bring on a headache or make an existing headache worse?

Bright lights? _____   Flickering lights? _____

Loud sounds? _____   Particular smells? _____

Exercise? _____   Weather changes? _____

Coughing? _____   Sneezing? _____

Straining in the bathroom? _____   Travel? _____

Changes in altitude? _____   Anything else? _____

The presence of these triggers helps guide the structure of the lifestyle changes and prevention strategies that may ultimately decrease the frequency and severity of your headaches.

Have there been periods in your life when your headaches were particularly:

Good? _____

Bad? _____

This question provides insight into your triggers, particularly hormonal and emotional, and can help guide the treatment plan.

Over time, have your headaches remained the same or become progressively better or worse?

_____

_____

For some people, migraine is a progressive disease, and in these cases, the strategy for managing the headaches is different from that for people with "stable" headaches.

Have you noticed any patterns to your headaches?

_____

_____

Such patterns can point to seasonal fluctuations, weather changes, stress responses, or environmental influences.

Are your headaches worse during a particular season?

_____

_____

Allergy season gets a lot of press, so it is good to address this issue up front.

Does a dramatic change in the weather affect your headaches?

_____

_____

Sometimes barometric changes that come with storm fronts, strong winds, or other severe weather can trigger a headache.

Does stress or other strong emotion play a role in your headaches?

_____

_____

It is important to know whether stress makes your headaches worse, because if it does, stress management must become a significant part of your lifestyle changes.

What kind of work do you do?

_____

_____

Hobbies?

_____

_____

If you work in a DDT factory or are chained to a computer eight hours a day, or if your hobby involves mold or airplane glue, this is obviously important information for your doctor.

List any MRI or CT scans of your head or neck, with dates:

_____

_____

If available, both the timing and results of such tests are important, for both your doctor's thoroughness and your reassurance.

List any other diagnostic tests for your headaches:

_____

_____

The most common of these would be spinal fluid analysis, blood work, and cardiac imaging.

List any other medical conditions you now have or have had in the past:

_____

_____

Many other conditions are more common in headache sufferers, and many medications can worsen head pain, so it is important to know what else is going on medically.

Have you had any surgeries?

_____

_____

Previous surgery, particularly of the neck, brain, or sinuses, can influence both diagnosis and treatment planning.

Do you maintain a regular sleep schedule?

_____

_____

Do you have problems with:
Falling asleep? _____ Staying asleep? _____
Early awakening? _____

Sleep is one of the most common triggers for headaches, so a careful consideration of improving sleep is a major part of developing an effective treatment plan.

Do you eat meals at regular times?

_____

_____

Erratic eating schedules and skipping meals are other common triggers, so these habits need to be addressed in the treatment plan.

Do you drink coffee or other caffeinated drinks?

_____

_____

If so, do you get caffeine at regular times, including weekends?

_____

_____

Caffeine consumption needs to be addressed, though not every migraineur is affected by caffeine in the same way, and controversy persists over regular versus sporadic versus no caffeine.

Do you exercise? _____
If so: How often? _____
For how long? _____ At the same time each day? _____

How does it affect your headaches?

_____

_____

In general, exercise makes an existing migraine worse but improves tension headache. Overall, though, exercise is important for headache sufferers, and every treatment plan needs to include a strategy for incorporating exercise without worsening the headaches.

If you are sexually active, does sex affect your headaches?

_____

_____

At its best, sex is a lot better than exercise, and at its worst, well, you know. But for headache sufferers, sexual activity can improve, worsen, or bring on a headache. How your head-aches respond to sexual activity can provide insight into what kind of headaches you have, and can be an important part of your treatment strategy.

What help do you need to manage your headaches better?

_____

_____

_____

_____

This is huge. It is important to know what your treatment goals are and, if you are seeking help from a doctor, to have this discussion so that you avoid misunderstandings about what is realistic and what is important to you with regard to your headaches.

Current Therapies

The idea is to create a "snapshot" of your current therapies. It should not include what you are supposed to be doing, what you meant to be doing, or what you intend to do. Be real and be thorough. Include all of your therapies—over-the-counter medicines, herbs, spices, alternative substances, supplements, and psychological, spiritual, and physical treatments— in addition to your prescription medicines.

What do you currently take to try to *prevent* your headaches?

Name	Dose	Frequency	Date started

List any other strategies you use to prevent your headaches:

_____

_____

_____

What do you take for rescue when you get a headache?

Name   Dose   Days per week (average)

_____

_____

_____

List any other strategies you use for rescue:

_____

_____

_____

List other medications, remedies, or strategies you currently use for any other conditions:

Name   Dose   Frequency   Date started   Used for

_____

_____

_____

Do you have any medication allergies?

_____

_____

Do you smoke? _____

Drink? _____

Use street drugs? _____

If we know where we have been, we can avoid going over old ground again. But when it comes to migraine treatment, very often we tried therapies in inadequate doses, for too short a time, or in combination with other therapies that negated the intended benefit. Sometimes, we terminate medications or other therapies because of presumed side effects that might actually have been a component of the headache or another medication. When well organized, this critical information can simplify and clarify future treatment options.

Record information for all prescriptions, over-the-counter medications, and nontraditional, nonmedication approaches you have tried for prevention and rescue. It is important that you include details—how long you tried the therapy, the dose(s) of medicines you tried, other concurrent therapies—and as much information as possible.

Name of Medication _____

Date started _____   Beginning dose _____

Date ended _____   Ending dose _____

What effect did this medication have on your headaches?

_____

What side effects did you experience from this medication?

_____

What other medications were you taking at the same time?

_____

Other notes about this medication: _____
_____

Name of Medication _____

Date started _____   Beginning dose _____
Date ended _____   Ending dose _____

What effect did this medication have on your headaches?
_____

What side effects did you experience from this medication?
_____

What other medications were you taking at the same time?
_____

Other notes about this medication: _____
_____

Name of Medication _____

Date started _____   Beginning dose _____
Date ended _____   Ending dose _____

What effect did this medication have on your headaches?
_____

What side effects did you experience from this medication?
_____

What other medications were you taking at the same time?
_____

Other notes about this medication: _____
_____

Appendix 3

Evaluation

Not only does migraine change over time, but common sense tells us that people change, environments change, and, therefore, triggers change. While vigilance is important, you don't want to make a career out of your headaches. This questionnaire will help you regularly monitor your progress and reassess your headache status in an efficient and purposeful way. Ultimately, the goal is to refine and modify your treatment plan to continually reduce the number and frequency of headaches.

How often you need to revisit this exercise depends on how well your lifestyle changes, medication management, and other strategies are working to prevent your headaches. Initially, you should complete this questionnaire every month or two, but as headaches become less frequent the interval can increase. However, this should never go beyond six months. Once you complete this form, compare it with the previous form to look at your trend. If the direction is wrong, go back to your trigger tracker and see if you can identify what is different. If the direction is positive, keep on keeping on.

Average number of headache days/month since last evaluation:

_____

Number of days "lost" to headaches each month:

_____

Average duration of headaches:

_____

Headache distribution by day of the week:

M	Tu	W	Th	F	Sa	Su

Headache distribution by time of day:

6 a.m.–10 a.m.   10 a.m.–2 p.m.   2 p.m.–6 p.m.

6 p.m.–10 p.m.   10 p.m.–midnight   midnight–6 a.m.

Number of exercise days per month: _____

Average daily duration of exercise per day: _____

Medications for prevention: _____

Changes in preventive medications: _____

Medications for rescue: _____

Changes in rescue medications: _____

Response to rescue medications: _____

Level of satisfaction with headache management:

_____

Index

aspirin with antiplatelet medications
(Plavix, Aggrenox), 273
aspirin with caffeine and butalbital
(Fiorinal), 193
aspirin with caffeine and orphenadrine
(Norgesic Forte), 175, 192
asthma, 150, 352, 353–54
Ativan (lorazepam), 202–3
aura, 37–40, 310–11, 316
Aventyl (nortriptyline), 156, 275, 294
Axert (almotriptan), 175, 188

baclofen, 175, 192
barometric pressure changes, 84, 142–43,
346
basilar migraine, 47
behaviors. *See* lifestyle, antimigraine
Benadryl (diphenhydramine), 198,
202, 293
benzodiazepines, 202–3
beta-blockers, 155, 275
biofeedback training, 168
Botox (botulinum toxin), 194–95
brain
during aura phase, 37
cortical spreading depression (CSD),
23, 27, 38–39, 152
damage from repeated headaches,
39, 117, 145
during headache phase, 40
increasing sensitivity, windup
phenomenon, 24, 44
of migraineur, 23–24, 26–28, 239
neurologic deficits, 46
pain messages, 25
response to regular exercise, 263–64
sensitivity adjustments, 86–87
tumors, 25, 34, 66, 68, 361, 363, 365
breast-feeding, 309–10
bupivacaine, 194
bupropion (Wellbutrin), 156
Burstein, Rami, 81
butalbital with caffeine and acetaminophen
(Esgic, Fioricet), 175, 193
butalbital with caffeine and aspirin
(Fiorinal), 193
Butazolidin (phenylbutazone), 273
butterbur, 160–61, 183, 275, 308

Cady, Roger, 61
caffeine, 198–99, 295–96, 344
caffeine with butalbital and acetaminophen
(Esgic, Fioricet), 175, 193
caffeine with butalbital and aspirin
(Fiorinal), 193
caffeine with orphenadrine and aspirin
(Norgesic Forte), 175, 192
calcium channel blockers, 155
cannibinoids (marijuana, Marinol),
183, 200
captopril, 155
carbonic anhydrase inhibitor, 349
caregivers. *See* doctors; support system
carisoprodol (Soma), 175, 192
Cataflam (diclofenac), 273
CDH (chronic daily headache)
causes, 51–52
medication overuse, 52–58, 174
progression from episodic headaches,
50–51
Celebrex (celecoxib), 155, 273, 274
central sensitization theory, 181
cephalagia, 33
CGRP antagonist, 156, 173
chamomile tea, 292
Charles, Andrew, 38
children, explanations to, 244
choline magnesium salicylate (Trilisate),
273
chronic daily headache (CDH)
causes, 51–52
medication overuse, 52–58, 174
progression from episodic headaches,
50–51
chronic pain syndromes, 358–59
clonidine, 314
cluster headaches, 65, 187, 195
coenzyme Q10, 161–62, 183, 275
comorbid conditions. *See also* headaches,
secondary
asthma, 150, 252, 353–54
considerations in migraine treatment,
351–52
depression, 354–55
irritable bowel syndrome, 357
obesity, 358
sleep apnea, 62

temporomandibular joint (TMJ)
syndrome, 61–62
Compazine (prochlorperazine), 196
complicated migraine, 46
computer use, 323, 325
cortical spreading depression (CSD), 23,
27, 38–39, 152
cortisol levels, 130, 281, 287
Cox-1 and Cox-2 inhibitors, 155, 191, 274
CSD (cortical spreading depression), 23,
27, 38–39, 152
CT scan, 35–36
cutaneous allodynia, 9–10, 45, 181–82, 192
cyclobenzaprine (Flexeril), 175, 192
Cymbalta (duloxetine), 153, 156

danger signs, 67–69, 216
D2 antagonists, 195
Daypro (oxaprozin), 273
dehydration, 196, 216
Depacon, Depakene, Depakote (valproic
acid, valproate, divalproate), 154–55,
196, 275, 307, 358
depression
antidepressants, 153, 156, 356
comorbidity with headaches, 166,
354–55
during midlife, 360–61
desipramine, 294
DHE (dihydroergotamine, Migranal), 194
diagnosis of headaches, 33–36
diary. See headache diary
diazepam (Valium), 202–3
diclofenac (Voltaren, Cataflam,
Voltaren-XR), 273
dietary habits. See foods and eating habits
dietary supplements, 159–63. See also
natural remedies and agents
diflunisal (Dolobid), 175, 273
dihydroergotamine (DHE, Migranal), 194
diltiazem, 155
diphenhydramine (Benadryl), 198, 202, 293
diphenhydramine with acetaminophen
(Tylenol PM), 293
Disalcid (salsalate), 273
diseases associated with migraines.
See comorbid conditions;
headaches, secondary

doctors
access to, 207, 212
arrangements for emergency room
treatment, 212–13
communication with, 225–26
early consultation with, 229–30
emergency room, 217
levels of help provided, 230–31
to locate, 135, 370
patient education, 372
preparation for consultation with, 231–33
review and evaluation of diary entries, 93
review of management progress, 369
working with, 233–35
Dolobid (diflunisal), 175, 273
duloxetine (Cymbalta), 153, 156
Duradrin (isometheptene/
dichloralphenazone with
acetaminophen), 193–94

eating habits. See foods and eating habits
Ecotrin (aspirin, acetylsalicylic acid), 197, 273
education
of nonmigraineurs, 237–40
for patients, 370–72
Effexor (venlafaxine), 153
Elavil (amitriptyline), 156, 294, 358
elderly migraineurs
late-life migrainous accompaniments,
48, 311, 361–62
nonmigraine headaches, 363–65
eletriptan (Relpax), 175, 189
emergency room visit
emergency room procedures, 216–17
headache as emergency, 215–16
narcotics, 212, 217–18
nonnarcotic rescues, 214–15
prearrangement for, 212–13
rehydration, 196, 216
employment. See workplace
encephalitis, 70
endorphins, 132, 265, 266–67, 314
environmental triggers
altitude changes, 84–85, 139, 349–50
brain's response to, 23–24, 44
external and internal triggers, 81–83, 125
hormone level fluctuations, 128, 141–42,
158, 303–4, 311–12

unique migraineur sensitivities, 77–79,
255–56, 257
Frova (frovatriptan), 175, 189–90, 274, 304,
306–7, 341, 349

gabapentin, 154–55
gastric stasis, 42–43
genetic factors
asthma-migraine comorbidity, 353
family headache history, 118–19
hemiplegic migraine, 47
menopausal patterns, 83, 297
predisposition to headaches, 25, 83
syndromes associated with migraine,
49–50
giant cell arteritis, 72–73, 364
glaucoma, 363

Harrington, Michael, 6
headache diary
guidelines, 94–100
pattern and trigger identification, 93–94,
256, 341
review and evaluation of data, 100–101,
369–70
sample headache calendar, 98–99
headache history, 117–20, 373–82
headache red flags, 67–69, 216
headaches, migraine
definition, 31
diagnosis, 33–36
future treatment prospects, 156,
173, 372
migraineur personality types, 177,
222–23
phases, 36–41
presentations, 30
progressive nature of, 50–51, 145, 367
research and study of, 9–10, 26–28,
181–82
symptoms, 41–45
types requiring special treatment, 51–58
variants, 46–50
headaches, nonmigraine primary
cluster headaches, 65
hemicrania continua, 65
paroxysmal hemicrania, 65
sinus headaches, 63–64

from sleep disorders, 62
SUNCT syndrome, 66
from temporomandibular joint (TMJ)
syndrome, 61–62
tension-type, 49, 58–61, 203, 264, 265,
267, 338
headaches, secondary. *See also* comorbid
conditions
cardiac disease, 364
chronic pulmonary disease, 364
following head trauma, 71–72
glaucoma, 363
hypertension, 364
from medications, 352, 365
during midlife, 361
red flags, 68–69, 216
spinal meningitis and encephalitis, 70
stroke, 66, 364
subarachnoid hemorrhage, 67, 69
as symptoms of diseases, 66–69, 216,
352, 361
temporal arteritis, 72–73, 364
tumors, 66, 365
headache specialists. *See* doctors
headache status questionnaire, 387–88
head trauma, 71–72
health care providers. *See* doctors
health maintenance, 164–65
heart, hole in, 27
hemicrania continua, 65, 155
hemiplegic migraine, 46–47
history
headache, 117–20, 373–82
previous therapies, 385–86
hops, 292
hormone-related headaches
cessation with menopause, 297, 310
changes with age, 318–19
familial patterns, 83, 297
hormone level fluctuations, 128, 141–42,
158, 303–4, 311–12
hormone questionnaire, 300–301
hormone replacement therapy, 158, 312,
315–17
hysterectomy and, 313, 317–18
menstrual headaches, 141–42, 298,
302–9
perimenopause, 310–15